The New Prescriber

The New Prescriber

An Integrated Approach to Medical and Non-medical Prescribing

Edited by

Joanne S Lymn BSc PhD
Dianne Bowskill RN BSc DHSci
Fiona Bath-Hextall BSc PhD
Roger D Knaggs BSc BMedSci PhD MRPharmS
University of Nottingham and
Nottingham University Hospitals NHS Trust

WILEY-BLACKWELL

A John Wiley & Sons, Ltd., Publication

This edition first published 2010
© 2010 John Wiley & Sons

Wiley-Blackwell is an imprint of John Wiley & Sons, formed by the merger of Wiley's global Scientific, Technical and Medical business with Blackwell Publishing.

Registered office
John Wiley & Sons Ltd, The Atrium, Southern Gate, Chichester, West Sussex, PO19 8SQ, United Kingdom

Editorial office
John Wiley & Sons Ltd, The Atrium, Southern Gate, Chichester, West Sussex, PO19 8SQ, United Kingdom

For details of our global editorial offices, for customer services and for information about how to apply for permission to reuse the copyright material in this book please see our website at www.wiley.com/wiley-blackwell.

Library of Congress Cataloging-in-Publication Data

The new prescriber : an integrated approach to medical and non-medical prescribing / edited by Joanne S. Lymn ... [et al.].
    p. ; cm.
  Includes bibliographical references and index.
  ISBN 978-0-470-51987-5 (pbk. : alk. paper) 1. Drugs–Prescribing. I. Lymn, Joanne S.
  [DNLM: 1. Drug Prescriptions. 2. Drug Therapy–methods. 3. Pharmaceutical Preparations–administration & dosage. 4. Pharmacological Phenomena. 5. Physician's Practice Patterns. QV 748 N532 2010]
  RM138.N457 2010
  615′.1–dc22   2010008439

A catalogue record for this book is available from the British Library.

Set in 10/12 pt Garammond-Book by Aptara® Inc., New Delhi, India
Printed and bound in Singapore by Markono Print Media Pte Ltd

2   2013

Contents

Contributors List

Dr Nick Allcock   Associate Professor in Pain Management, University of Nottingham

Dr Sarah Armstrong   Associate Professor in Statistics, University of Nottingham

Dr Fiona Bath-Hextall   Associate Professor and Reader in Evidence-Based Healthcare, University of Nottingham.

Dr Dianne Bowskill   Lecturer in Non Medical Prescribing, University of Nottingham.

Dr Frank Coffey   Consultant in Emergency Medicine, Nottingham University Hospitals NHS Trust Associate Professor, University of Nottingham

Dr Richard Cooper   Lecturer in Public Health, University of Sheffield

Dr Finola Delamere   Centre of Evidence-Based Dermatology, University of Nottingham.

Fiona Dobson   Staff Tutor, Open University

Judith Gregory   Renal Pharmacist, Nottingham University Hospitals NHS Trust

Tim Hills   Senior Pharmacist - Microbiology & Infection Control, Nottingham University Hospitals NHS Trust

Dr Sarah Jones   Specialist Registrar, Nottingham University Hospitals NHS Trust

Dr Martyn Kingsbury   Lecturer in Medical Education, Imperial College London

Dr Roger Knaggs   Specialist Pharmacist - Anaesthesia & Pain Management, Nottingham University Hospitals NHS Trust

Briony Leighton   Trust Principal Pharmacist, United Lincolnshire Hospitals NHS Trust

Dr Jo Leonardi-Bee   Associate Professor in Medical Statistics, University of Nottingham.

Dr Joanne Lymn   Associate Professor in Pharmacology, University of Nottingham

Dr Alison Mostyn   Lecturer in Biological Sciences, University of Nottingham

Richard Pitt   Associate Professor in Inter-professional Learning, University of Nottingham

Dr Nigel Plant   Associate Professor (healthcare law and mental health), University of Nottingham

Dr Michael Schachter   Senior Lecturer in Clinical Pharmacology, Imperial College London

Dr Dave Skingsley   Senior Lecturer in Physiology & Pharmacology, Staffordshire University

Margaret Stone   Joint Head of Postgraduate Pharmacy and CPD, De Montfort University

Dr Michael Watson   Lecturer in Public Health, University of Nottingham

Professor Joy Wingfield   Special Professor in Pharmacy Law and Ethics, University of Nottingham.

Preface

While there are a number of current textbooks which deal with individual aspects of prescribing, this is the first to pull together all key elements of prescribing using an integrated approach.

This book is divided into three sections dealing with the patient, evidence-based practice and pharmacology. The initial section, the patient, explores the consultation and outlines legal, professional and ethical frameworks which guide medical and non-medical prescribing. The second is devoted to evidence-based practice, highlighting key skills essential to all clinicians. This section encourages the reader to identify why evidence-based practice should underpin prescribing decisions. The third and final section is concerned with pharmacology. Here, the reader is introduced to basic concepts of pharmacodynamics and pharmacokinetics, adverse drug reactions and variability of response. These concepts are important as the reader progresses to the major body systems and drugs used to treat infection.

Throughout the text, the reader will find 'Stop and Think' and 'Practice Application' boxes. These are intended to help the reader link theory to practice but in different ways. The 'Stop and Think' boxes are designed to do exactly what they say and encourage the reader to stop and reflect on the knowledge gained and how this might be applied in practice, thus developing greater understanding. Ideal answers to the questions in these boxes are not presented in the book but should be drawn from an integration of all the relevant information presented within the chapter itself, previous chapters of the book and clinical practice. 'Practice Application' boxes take a more factual approach by providing a direct link from theory to clinical practice.

Key terms used in the book are highlighted in blue font when they first appear in the text. Definitions of these terms can be found in the relevant section glossary.

Section 1

The Patient

Section introduction

In this first section we focus on the practical aspects of prescribing for patients. As a new prescriber, you will find there are many factors specific to your patient, your profession and your employer which influence both your decision to prescribe and the prescribing decisions you make. Throughout this chapter you will be encouraged to think about prescribing in practice and we begin with the consultation, the starting point for prescribing. All prescribers must practise within the law and in a manner consistent with professional and public expectations of a prescriber. The legal framework of medical and non-medical prescribing are defined in this section and new prescribers are encouraged to think about their prescribing role in relation to these aspects. Your actions as a prescriber will reach far beyond the patients you prescribe for and this section encourages you to explore the ethical and public health issues associated with prescribing authority. As your prescribing experience grows, you will find it useful to revisit the definitions and the questions raised in this section.

The term non-medical prescriber is used throughout the book and refers to nurses, pharmacists and allied health professionals who, following successful completion of a programme of formal prescribing education, are on the professional record as a prescriber.

1 The consultation

Learning outcomes

By the end of this chapter the reader should be able to:

- recognise and analyse the important elements of a consultation
- identify the components of the traditional medical history
- appreciate the diagnostic process and distinguish between the treatment of symptoms and the treatment of a disease or condition
- identify the elements of the consultation essential for safe prescribing ('bottom liners')
- refine their professional assessment/consultation for the prescribing role.

As you begin your prescribing education you already have a wealth of professional experience in your own area of practice. The assessment and consultation skills learnt as part of professional registration are well practised but may need to be refined as you take on prescribing. We are not suggesting that you need to adopt a new or medical model of consultation, although this might be desirable in certain advanced practice roles. For the majority of new prescribers, the focus will be on analysing their current framework of assessment or consultation and identifying adaptations required to support prescribing decisions. In this chapter we will ask you to think about the elements of the consultation that you may need to adapt or work on. We will give practice tips and point out common errors that can affect the quality of a consultation.

Prescribing inherently brings with it a greater requirement to make a diagnosis. This responsibility may be new and quite daunting. Prescribers need to have an understanding of the diagnostic process. In most circumstances, the key factor for accurate diagnosis is eliciting a good history. For this reason we will look in detail at the elements of a history. Examination and investigations are directed by and supplement the history. The depth and focus of the history and examination will vary depending on the setting and your role. Wherever you work, however, it is essential to be thorough and systematic and above all to know the bounds of your competence. History taking, examination and clinical decision making are skills that need to be continuously practised under expert supervision.

The New Prescriber. Edited by J Lymn, D Bowskill, F Bath-Hextall, R Knaggs, © 2010 John Wiley & Sons.

Ideally your prescribing will be effective but above all it should be safe. The primary dictum of all healthcare practice is 'primum non nocere (above all do no harm)'. In the final part of the chapter we will outline the elements of the consultation that are essential for safe prescribing, the 'bottom liners' of a prescribing consultation.

The consultation

There are many factors that influence consultations and no two encounters between a practitioner and a patient are the same. The nature of your role will influence the types of patients you treat and the environment in which you see them. Other factors include the purpose of the consultation, the urgency and seriousness of the presentation, time constraints and the personalities, culture, language and medical knowledge of both the patient and the clinician. Previous contact with the patient, autonomy and confidence are other clinician factors. Communication and consultation skills are inextricably interlinked. There are many excellent textbooks available for prescribers who wish to enhance their communication skills (Silverman, Kurtz and Draper, 1998; Berry, 2004).

Elements of a consultation

Although consultations differ in the specifics, there are common elements and generic skills that are applicable in varying degrees to any given situation. Numerous consultation models have been developed over the years, for example Neighbour (2005), Pendleton et al. (2003), Calgary Cambridge in Silverman, Kurtz and Draper (1998). Rather than dwelling on the theory underpinning consultations, we will describe a practical framework, the elements of which can be applied in varying degrees to all consultations – see Box 1.1.

Box 1.1　Elements of a Consultation

(a)　Preparing for the consultation and setting goals for it.
(b)　Establishing an initial rapport with the patient.
(c)　Identifying the reason(s) for the consultation.
(d)　Exploring the patient's problem(s) and ascertaining their ideas, concerns and expectations (ICE) about it.
(e)　Focusing questions to obtain essential information.
(f)　Gathering sufficient information relating to the patient's social and psychological circumstances to ascertain their impact.
(g)　Coming up with a diagnosis or a number of differential diagnoses in order of likelihood.
(h)　Performing a focused physical examination and near-patient tests to support or refute the differential diagnoses.
(i)　Interpreting the information gathered and re-evaluating the problem.
(j)　Reaching a shared understanding of the problem with the patient.
(k)　Considering further investigations if necessary.
(l)　Deciding what treatment options, pharmacological and non-pharmacological, are available.
(m)　Advising the patient about actions needed to tackle the problem.

(n) Explaining these actions and the time of follow-up if required.
(o) Inviting and answering any questions.
(p) Summarising for the patient and terminating the consultation.
(q) Making a written record of the consultation.
(r) Presenting your findings to another health professional.

It is important for consultations to have a degree of structure. The skill in consulting is to maintain a structure and system that includes all the vital elements and yet does not feel like a straitjacket for the patient or clinician. In the following section we will analyse the different elements of the consultation in more detail and highlight those that are likely to change or need more emphasis for you as you take on prescribing.

 Stop and think

Using Box 1.1 as a framework, reflect on your current consultations. What learning and development needs do you have?

(a) Preparing for the consultation and setting goals

Take time to study all the information available to you about the patient prior to the consultation. Study referral letters and available medical records for vital information, including the patient's past history, medications and allergies. Set goals for the consultation and ensure that the environment is set up appropriately with adequate lighting and privacy.

(b) Establishing the initial rapport

First impressions are very important and will influence your subsequent relationship with the patient. If you have not encountered the patient before, introduce yourself by name and explain your role. Check the patient's details (name, date of birth, address). Observe the patient's demeanour and physical appearance. The patient will invariably be feeling nervous. Put them at ease by projecting confidence and warmth and they are more likely to open up to you during the consultation.

(c–g) History taking/diagnosis hypothesis

Elements 'c–g' in Box 1.1 are primarily concerned with the taking of a history and the consideration of differential diagnoses. The importance of the history cannot be overstated. In the vast majority of cases (>70%) the history will provide an accurate diagnosis or differential diagnosis even before the examination and investigations are performed. A good history will therefore facilitate effective prescribing. Certain minimum information *must* be elicited to ensure safe prescribing,

The history is two-way process. In reality, we do not 'take' a history. Rather, we 'make' a history with the patient. The result is influenced by both the practitioner's and the patient's prior knowledge, experiences and understanding of language. Where understanding of language is a barrier, clinical risk is significantly increased and an interpreter should be considered. There are psychodynamic processes at play during any consultation which the practitioner needs to be aware of. These are explored in detail in other publications (Berry, 2004; Stewart *et al.*, 2003).

The scope and depth of the history will depend on the role of the practitioner and the circumstances surrounding the consultation. Whatever the nature of the history, it is essential to be systematic and as far as possible follow the same sequence of questioning each time. In this way vital information will not be overlooked. This becomes particularly important when the patient has multiple symptoms and/or a complicated medical history.

The majority of histories will contain some or all of the elements of the traditional medical history. This structure has limitations and has been criticised for being practitioner rather than patient centred. A full history is too time-consuming in most situations. However, we believe that it is important for prescribers to have an understanding of the elements of the traditional history before considering some of the modified and/or abbreviated versions that are used in practice.

The traditional medical history

Presenting complaint (PC)

Consider the symptom(s) or problem(s) that has brought the patient to seek medical attention and its duration. The presenting complaint should ideally be written or presented orally in the patient's own words, for example 'tummy ache for 3 hours' 'dizzy spells for 2 years'.

Remember that the complaint that the patient seeks medical advice about might not be their main concern, for example a man concerned about impotence might attend on the pretext of back pain. The true presenting problem will be elucidated by an empathetic and skilled interviewer.

History of the presenting complaint (HxPC)

This is where you clarify the presenting complaint. It is the most important part of the history and is essential for the formulation of a differential diagnosis. Explore the patient's symptoms and try to build a clear picture of the patient's experience. Avoid leading questions as far as possible. At some point, however, you will need to move to focused questioning to elicit essential information and fill in gaps in the patient's story. When there are a number of symptoms, it is important to complete the questioning around each symptom in a systematic fashion before moving on to the next one. Pain is the one of the most common presenting symptoms. The following information should be elicited about pain – its onset (gradual or sudden), location, radiation, character, periodicity (does it come and go?), duration, aggravating and relieving factors and associated features (secondary symptoms). Similar questioning with modifications can be applied to most symptoms, for example for diarrhoea – the character (amount, colour, etc.), timing, aggravating and relieving factors and associated symptoms (e.g.

Box 1.2   Symptom Analysis Mnemonic

PQRST

P – provocation or palliation.
Q – quality and quantity: what does the symptom look, feel, sound like?
R – region/radiation.
S – severity scale. May be rated on a scale of 1–10 which is useful for subsequent evaluation and comparison.
T – timing.

SQITARS	SOCRATES
S – site and radiation	S – site
Q – quality	O – onset
I – intensity	C – character
T – timing	R – radiation
A – aggravating factors	A – associated symptoms
R – relieving factors	T – time intensity relationship
S – secondary symptoms	E – exacerbating/relieving
	S – severity

---

abdominal pain) are all relevant. A number of mnemonics have been created as an *aide mémoire* for symptom analysis (see Box 1.2 for examples).

Always ask about the cardinal symptoms in any system potentially involved, for example for chest pain, ask about the cardinal symptoms relating to the cardiovascular and respiratory systems. The cardinal respiratory symptoms are cough, dyspnoea, wheeze, chest pain, sputum production and haemoptysis. Include within the history of the presenting complaint the presence of risk factors for conditions that may be the cause of the presenting symptom(s), for example if ischaemic chest pain is in the differential, hypertension, smoking and a positive family history are examples of such risk factors. Similarly, oral contraceptive pill (OCP) therapy or prolonged immobilisation would be risk factors for pulmonary embolism.

Past medical and surgical history (PMHx)

The past medical history, along with 'medications, drug history and allergies', provides the background to the patient's current health or disease. Record previous illnesses, operations and injuries in chronological order. Include the duration of chronic conditions, for example diabetes mellitus or asthma, in your record and where appropriate, the location of treatment and the names of the treating clinicians. Remember that many medical conditions may impact on your choice and/or dose of drug treatment.

Family history (FamHx)

Information regarding the age and health or the cause of death of the patient's relatives can be invaluable and provide vital clues in the diagnostic process. Many conditions have a well-defined mode of inheritance. Enquire specifically about the following common conditions – hypertension, coronary artery disease, high cholesterol, diabetes mellitus, kidney or thyroid disease, cancer (specify type), gout, arthritis, asthma, other lung disease, headache, epilepsy, mental illness, alcohol or drug addiction and infectious diseases such as tuberculosis. Depending on the clinical area, you may need to explore the family history of sensitive areas such as mental health, drug misuse or sexual health in more detail. The family history may also throw light on the patient's ideas, fears and expectations, for example a patient whose sibling has died from a brain tumour is likely to be very concerned about a headache that is persisting.

Medications, drug history and allergies

The drug and allergy history is an extremely important part of the medical history. The presenting symptoms may result from the side effects or complications of drug therapy. Current medications and previous allergies will influence prescribing. Ask the patient to list the medications that they are taking on medical advice or otherwise. Ask to see a recent medication list or prescription. Ideally you should see the medications. Note the name, dose, route, frequency of use and indications for all medications. It is also important to establish if the patient is taking the medicines prescribed. List over-the-counter (OTC) drugs, complementary and herbal medicines. The oral contraceptive pill is often not perceived as a medication. Ask specifically about it in women of the appropriate age. Patients may omit to mention medications that are not tablets (e.g. inhalers, home oxygen, creams, eye or ear drops, pessaries, suppositories). Ask specifically about such agents.

Enquire about allergies or adverse reactions to medications, foods, animals, pollen or other environmental factors. If the patient gives a history of allergy, record the exact nature and circumstances of the reaction and the treatment given.

Personal and social history

The personal and social history is a critical aspect of the history. All illnesses, treatments and rehabilitation must be seen in the context of the patient's personality, spirituality and personal and social circumstances. Occupation, habitation, hobbies and lifestyle habits can have a profound impact on health and disease. Where appropriate, do not neglect to ask about recent travel abroad and sexual history. Ascertain whether the patient smokes or has smoked in the past and quantify their smoking. Enquire about alcohol intake and, where appropriate, the use of illicit drugs. Some patients may be reluctant to reveal the full extent of their smoking, alcohol consumption or recreational drug use. Maintain a non-judgemental attitude to encourage such patients to share information.

Systems review

The systems review (SR), which is undertaken at the end of the history, involves a series of screening questions that systematically cover all the body systems. It is usually done in a head-to-toe sequence. Its purpose is to elicit any further information that might be relevant to the current illness or to uncover present or past problems that the patient has overlooked. The SR may provide information that leads you to suspect a multisystem disease process such as systemic lupus erythematosus or may demonstrate associated symptoms in another system, for example arthritis associated with inflammatory bowel disease. A comprehensive list of SR questions can be found in Randle, Coffey and Bradbury (2009).

(h) Physical examination/near-patient tests

The purpose of the physical examination and 'near-patient tests' is to supplement your findings from the history and to support or refute your diagnostic hypotheses. The extent of your examination will depend on your training and experience. It is not essential to be able to perform a physical examination to be a competent prescriber in a specialised area. Increasingly, however, healthcare practitioners (HCPs) are taking on advanced examination skills. It is important that these are taught and assessed appropriately.

Perform vital signs including temperature. Consider vital signs in the context of the patient's age, physical fitness and medication and always seek a reason for abnormal vital signs. Perform a thorough examination and avoid taking shortcuts. In most cases, your examination will be a focused one, concentrating on a specific area of the body. It is important to expose adequately the area to be examined and always compare limbs with the contralateral one.

Near-patient tests are essentially tests that produce immediate results, for example electrocardiograms, urinalyses, arterial blood gases, blood glucose. Increasingly other investigations such as the full blood count and urea and electrolytes are becoming available as near-patient tests. These tests can be invaluable for diagnosis and can also direct or influence the prescription of medications. Remember always to check glucose level in a patient with confusion or altered consciousness.

(i–k) Diagnosis

Diagnosis is the process of ascertaining the nature and cause of a disease. This enables the practitioner to target treatments effectively. The diagnosis is made by evaluating the symptoms, signs and investigation results which together constitute the 'diagnostic criteria'. The information is considered in the context of the patient's physical, social and psychological status. A treatment plan is then formulated, ideally in partnership with the patient who should be kept informed throughout the diagnostic procedure.

Increasingly healthcare practitioners other than doctors are involved in the diagnostic process. The advent of non-medical prescribing has accelerated this trend. Practitioners moving into the diagnostic arena need to understand the process and be aware of potential pitfalls. The way clinicians diagnose alters as they become more experienced .The word *diagnosis* comes from the Greek words 'through' (*dia*) and knowledge (*gnosis*) and fundamental to the process for any practitioner is a thorough knowledge of the presenting features, examination and investigation findings of conditions likely to present to their area of practice. Some of this knowledge is gained through experience with patients (pattern recognition) and much of it is 'book learned'. The practitioner must apply their knowledge to extract information from the patient that will make conditions in the potential differential diagnosis more or less likely, for example eliciting the presence of haemoptysis, oral contraceptive pill therapy and a previous deep vein thrombosis in a 39-year-old woman presenting with pleuritic chest pain would make the diagnosis of pulmonary embolism extremely likely. If these features were absent and the same patient with pleuritic chest pain had fever and cough with purulent sputum, chest infection or pneumonia would be a more likely diagnosis. The presence of breathlessness, while an important symptom, would not help to differentiate between these two diagnoses. The speed of onset of the breathlessness might help, however, as an acute onset would be more typical of a pulmonary embolism.

Practitioners should know the 'red flag' features, suggesting serious pathology or high risk, in conditions likely to present to them. Examples of these would be new onset of back pain with urinary incontinence, warfarin therapy in a patient with a head injury or a suicide note written by a patient who has overdosed. Examples of generic red flag symptoms are unexplained weight loss, night sweats, unexplained chronic pain or pain that keeps the patient awake at night. You should also be aware of classic atypical presentations in your area of practice, for example myocardial infarction presenting with jaw, arm or abdominal pain or ectopic pregnancy masquerading as shoulder tip pain and collapse.

One of the common errors made by practitioners new to diagnosis is 'premature closure', that is, establishing a diagnosis early in the consultation and being blinkered to evidence that might refute that diagnosis or suggest an alternative, for example deciding that colicky abdominal pain with loose stools is due to gastroenteritis and ignoring the radiation of the pain to the scrotum which might suggest a urological cause. It is important to weigh up *all* the evidence from the history, examination and any investigations performed. The consideration of risk factors is also an important part of this process. Even though the chest pain of a 40-year-old man may not sound typical for cardiac pain, the fact that his brother died of a heart attack aged 38 will significantly alter your index of suspicion and consequently your management.

 Stop and think

What is the difference between treating a symptom and a disease? Identify examples from your practice.

Symptom versus disease/condition

In the context of diagnosis, prescribing practitioners should have a clear understanding of the difference between a symptom and a disease or condition. A *symptom* is a manifestation of a disease described by the patient, for example chest pain, breathlessness and haemoptysis are symptoms associated with pneumonia. A symptom may give a clue as to the nature of the disease but it is not in itself a diagnosis. A *diagnosis* is the recognition of a disease or condition by its outward symptoms and signs. These are supplemented by the findings from near-patient testing, imaging and other investigations. A pneumonia, for example, might be diagnosed on the basis of symptoms (cough, dyspnoea, pleuritic chest pain, rusty coloured sputum), signs (tachypnoea, pyrexia, decreased breath sounds, crackles, bronchial breathing) and imaging (CXR).

Medications can be prescribed to treat symptoms or conditions/diseases, for example morphine can be used to treat the symptom of severe chest pain without knowledge of the underlying diagnosis. An ECG might reveal the diagnosis of myocardial infarction which may then be treated with a range of pharmacological and non-pharmacological interventions.

In many situations the diagnosis also includes the underlying physiological, biochemical or microbiological cause(s) of a disease or condition, for example pneumococcal pneumonia suggests not only the diagnostic criteria for pneumonia but also the causative micro-organism. Where causality is known, it is usually possible to target prescribing more effectively to treat or cure the condition. There are conditions, however, where the underlying cause has yet to be discovered. In such situations, palliative treatment targeted at reducing the symptoms may be the best that the clinician can achieve. It is vital, however, that symptoms are not treated without looking for an underlying diagnosis. Pain, the most common symptom for which patients seek healthcare advice, is frequently treated before the underlying diagnosis is identified. Constipation is another example of a symptom that may be treated without an effort being made to find a cause for it. You need to understand as a prescriber that it is not sufficient to treat a symptom. If for example the underlying diagnosis is bowel cancer for a patient who presents with constipation, failing to seek a cause may have disastrous consequences. You must seek to make a diagnosis and if the diagnostic reasoning lies outside your area of expertise, you must refer on to another appropriate health professional.

(l) Treatment

When you have made a diagnosis consider the various treatment options. Non-pharmacological options, for example weight loss and salt reduction for hypertension, should be considered before prescribing drugs with potentially debilitating side effects. Take into account the patient's age, lifestyle, mobility, dexterity and potential compliance when prescribing. Ensure that the patient is not allergic to the treatment that you are considering and that it does not interact with other medications or worsen any existing medical conditions.

(m–p) Summarising and closing the consultation

When you have all the information required, share your conclusions with the patient in language appropriate to their intellectual and educational level, avoiding medical 'jargon'. Ensure that the patient has understood the information that you have given and agreed the treatment plan. This will improve concordance. Give the patient verbal and ideally written information about the administration and common side effects of any prescribed medications.

Illnesses evolve. Initial mild viral-like symptoms may develop rapidly into a full-blown meningococcal septicaemia. A patient may progress from having abdominal pain with minimal abdominal tenderness to obvious appendicitis with peritonism a few hours later. Give the patient a realistic timeframe for the resolution of symptoms and ask them to return or contact you if things deteriorate or do not improve as anticipated. Record this advice clearly in your notes.

Always offer the patient the opportunity to ask questions. If you are unable to answer, be honest. Tell the patient that you will need to look up the answer or consult with another colleague. Finally summarise the findings and treatment for the patient and finish the consultation.

(q and r) The recording and presentation of consultation findings

The written record is a medico-legal document that may be required to justify your diagnosis and choice of treatment. A satisfactory record of a consultation should include the presenting problem, the main features including important negatives (e.g. haemoptysis or the absence of risk factors for thromboembolic disease for a patient with pleuritic chest pain). The examination findings should also contain relevant negatives. It is good practice to write an impression after the history and examination with a list of differential diagnoses in order of likelihood. The investigations (and findings if available) should then be recorded followed by a final diagnosis and management plan. When prescribing medication(s), document the names of the drug(s), the dosage and the length of prescription. It is a useful exercise to critique your documentation, imagining that you are standing in a courtroom defending the contents 2 or 3 years after you have written them.

The ability to present the findings from a consultation in a systematic and concise fashion is vital in a busy practice area and when making referrals or requesting advice over the telephone. It is a difficult skill, which requires a great deal of practice. As you take on the role of prescribing, encourage your medical mentors and colleagues to critique your oral presentation skills.

 Stop and think

What do you consider to be the essential components of a consultation to ensure *safe* prescribing?

'Bottom liners' when prescribing

Much of this chapter has related to factors that contribute to effective prescribing, for example the formulation of an accurate diagnosis. In this section we will highlight the elements of the consultation that are essential for *safe* prescribing.

(a) Ascertain that you have the right patient, by checking name, date of birth, address, hospital or NHS number.
(b) Check weight where appropriate, particularly when prescribing for children.
(c) Ascertain that the patient is not allergic to the medication and that there are no interactions with other medications that the patient is taking.
(d) Ensure that the patient is not suffering from any medical condition that might be exacerbated by the medication (e.g. peptic ulcer disease by NSAIDs) or require a different dosage (e.g. antibiotics in patients with renal failure).
(e) Inform the patient of both nuisance and serious side effects of the medication and advise them to return if serious side effects occur or if the medication is not working as anticipated.

Summary

- The consultation is made up of a number of elements. As a prescriber, you need to analyse your professional assessment, refine current skills and, where appropriate, develop new ones.
- The history is central to making a diagnosis. Incorporate the elements of the traditional medical history to your consultation. A systematic approach is required for gathering essential information. Combine this with a collaborative patient-centred approach.
- Diagnosis is important in prescribing. To diagnose, you should have an in-depth knowledge of conditions presenting to your practice. You need to integrate this knowledge with information systematically obtained from the history, examination and investigations. Be aware of red flags and early diagnostic closure.
- Both symptoms and conditions or diseases can be treated. It is important to understand the difference and to seek the underlying cause of any symptom you treat.
- 'Bottom liners' for safe prescribing are the reason for the prescription, date of birth/(weight), past medical history, medications, allergies and the provision of appropriate information to the patient.

 Activity

1. What sort of preparation should you make in advance of a patient consultation?
2. List the seven elements of a traditional medical history.
3. The purpose of the physical examination and near-patient tests is diagnosis. Is this statement true or false?
4. Identify two generic 'red flag features'.
5. There are a number of 'bottom liners' which are considered essential elements for safe prescribing. List as many bottom liners as you can.

References

Berry, D. (2004) *Risk, Communication and Health Psychology*, Open University Press, Berkshire.

Neighbour, R. (2005) *The Inner Consultation. How to Develop Effective and Intuitive Consulting Styles*, Radcliffe Medical Press, Oxford.

Pendleton, D., Schofield, T., Tate, P. and Havelock, P. (2003) *The New Consultation. Developing Doctor–Patient Communication*, Oxford University Press, Oxford.

Randle, J,. Coffey, F. and Bradbury, M. (2009) *Oxford Handbook of Clinical Skills in Adult Nursing*, Oxford University Press, Oxford.

Silverman, J., Kurtz, S. and Draper, J. (1998) *Skills for Communicating with Patients*, Radcliffe Medical Press, Abingdon.

Stewart, M., Belle Brown, J., Weston, W.W. *et al.* (2003) *Patient-Centred Medicine: Transforming the Clinical Method*, 2nd edn, Radcliffe Medical Press, Abingdon.

Further reading

Donovan, C., Sucking, H. and Walker, Z. (2004) *Difficult Consultations with Adolescents*, Radcliffe Medical Press, Abingdon.

Edwards, C. and Stillman, P. (2006) *Minor Illness or Major Disease? The Clinical Pharmacist in the Community*, 4th edn, Pharmaceutical Press, London.

Hastings, A. and Redsel, S. (2006) *The Good Consultation Guide for Nurses*, Radcliffe Medical Press, Oxford.

Pollock, K. (2005) *Concordance in Medical Consultations. A Critical Review*, Radcliffe Press, Abingdon.

2 Accountability and prescribing

Learning outcomes

By the end of this chapter the reader should be able to:

- define professional accountability and responsibility
- identify the spheres of accountability which underpin clinical practice
- discuss how clinical governance and frameworks of accountability may be used to ensure good prescribing practice
- apply the principles of accountable practice to the prescribing role.

As a registered healthcare practitioner, you will already be familiar with the fact that you are accountable for the care provided to your patients. In developing your role to include prescribing, it is appropriate to consider your accountability in the context of prescribing. This chapter will explore definitions of responsibility and accountability and consider the relationship between accountability, quality and clinical governance. Having determined what accountability is, the chapter will analyse the spheres of accountability and the process by which the practitioner is held to account. We present a model of this process which we use to stimulate your professional thinking about accountability and prescribing.

With accountability comes responsibility. There are those who will argue that they are one and the same; even so, you could be responsible for an action but may not be held accountable. For example, a learner may be responsible for the care they provide the patient, but the registered practitioner supervising the learner is likely to be professionally accountable for the care provided. At this point it is appropriate to consider what we mean by accountability.

Defining accountability

Accountability is a difficult concept to define. Many will state that it is an ethical concept associated with other concepts such as liability, responsibility, answerability or in terms

---

of an expectation to give account of one's actions or omissions. In this way practitioners may associate accountability with a culture of blame. However, accountability is not necessarily a negative concept (Savage and Moore, 2004) and should promote good practice.

 Stop and think

Spend a few moments developing your definition of accountability. You may find it helpful to identify what you consider to be the key attributes of accountable practice.

As a prescriber you will be required to assess, diagnose and prescribe within your scope of practice and area of competence. To fulfil this, you need to be able to foresee probable or possible consequences of your actions, non-actions or omissions and have the freedom to act on the basis of your clinical decision making (Batey and Lewis, 1982). Accountability is the cornerstone of professional practice; it is in being accountable that health professionals are able to respond to patient needs, ensuring that their practice is evidence based, efficient and effective (McSherry and Pearce, 2002).

 Stop and think

Identify the factors which will assist you in becoming an accountable prescriber. Are there potential challenges you may face in taking on the role of prescriber?

Assuring quality

Health professionals through their regulatory bodies are held accountable to be responsible to deliver safe and effective care based on current evidence, best practice and where appropriate validated research. There are a variety of different authorities and organisations that create structures and standards of accountability, for example the National Institute for Health and Clinical Excellence, National Service Frameworks, NHS Litigation Authority, National Patient Safety Agency, Healthcare Commission. These organisations evolved as a response to the public's perception of systemic failings in the National Health Service, such as Victoria Climbié (Laming, 2003), Bristol Royal Infirmary Enquiry (Kennedy Report, 2001), Shipman (2002, 2003a,b), Alder Hey (Redfern, 2000), and a consequent lack of confidence in professional self-regulation. These organisations act to ensure that both practitioners and their employers are accountable for the care they provide.

Clinical governance

Clinical governance is the means by which NHS trusts ensure that patients receive good quality care. It was first defined in the consultation document 'A First Class Service: Quality in the

New NHS' (DH, 1998) as a framework through which NHS organisations are accountable for continuously improving the quality of their services and safeguarding high standards of care by creating an environment in which excellence within clinical care will flourish. Scally and Donaldson (1999) recognise clinical governance as a framework through which NHS organisations are accountable for quality assurance activities which ensure that the predetermined clinical standards that have been set are seen to be maintained by practitioners, and are evident within the health and social care settings.

This highlights the importance of ensuring that prescribing practice is in keeping with governance principles. These include ensuring patients are involved in decisions about their care, that clear procedures are in place for risk reporting, and that as a prescriber you maintain your knowledge and competence (NMC, 2006; RPSGB, 2007; HPC, 2009).

 Stop and think

Not all patients wish to be involved in making decisions about their care. Identify the strategies you may use to manage these situations when prescribing.

All professional regulatory bodies clearly identify that patient safety and protecting society are the fundamental principles that can only be achieved through acknowledgement and working to legislative and regulatory body guidance. For further discussion on policy and the legal framework for prescribing see Chapters 3 and 6.

The five spheres of accountability

In undertaking your professional clinical practice you are accountable to:

- your profession
- your patient
- the wider public and society
- your employer
- yourself.

These five spheres of accountability provide a framework by which we may analyse accountable prescribing practice.

Professional accountability

All prescribers are accountable to their professional body; this will be the Nursing Midwifery Council for nurses, the Health Professions Council for other non-medical professionals, the Royal Pharmaceutical Society of Great Britain or the General Medical Council. All these regulatory bodies work to protect the well-being of people who use the services of nurses, midwives, occupational therapists, physiotherapists, pharmacists, orthoptists, dieticians, operating department practitioners, clinical scientists, chiropodists/podiatrists, radiographers, prosthetics and orthotists, art therapists, biomedical scientists and speech and language therapists. These regulatory bodies set standards of education for entry to the professions and standards of conduct for their members. It is against these standards that 'fitness for practice' is judged. These standards are applicable to all aspects of the practitioner's work, including prescribing. For nurses, the NMC has produced specific standards of proficiency for nurses and midwife prescribers (NMC, 2006).

Issues of professional competency are appropriate to all practitioners. While the legal framework for prescribing is discussed elsewhere, practitioners should only prescribe within the sphere of their own competence; for many prescribers this will mean prescribing from a limited formulary of drugs which are familiar to you from your clinical experience. The RSPGB (2007) produced 'Professional Standards and Guidance for Pharmacist Prescribers' focusing on the seven principles from the Code of Ethics. These principles are similar to those identified by the NMC (2006, p. 5) who determine that prescribers must have sufficient knowledge and competence to:

- assess a patient's/client's clinical condition
- undertake a thorough history, including medical history and medication history, and diagnose where necessary, including over-the-counter medicines and complementary therapies
- decide on management of presenting condition and whether or not to prescribe
- identify appropriate products if medication is required
- advise the patient/client on effects and risks
- prescribe if the patient/client agrees
- monitor response to medication and lifestyle advice.

What is evident is that your accountability extends to the whole of the prescribing process from assessment to diagnosis, as well as the decision as to whether to prescribe or not. The decision not to prescribe can in practice be a difficult one for the practitioner when faced with a patient who expects a prescription. We will consider this issue again later in this chapter, but the example serves to highlight the fact that as a practitioner you are accountable for not only your actions but also your omissions to act, your decision making and your clinical skills. This brings us to your responsibilities in law and your responsibilities to your patient.

Accountability to your patient

All practitioners would accept that the patient or client is central to healthcare provision. As such, clinicians are accountable to their patients but the issue is how patients hold members of the professions to account for their actions or their failure to act. The answer lies in two specific frameworks. The first is the NHS complaints procedure which facilitates the patient or family in making a complaint to the trust about the care provided. While the process is somewhat formal, the emphasis is placed on the local resolution of complaints but facilitates a process by which patients may ultimately complain to the Health Service Commissioner.

The second process entails the patient taking a civil legal action under the tort of negligence. It is worth noting that patients who purchase their health services privately would pursue a similar action under contract law. The basis of the civil action in negligence is that there has been a breach of the duty of care owed to the patient which has caused foreseeable damage. It is important to recognise that to the lawyer, negligence is therefore something very specific and as such, the term should not be used by the clinician in its lay meaning, that is, as a mistake or error of judgement.

The relationship between the practitioner and patient is significant in determining whether a duty of care exists. Indeed, it is this duty of care which is the basis of healthcare law. For the purposes of this chapter, we can assume that the clinician who is prescribing for their patient owes that patient a duty of care. What is more appropriate is to identify the standard of care that is to be associated with prescribing practice. The case of Bolam v Friern Barnet Hospital Management Committee (1957) 2All ER 118; 1 WLR 528 set the test for the standard of care owed to the patient. This case concerned a mental health patient who was to have ECT for treatment of his depressive illness. At the time of the ECT, there were two different but recognised approaches to providing the treatment: the first involved using practitioners to hold the patient while the fit was induced while the second and more recent method involved the use of paralysing agents or muscle relaxants and anaesthesia. Mr Bolam received his ECT using the traditional method and in doing so received fractures to his hips. In determining whether the doctor had breached the duty of care, there is no breach of the standard of care if a responsible body of professional opinion would accept the practice as being proper even if they would have adopted a different practice.

The test has been criticised as favouring the professional who may only need to find others who would be supportive of their practice. The more recent case of Bolitho v City & Hackney Health Authority (1996) identified that it is no longer sufficient for healthcare professionals to rely solely on the Bolam test. Rather, evidence needs to be presented to the court. In rare cases where it can be demonstrated that professional opinion is not capable of withstanding logical analysis, the judge is entitled to conclude that the body of opinion is neither responsible nor reasonable. What we can therefore conclude is that prescribing practice must be responsible and reasonable and to the standard normally associated with a prescriber. The prescriber should consequently be able to provide evidence for their prescribing practice to a court if required to do so.

The final aspect of the negligence action is that the breach of damage caused the damage which is to be compensated for. This is often considered using the 'but for' your actions (or omissions to act) test or the material contribution test; that is, the actions or omissions of the practitioner materially contributed to the damage sustained by the claimant.

Accountability to the public/society

Society has expectations about the role of professional healthcare staff. While generally the standard of care provided by healthcare professionals is an issue for the civil courts, there are occasions where the health professional's conduct may attract criminal liability. One example of this is a drug error which results in the death of a patient. In this situation the coroner would in the first instance undertake a postmortem and hold an inquest into the patient's death. Following this, the police may investigate the death and refer their findings to the Crown Prosecution Service which would consider whether there were grounds to prosecute the health professional in connection with the patient's death.

Accountability to the employer

Healthcare professionals are accountable in contract to their employers. There is an implied term in the employment contract that employees will follow the reasonable instructions of their employee and will use care and skill in carrying out their duties (Dimond, 2005). The policies and procedures of the employer are implied in the contract of employment; therefore a failure to follow policy could amount to a breach of the employment contract and result in disciplinary action. It is therefore important that prescribers follow the procedures of their employers who are ultimately vicariously liable for the torts or wrongs of their employees as long as the employee is acting in the course of their employment and doing the job they are paid to do. Further discussion on working with policies and procedures can be found in Chapter 6.

Accountability to self

While we have left this issue until last, in many ways this aspect of accountability may be the most important to the practitioner providing care, in that it brings into the arena the issue of one's own moral and ethical viewpoints. Beauchamp and Childress (2001) advocate four principles of medical ethics, as follows.

Autonomy

Autonomy is the principle that patients should be self-directing or self-determining about what happens to them. As we will see in the following case studies, the concept of autonomy encapsulates issues of consent, information giving and decision making. The prescriber is therefore engaging the patient or client in the decision-making process, sharing information with the patient who themselves understands their symptoms in order to arrive at a prescribing decision (or not).

Beneficence

Beneficence implies that healthcare should be provided for the benefit of the patient or client. While this in itself may not be controversial, in practice identifying the patient's best interest can be difficult, especially when patients may choose to exercise their autonomy in a way which the practitioner believes compromises their interest, for example by not taking drugs which have been prescribed.

Non-maleficence

Non-maleficence is the duty not to harm the patient. Again, on first sight the prescriber may feel that this does not apply to them but many of the drugs in everyday use have side effects which may be viewed as being harmful to the patient.

Justice

The principle of justice suggests that health professionals should provide care that is equitable. While we are familiar with the notion of the 'postcode lottery', prescribers may have to consider what 'just' prescribing entails. We find that these concepts are helpful in determining the nature of ethical dilemmas in practice and in recognising the complexities involved in meeting the needs of a diverse population with diverse needs. Further discussion on the principles of ethical decision making can be found in Chapter 4.

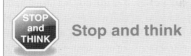

Stop and think

Having explored the five spheres of accountability, how will you ensure that your prescribing practice meets the required professional standards?

Using the five spheres of accountability

We need to recognise that the different spheres of accountability may at times conflict with one another. It is possible (though unlikely, perhaps), for instance, that what your employer wants you to do in a particular instance would not be in keeping with your professional code. Or that your patient requests treatments which are not in keeping with your professional judgement. We find it useful in these instances to recognise the different demands being placed on the practitioner. We have represented the process of accountability in Figure 2.1.

The process of accountable practice

Figure 2.1 represents the elements of accountable practice. While prescribers need to ensure their practice is lawful, this in itself does not mean that practice atuomatically meets accepted standards. As we have seen in this chapter, ethics plays an important part in accountable

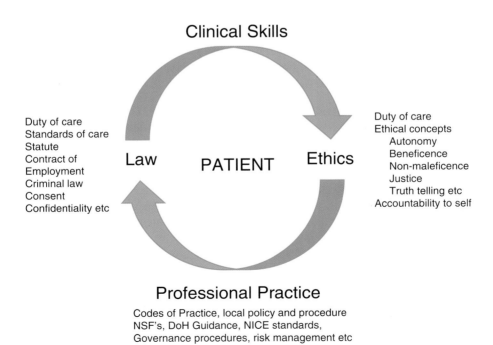

Figure 2.1   A model for accountable practice.

practice. What the practitioner considers to be ethical may, however, be unlawful and vice versa. Professional accountable practice is also influenced by national and local policy, clinical guidelines, codes of practice and clinical standards, all of which influence clinical decision making. However, the clinical skills the practitioner uses in implementing the prescribing decision are not to be underestimated; for example, in prescribing for your patient it is important that you share information with them about the dosage, route of administration and potential side effects. The challenge for the prescriber is to provide meaningful information to the patient who may be anxious and in pain. This process all takes place in the context of the relationship that is evolving between the patient and the prescriber.

As an accountable prescriber you will need to use your knowledge, skills and attitudes in determining the most appropriate professional practice that is both lawful and ethical to meet the needs of your patient.

Accountable prescribing

The following scenario will be familiar to many practitioners who are not prescribers. We are sure many of us have asked a doctor to prescribe something for our patient based on our own professional judgement and s/he may or may not have done so. The question is, how will you respond when a colleague, recognising that you can now prescribe, requests that you prescribe a drug for their patient?

While you may feel that your answer is going to be 'no', it is perhaps the process of considering your accountability that is of particular interest. Perhaps a good starting point is to consider the law. Is the drug you are being asked to prescribe authorised under independent and supplementary prescribing? You will find further discussion of the prescribing framework in Chapter 5. Certainly your colleague holds a duty of care to their patient but it is perhaps debatable as to whether at this time you share that duty, though it is conceivable that in fact you do. As such, you have a legal responsibility to the patient for the decision you make.

In making your decision, you should also consider the relevant codes of practice, appropriate clinical guidelines and local policies that are in place to guide your decision making.

If you were to refuse to prescribe, some thought would need to be given to the consequence of your actions. This may include the effect on the patient and how you can ensure that their health needs are met. Here we are in the domain of healthcare ethics as discussed in Chapter 4. Perhaps a more appropriate approach would be to recognise the clinical judgement of your colleague and your responsibilities for team working and see the patient with them to make your clinical judgement. Of course, there are at least three options available to you: to prescribe the drug your colleague thinks appropriate, to prescribe a different drug or not to prescribe at all. In any event, it is you who is accountable for the decision you take. Similarly, you will need to give thought to the skills you use not only to make your prescribing decision but also in exercising your accountability; that is, in maintaining your professional relationship with your colleague, respecting the relationship between your colleague and their patient, and in involving the patient who is now also your patient in the decision-making process.

Conclusion

It can be seen that in exercising your accountability as a prescriber, it is necessary to view accountability as a process that requires each prescribing situation to be considered on its own merits. We have presented here the five spheres of accountability that provide a means for analysing your responsibility as an accountable prescriber. While it is evident that defining accountable practice is in itself difficult, we have presented a process of accountable practice that may provide you with a framework to analyse your accountability in your day-to-day practice.

Summary

- As a practitioner, you are accountable for both your actions and omissions to act.
- There are five spheres of accountability. You are accountable to your employer, your professional body, your patient, the public and yourself.
- You are accountable professionally, ethically and legally for your prescribing practice.
- As a prescriber, you owe your patient a duty of care. Your duty is to act as the reasonable prescriber and you should be able to provide evidence to support your prescribing decisions.
- Maintaining your competence and updating your knowledge is a legal, ethical and professional responsibility.
- Accountable practice empowers the practitioner to meet patient need and improves patient outcomes.

 Activity

Answer true or false to each of the following:

1. The HPC, NMC and GMC all act to protect the interests of the profession they represent.
2. You cannot be held accountable for omissions in your prescribing.
3. Maintaining your clinical knowledge and competence is only a professional requirement.
4. The Bolam test means that as a prescriber, you have not breached your duty of care if other prescribers would have done the same thing.
5. An error in prescribing resulting in a patient's death may result in criminal proceedings against the prescriber.
6. Tort of negligence is covered by criminal law.
7. In ethical practice I can always act with no harm to the patient.

Useful websites

The website of the Medicines and Healthcare Products Regulatory Agency (MHRA) provides information about medicines regulation: www.mhra.gov.uk.

The National Prescribing Centre provides some helpful information about prescribing and patient group directions: **www.npc.co.uk**.

The relevant legislation is available from the Office for Public Sector Information's website: www.opsi.gov.uk.

The Health Professions Council is an independent, UK-wide health regulator. It sets standards of professional training, performance and conduct for 13 professions. It maintains a register of health professionals that meet its standards, and take action if registered health professionals do not meet those standards. Its website is: www.hpc-uk.org.

Patient Group Directions is a webpage where a centrally maintained archive of approved PGDs can be found; visit www.druginfozone.nhs.org.uk

References

Batey, M.V. and Lewis, F.M. (1982) Clarifying autonomy and accountability in nursing service. Part 1. *J Nursing Admin*, **12**, 13–18.

Beauchamp, T.L. and Childress, J.K. (2001) *Principles of Biomedical Ethics*, 5th edn, Oxford University Press, Oxford.

Bolam v *Friern Barnet Hospital Management Committee* (1957) 2All ER 118; 1 WLR 528.

Bolitho v *City & Hackney Health Authority* (1996) 7 Med LR 1; (1997). 3WLR 1151; (1998) AC 232.

Bristol Royal Infirmary Inquiry [Kennedy Report] (2001) *Learning From Bristol: the Report of the Public Inquiry into Children's Heart Surgery at the Bristol Royal Infirmary 1984-1995, Cm5207*, Stationery Office, London.

Department of Health (1998) *A First Class Service: Quality in the New NHS*, Department of Health, London.

Dimond, B. (2008) *Legal Aspects of Nursing*, 5th edn, Pearson Longman, Harlow.

Health Professions Council, Medicines and Prescribing (2009) www.hpc-uk.org/aboutregistration/medicinesandprescribing.

McSherry, R. and Pearce, P. (2008) *Clinical Governance: A Guide to Implementation for Healthcare Professionals*, 2nd edn, Blackwell Science, Oxford.

Nursing and Midwifery Council (2006) *Standards of Proficiency for Nurse and Midwife Prescribers*, Nursing and Midwifery Council, London.

Redfern, M. (2000) Report of The Royal Liverpool Children's Inquiry, Stationery Office, London.

Royal Pharmaceutical Society of Great Britain (2007) *Professional Standards and Guidance for Pharmacist Prescribers*, Royal Pharmaceutical Society of Great Britain. London.

Savage, J. and Moore, L. (2004) *Interpreting Accountability*, Royal College of Nursing, London.

Scally, G. and Donaldson, L. (1999) Clinical governance and the drive for quality improvement. *BMJ*, **317**, 61–65.

Shipman Inquiry First Report: Death Disguised, www.the-shipman-inquiry.org.uk/reports.asp.

Shipman Inquiry Second Report: The Police Investigation of March 1998, www.the-shipman-inquiry.org.uk/reports.asp.

Shipman Inquiry Third Report: Death and Cremation Certification, www.the-shipman-inquiry.org.uk/reports.asp.

Victoria Climbié Inquiry Report (2003) Report of Inquiry by Lord Laming, Cm 5730. Department of Health, Norwich.

Further reading

Caulfield, H. (2005) *Accountability*, Blackwells, Oxford.

Health Professions Council, Medicines and Prescribing (2009) www.hpc-uk.org/aboutregistration/medicinesandprescribing.

Ieraci, S. (2007) Responsibility versus accountability in a risk-averse culture. *Emerg Med Australasia*, **18**, 63–64.

Nursing and Midwifery Council (2008) *Standards for Medicines Management*, Nursing and Midwifery Council, London.

Royal Pharmaceutical Society of Great Britain (2007) *Code of Ethics for Pharmacists and Pharmacy Technicians*, Pharmaceutical Press, London.

Royal Pharmaceutical Society of Great Britain (2007) *Professional Standards and Guidance for Pharmacist Prescribers*, Pharmaceutical Press, London.

Section 1

3 Legal aspects of prescribing

Learning outcomes

By the end of this chapter the reader should be able to:

* define the differences between licensed, off-label and unlicensed medicines and how this affects your liability for harmful effects when you prescribe them
* identify the four legal categories of medicines and outline the controls on the prescribing and supply of each category
* describe the difference between independent and supplementary prescriber status and outline what each can prescribe, under what circumstances and what information must appear on their prescriptions
* describe the supply of medicines through the use of Patient Group Directions (PGDs) and written directions in hospital
* Outline how non-medical prescribers could be held liable for the quality of their prescribing.

Perhaps the first thing to note is that the law generally makes no distinction between health-care provided within the NHS and that provided elsewhere, in the private or voluntary sectors. The law controlling the supply of medicines applies within hospitals, clinics, GP surgeries, prisons, the armed forces, care homes, pharmacies, newsagents and even supplies to a patient in their own home. However, administrative law (see below), which underpins the structures and operation of the NHS, now does vary significantly between the home countries of England, Scotland, Wales and Northern Ireland, although the broad principles remain very similar.

The law relating to prescribing

We should first of all distinguish between several types of law; the distinctions are important because they dictate the nature of the sanction if you break the law! The form of law familiar

---

The New Prescriber. Edited by J Lymn, D Bowskill, F Bath-Hextall, R Knaggs, © 2010 John Wiley & Sons.

to most of us is statutory criminal law which can be characterised by the penalty for breach of the law. Statutory law comprises one of two main divisions of law: statute law and civil law. A statute is, strictly speaking, an Act of Parliament. In the context of prescribing, the two Acts you should be familiar with are the Medicines Act 1968 and the Misuse of Drugs Act 1971. An Act constitutes the 'bones' of a body of law; the 'flesh' is then added in the form of Regulations, which provide the detail of how the Act will be implemented. Breach of the Medicines Act, Misuse of Drugs Act or their Regulations attracts criminal sanctions such as fines or prison. Almost all health professionals are now regulated by a regulatory authority such as the Nursing and Midwifery Council or the General Medical Council. Such bodies have legal powers, developed and approved by Parliament, set out in statutes. The sanctions for breach of this statutory professional law may not be fines or prison but are more likely to be orders for supervised practice, suspension or removal from a professional register.

The other form of statutory law relevant to prescribers is called statutory administrative law. Every body that carries out public services – be it an ambulance trust, a primary care organisation, a hospital or your local education authority or borough council – has its powers set out in statute. Law is needed to give the public body the right, for example, to manage property, employ staff and pay them and contract for services. A public body needs to hold those who work for it or contract with it accountable for the services they provide on its behalf, usually through tribunals rather than the criminal courts. The sanctions for breach of this kind of statutory law could be through internal disciplinary processes, loss of job or the contract or in some case fines that are paid to the public body rather than the state.

Breach of the statutory law relating to prescribing therefore could put you at risk of criminal sanctions, such as a fine or a prison sentence, could jeopardise your professional registration or could result in a challenge to your employing body or jeopardy to your job.

Before going into more detail, we should consider the other major branch of law: the civil law. This term derives from the notion of duties and responsibilities owed between citizens to each other. Action under civil law (a suit or being sued) allows an aggrieved party to sue for compensation from another citizen who is alleged to have 'wronged' them. In healthcare terms, the action is likely to be for clinical negligence in that the provider of the health service did not exercise the proper duty of care and hence caused harm to the patient.

The Medicines Act 1968 and the Misuse of Drugs Act 1971

All prescribers should be aware of the legislation covering the commodities they are prescribing for others and even pharmacists may welcome an update on the legal framework for non-medical prescribing. The Medicines Act has two main purposes: to assure the quality, safety and efficacy of medicines that are marketed in the United Kingdom and to maintain the safety of the public by controlling routes of access to potentially dangerous commodities like medicines. The Misuse of Drugs Act and its subordinate legislation add an additional layer of tougher supply controls for a number of medicines with a high potential for abuse – the so-called controlled drugs. We look first at the licensing process which applies to all medicines, including controlled drugs.

Medicinal products and the licensing system

The thalidomide tragedy in 1961 precipitated a demand for legislation to define precisely what is a medicine, as opposed to a poison, and to control the safety, quality and efficacy of medicines (the law calls them medicinal products) marketed in the UK. Under the Medicines Act, the definition of a medicinal product is, broadly speaking, something that is marketed for a 'medicinal purpose'. Thus a medicinal product is (paraphrased):

> Any substance or combination of substances marketed for the purpose of treating or preventing disease or administration with a view to making a medical diagnosis or to restoring, correcting or modifying physiological functions.

Claims that a substance or product is a medicine will depend upon whether medicinal claims are made for it. Before a medicinal product can be marketed in the UK, it must first be granted a marketing authorisation (MA) by the relevant licensing body, the Medicines and Healthcare products Regulatory Agency (MHRA). The term marketing authorisation replaced the earlier term product licence (PL) but PL still frequently appears on packs of medicines sold in the UK. Before granting an MA, the MHRA must be satisfied of the safety, quality and efficacy of the medicinal product. Once the MHRA is satisfied (which can take many years from the development of the drug), the medicine is licensed.

The importance of a medicine being licensed

We have drawn particular attention to the process of licensing because it affects the risks surrounding the prescribing of medicines. If a medicine is licensed, then provided the medicine is prescribed for the purposes, conditions and patients specified in the licence, the MA holder will be liable for any adverse effects that the medicine may have on the patient who takes it. The licence is, in effect, a guarantee from the MA holder direct to the patient that the MA holder will be liable for compensation for any unexpected harm (if proven) that arises when the medicine is prescribed and used according to the conditions of the MA. Note that this guarantee only applies when the medicine is prescribed and used 'within' the licence. You, as the prescriber, can rely on the MA holder for this protection.

It therefore follows that if you depart from the conditions specified in the MA (variously called off-label, off-licence or outwith the licence), or prescribe something without a MA at all (that is, unlicensed), you as prescriber will carry liability for any harm that may result. For this reason it is very important that you are aware of the licensing status of any medicines that you prescribe. The important details of a MA or PL for most UK licensed medicines are set out in the Compendium of Data Sheets and Summaries of Product Characteristics (SPC) published by the organisation representing the pharmaceutical industry, the Association of the British Pharmaceutical Industry (ABPI). The SPC covers a great many matters: the presentation (tablet, capsule, liquid, cream, colour, shape, markings plus strength and dose volume); the indications or uses (which diseases in which patients); the recommended dosages and methods of administration; the contraindications (when not to use it) and warnings about side effects as well as the legal category and the product licence number. If you prescribe any medicine in circumstances which are not clearly covered in this detailed specification, then the liability for safety of that medicine becomes yours. Such 'off-label' usage is actually quite common, say on paediatric wards, in palliative care or in dermatology.

In some circumstances (see later) non-medical prescribers can also prescribe unlicensed medicines – that is, products or substances that have not been subject to any licensing process in the UK. This means that not only may their safety be suspect but also their quality and efficacy. One of the drawbacks of acquiring medicines over the internet is the heightened danger of receiving medicines which are not in fact what they claim to be or, worse, they may contain either no active ingredient or harmful ingredients.

Before moving on to the supply of medicines, you should be aware that the MHRA is responsible for enforcing adverse drug reaction (ADR) reporting by MA and PL holders and for dealing with reports under the 'Yellow Card scheme' (samples are bound into the back of the British National Formulary – BNF). This is a system available to doctors, pharmacists, nurses and patients to report any ADRs associated with medicines, both prescribed and purchased over the counter and with complementary medicines and traditional remedies. Virtually all pharmaceutical companies belong to the ABPI which has a code of practice for the marketing of medicines. This is published in the SPC Compendium. You should recognise that, as a non-medical prescriber, you may be a target for promotional literature and visits by representatives of pharmaceutical companies.

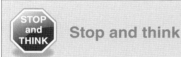 **Stop and think**

Before making a prescribing decision make sure that you know the licensing status of what you intend to prescribe.
   Is it fully licensed, outside its licence or completely unlicensed?
   Reflect on the consequences for yourself if a patient suffers harm from your prescribing; how does the licensing status affect this liability?

Legislation covering the supply of medicines

The three categories of medicines under the Medicines Act are shown in Table 3.1.

Table 3.1   Categories of medicines under the Medicines Act.

Category	Restrictions on availability
General Sales List medicines (GSL)	There are no restrictions on sale of these medicines except that they must be sold in the original manufacturer's packaging, there may be limits on the pack size and the sale has to be made from permanent premises, not from a market stall or van.
Pharmacy medicines (P)	These can only be sold from a registered pharmacy under the supervision of registered pharmacists. Proposals have been made to change these restrictions but they should have little impact on non-medical prescribers.
Prescription-only medicines (POM)	These can only be supplied or authorised for supply by an 'appropriate practitioner' (see below).

> **Box 3.1** **The Controlled Drugs Schedules**
>
> - **Schedule 1**: Includes drugs with virtually no current therapeutic use, which are licensed solely for research purposes. An example would be cannabis or LSD. A Home Office licence is required for prescribing, possession and supply.
> - **Schedule 2**: Includes opiates (e.g. diamorphine, morphine, pethidine and methadone) and major stimulants (e.g. amphetamine).
> - **Schedule 3**: Drugs such as temazepam, buprenorphine and flunitrazepam which are thought to be less likely to be abused than those in Schedule 2 and, if abused, are considered less harmful.
> - **Schedule 4**: Contains two classes of drugs – benzodiazepines and anabolic steroids.
> - **Schedule 5**: These are preparations containing CDs exempted from controls because of their low strength or concentration. Some are even exempted from POM controls and are P medicines. They have no special requirements as far as prescribers are concerned.

Controlled drugs (CDs)

All controlled drugs are prescription-only medicines (POM) *and* CD. Mere possession of a controlled drug is a criminal offence unless you are covered by one of the exemptions in the legislation. The Misuse of Drugs Act classifies drugs into Classes A, B and C; this has no relation to their use as medicines but relates to their relative harmfulness as illicit drugs, and is used to determine the scale of penalties for offences under the Act. CDs are permitted to be used lawfully for medical purposes but are subject to further controls (in addition to those in the Medicines Act) depending on the category or Schedule in which they are listed. The five categories are described in Box 3.1.

Only those drugs in schedules 2 and 3 have relevance for non-medical prescribers. The legislation covering CDs requires meticulous attention to detail and covers registers and safe custody, inspection and monitoring, destruction (see Box 3.2) and prescription writing requirements (see Box 3.3).

Appropriate practitioner

In the original Medicines Act Regulations there were only three appropriate practitioners:

- doctor
- dentist
- vet.

Since the advent of non-medical prescribing four more categories have been added:

- a community nurse practitioner (formerly called district nurse or health visitor prescribers)
- a nurse independent prescriber
- a pharmacist independent prescriber
- a supplementary prescriber (includes nurses, pharmacists, physiotherapists, podiatrists and radiographers).

Box 3.2	**Details of Relevant Legislation on Controlled Drugs**
Records	For Schedule 2 drugs, all transactions, both receipts and supplies, must be recorded in an official CD Register which may be computer produced as well as written and, although not yet a legal requirement, a running balance of the stock of each drug should be maintained.
Safe custody	All Schedule 2 drugs (except quinalbarbitone) and some Schedule 3 drugs must be kept in safe custody in a locked cabinet of a design approved by the police or, in the community pharmacy, in accordance with the specifications in the Safe Custody regulations.[1]
Safe Management	Since 2007[2] all NHS and private health organisations must have appointed an 'Accountable Officer' who is responsible for the safe management of CDs within that organisation. All healthcare providers who hold stocks of CDs have to comply with standard operating procedures for their management and to make 'periodic' declarations that they have CDs on their premises and the stock levels. Each primary care contractor (GPs, pharmacies, opticians and dentists) is subject to a formal CD review once a year.
Destruction	Stocks of CDs that are unwanted, out of date or obsolete may only be destroyed in the presence of an 'authorised person'. The groups of people who are authorised to witness destruction of CDs expanded in 2007 to include any officer of a healthcare organisation, including strategic health authority pharmacy leads, medical directors and clinical governance leads provided they are not themselves routinely involved in the management or use of CDs.

[1] Misuse of Drugs Act (Safe Custody) Regulations 1973 SI 1973 No. 798
[2] The Controlled Drugs (Supervision of Management and Use) Regulations 2006 SI 2006 No. 3148

The first six categories of practitioners are independent prescribers. Using their personal professional judgement, they can prescribe for patients under their care any medicinal product that the law allows them to. Supplementary prescribers prescribe within a treatment plan – the clinical management plan (CMP) – in partnership with the doctor *and* the patient. As we said at the outset, the Medicines Act and Misuse of Drugs Act apply both to NHS and private supplies of medicines. Thus doctors can and do write private prescriptions in all classes of medicines for patients who choose or are obliged to pay for their medicines privately, P and General Sales List (GSL) are available for sale in community pharmacies and GSL medicines are available from a wide range of shops, newsagents, petrol forecourts and the like. Moreover, doctors and dentists are allowed to supply all drugs, including CDs, to their own patients directly. The law does not, however, allow them to sell medicines to the general public.

Since 1992 a series of new laws have facilitated and set conditions for the development of 'non-medical prescribers' in England. Community nurse practitioners (CNP) must be first-level nurses or registered midwives, be annotated as a CNP in their professional register and are limited to the CNP formulary. Nurse and pharmacist independent prescribers must be similarly qualified and entered in their register and after a course of training may prescribe from the relevant formulary in the BNF. A supplementary prescriber must be a first-level nurse, a pharmacist, a registered midwife or a chiropodist, podiatrist, physiotherapist or radiographer and annotated as such in their respective professional registers. In addition, the law requires that where non-medical prescribers are treating NHS patients, they must be employed by an NHS body such as a primary care trust (in England), an NHS trust or a GP practice.

The above account describes the underpinning framework for the prescription of medicines in the UK. Before turning to the detail of those arrangements for non-medical prescribers, we should briefly consider the role of the NHS in medicines supply.

NHS regulations

Supplies of medicines within the NHS must comply with the criminal statutory law in the Medicines Act and the Misuse of Drugs Act but the NHS can also impose restrictions (through administrative law supplemented by internal policies and guidelines) on the use of some medicines by professionals who are employed by or contract their services to the NHS. The most common form of exclusion is the 'black-list' – a list of drugs and other substances not to be prescribed under NHS Pharmaceutical Services. Writing a prescription for a black-listed product is a breach of the NHS contract terms of service for the prescribing doctor and means that a pharmacist who dispenses the item will not be reimbursed by the NHS. Black-listed drugs are marked in the BNF by a symbol representing the word 'NHS' with a line through it.

Exclusion is also achieved through the use of formularies. Restrictions upon prescribing to NHS patients by CNPs or nurse or pharmacist independent prescribers are set out in the relevant formulary in the BNF publications. The BNF also lists 'borderline substances' which the NHS will only pay for if they are prescribed in circumstances when the Advisory Committee on Borderline Substances has advised that they may be regarded as drugs. Examples include specialised food supplements for malabsorption syndromes or enteral feeds. You should also note the use of the 'black triangle' against some BNF entries which denotes a newly licensed medicine that is being intensively monitored; you should take particular care to monitor and report any adverse effects if prescribing these medicines.

 Stop and think

When monitoring the progress of a patient's medication regimen, how will you ask about possible side effects or interactions with other medicines or food? Make sure you understand the sections of the BNF that set out this information. How and when would you use the Yellow Card notification forms at the back of the BNF?

Who can prescribe what in non-medical prescribing?

At this point we must stress that the legislation in this area is constantly changing, though not as rapidly as it did in the first few years of non-medical prescribing. Readers are strongly advised to download the latest version of guidance from the Department of Health website to supplement the information below.

Community nurse practitioners

The formulary available to community nurse prescribers comprises a small range of medicines with a larger range of dressings and appliances. All medicinal products must be prescribed by their generic names but dressings and appliances can be prescribed by their trade names.

Independent prescriber

The definition offered by the Department of Health is that 'independent prescribing is prescribing by a practitioner (e.g. doctor, dentist, nurse or pharmacist) responsible and accountable for the assessment of patients with undiagnosed or diagnosed conditions and for decisions about the clinical management required, including prescribing'(DH 2006). Providing you have successfully completed the appropriate training and you are working within your own competency, then as a nurse or pharmacist independent prescriber you may prescribe almost any medicine that you believe to be appropriate for your patients. There are two limitations: you may not prescribe black-listed medicines and you may only prescribe controlled drugs in certain circumstances (see the relevant formulary in the current BNF).

Supplementary prescriber

The definition offered by the Department of Health is 'a voluntary partnership between an independent prescriber (a doctor or dentist) and a supplementary prescriber to implement an agreed patient-specific Clinical Management Plan with the patient's agreement'. Supplementary prescribing differs from independent prescribing in that the treatment regime is initiated or suggested by a clinician or other independent prescriber (but not a nurse or pharmacist) who is responsible for determining what is wrong with the patient (DH 2005). As a supplementary prescriber, you may only prescribe medication within a patient-specific CMP which may include authority to alter doses or to stop medicines that are no longer needed. You may prescribe off-label, unlicensed medicines or controlled drugs if they are specified in the CMP, but not black-listed medicines.

Supply under patient group directions

Patient Group Directions (PGDs, formerly called group protocols) allow a wide range of health professionals to authorise supply of POMs to specified groups of patients without the usual need for an individually prepared prescription. The most common example of this would be the supply and administration of 'flu vaccine'. Here, all patients identified as needing this treatment are grouped together as a whole and are defined by their need for treatment, not their medical condition. A practitioner working under a PGD can therefore only supply a flu vaccination to the category of patient defined in the direction. PGDs are written documents which must be signed by a member of the healthcare profession supplying the medicine and a senior doctor and pharmacist. The legislation clearly defines what must be included in a written direction. When supplying medicines using PGDs, healthcare professionals must supply exactly as per the written direction. PGDs may authorise supply of GSL, P, POM and CD medicines in certain circumstances but they must be followed to the letter; there is no clinical freedom to change the specifications. It would be a criminal offence if a POM other than that stipulated in the PGD is supplied or if a condition is treated that is not specified in the PGD.

Supply against 'written directions' to supply

In hospitals only, sometimes called standing orders or bed charts. The legislation allows hospitals to supply a POM in the course of its business against a patient-specific written direction of a doctor. The written direction does not need to comply with the requirements specified for prescriptions (see below), but does need to relate to a specific patient. Most entries on a patient's bed card are directions to administer but providing the wording is clear, they can be used as an authority to supply, for example, take home medication.

 Stop and think

When you are considering authorising the supply of a medicine, make sure you understand the options available and the legal category of the medicine in mind. Will you be using your qualification as an independent or supplementary prescriber? If supplementary, are you familiar with the terms of the relevant CMP? Or is there a PGD in place that would be more appropriate? Is the medicine classified as a CD with special conditions? Or is it a POM, P or GSL? What difference does the legal category make to your prescribing?

Legislation on prescription writing

To be legally valid, prescriptions must comply with regulations made under the Medicines Act. If an invalid prescription is dispensed, the dispensing pharmacy or pharmacist commits a criminal offence. The Misuse of Drugs Act adds further legal requirements for CDs; both the writer and the dispenser of an invalid prescription for CDs commit a criminal offence. Box 3.3 sets out information which must appear on valid NHS or private prescriptions for POMs and CDs.

These are the only legal requirements. Surprisingly, essential information for prescribing POMs, such as the name of the drug, the strength, dose and quantity and the name and address of the patient, are not required by the Medicines Act!

Although not in the legislation, you should be particularly aware of the need to keep prescriptions and prescription pads secure. They should be treated like cheques in a cheque-book – never pre-sign prescriptions. Records should always be made, ideally at the time of writing, of the prescriptions you write. The record should clearly indicate the date, name of prescriber, name of item prescribed, quantity or dose, frequency and duration of treatment and, if appropriate, strength, dosing schedule and route of administration. Details of the consultation with the patient and your prescribing authority should also be included. For guidance on prescription writing please refer to the British National Formulary.

Box 3.3   **Legal Requirements for Prescriptions**

For prescription-only medicines

Requirement	Additional information
A signature (in ink) from the prescriber	This is the only part of the prescription that must be written personally by the prescriber *(except for handwritten prescriptions for CDs, see below)*; everything else can be written by someone else, computer generated, and so on. The law also permits the use of electronic signatures in preparation for an electronic prescription service.
The (practice) address of the prescriber	
The date the prescription was written	Prescriptions for POMs are valid for 6 months from the date of writing
Particulars indicating that the prescriber is an 'appropriate practitioner'	NHS forms will normally bear your pre-printed details; a private prescription should indicate the qualifications of the prescriber.
The age of the patient if under 12 years	

In addition for prescriptions for Schedule 2 (except temazepam) and Schedule 3 CDs	
The total quantity to be supplied must be specified in words and figures	Prescribing quantities solely by dose and length of treatment is not valid.
The form of the medicine (e.g. tablets) must be specified.	This applies even when there is only one form of a medicine and/or the form is implied in the name, for example MST Continus, Sevredol, Morcap SR, MXL
The strength of the medicine, if there is more than one, must be specified	
A dose must be specified	'As directed' or 'when required', and so on are not acceptable as doses, but 'one as directed' or 'two when required', and so on, are.
Prescriptions are only valid for 28 days	From the date written on the prescription by the prescriber – or can be a specified later date if initialled by the prescriber
The quantity of CD prescribed should not exceed 30 days' supply	
Repeat prescriptions are not permitted.	
Private prescriptions for CDs must be written on the official form	
The private prescriber's identification number should appear on the prescription (not the professional registration number)	

Accountability and non-medical prescribers

We have seen above that there is a significant quantity of complex statutory criminal law to observe as a non-medical prescriber. However, the criminal law cannot ensure that you are competent in your prescribing practice; other mechanisms are needed. We have already described how, if you are employed in the NHS, your employer will expect you to work within your competence and within any internal directions, policies, formularies, standard operating procedures, and so on that your employer expects to be followed. If you do this, then your employer will have vicarious liability for any harm to patients that may result from your practice. This means that in the event of a successful civil law action for negligence, your employer will meet any compensation payments to the patient. If, however, you depart (without good reason) from these requirements, or if you are carrying out work that your employer does not know about, then you may be personally liable for any compensation payments. Even if the consequences are not this serious, you may find that you will still be subject to internal disciplinary measures or may jeopardise your promotion or even your job. If you undertake prescribing in private practice then you should always check what professional insurance is available to you and consider taking out your own.

All non-medical prescribers will have their own professional regulatory (registration) body. Such bodies can also hold you accountable for the quality of your prescribing. They will also expect you to observe any ethical or good practice codes relevant to your profession. Any departure from these may be regarded as indicating that your fitness to practise should be investigated and all professional regulatory bodies have powers to convene professional tribunals which can order suspension, restricted practice or removal from the register. The standards that the regulatory body will apply will accord with the standard of proof in a civil action for negligence.

Conclusion

We hope the above account is not seen as a deterrent to non-medical prescribing! Only by knowing what the rules and risks are can you manage them and feel confident that you are a competent and safe prescriber.

Summary

● Non-medical prescribing is affected by statutory criminal law such as the Medicines and Misuse of Drugs Act and by NHS regulations
● Non-medical prescribers could be held to account for their prescribers by their professional regulator and by the patient under the civil law duty of care.
● If a medicine is fully licensed, then liability for adverse effects falls upon the holder of its marketing authorisation.
● If a medicine is used outside its licence (off-label) or is completely unlicensed, then the prescriber may be liable for its adverse effects.
● Medicines are legally categorised as GSL, P, POM or CD.
● Independent prescribers are solely responsible for their prescribing decisions.
● Supplementary prescribers share responsibility for their prescribing with the prescribing doctor, as set out in the clinical management plan.
● Patient Group Directions may be used where specific groups of patients and their conditions can be clearly defined in advance of supply.
● Prescriptions must comply with the relevant regulations to be legally valid.

 Activity

1. There is no real difference between off-label medicines and unlicensed medicines.
   True/False
2. Nurse independent prescribers can prescribe a limited range of controlled drugs.
   True/False

3. A clinical management plan can only contain fully licensed medicines. True/False
4. As long as I am employed, my employer is liable for any mistakes I make. True/False
5. It would be a criminal offence for me to supply a different POM from that specified on a PGD. True/False
6. Pharmacist independent prescribers cannot prescribe black triangle medicines. True/False
7. All transactions in Schedule 2 CDs must be recorded in a register. True/False
8. Medical prescribers can prescribe medicines that are on the NHS black-list. True/False
9. Nurse prescribers should not be reporting adverse drug reactions via the Yellow Card scheme. True/False

Useful websites

The National Patient Safety Agency leads and contributes to improved, safe patient care. www.npsa.nhs.uk.

The Medicines and Healthcare products Regulatory Agency safeguards the public by ensuring that medicines and medical devices work and are acceptably safe. www.mhra.gov.uk.

The Patient Group Direction website provides support to all healthcare professionals who work with PGDs or are involved in their development and review. www.portal.nelm.nhs.uk/PGD.

References

Department of Health (2005) *Supplementary Prescribing by Nurses, Pharmacists, Chiropodists/Podiatrists, Physiotherapists and Radiographers within the NHS in England. A Guide for Implementation*, Stationery Office, London.

Department of Health (2006) *Improving Patients' Access to Medicines: A Guide to Implementing Nurse and Pharmacist Independent Nurse and Pharmacist Independent Prescribing within the NHS in England*, Stationery Office, London.

Further reading

British Medical Association and Royal Pharmaceutical Society of Great Britain (2010) *British National Formulary*, 59th edn, BMJ Publishing, London.

Appelbe, G.E. and Wingfield, J. (2009) *Dale and Appelbe's Pharmacy Law and Ethics*, 9th edn, Pharmaceutical Press, London.

Department of Health (2006) *Medicines Matters*, Stationery Office, Department of Health London.

Dimond, B. (2009) *Legal Aspects of Consent*, 2nd edn, Quay Books, London.

Dimond, B. (2005) *Legal Aspects of Medicines*, Quay Books, London.

Dimond, B. (2008) *Legal Aspects of Nursing*, 5th edn, Pearson Education Limited, Harlow.

Herring, J. (2008) *Medical Law and Ethics*, Open University Press, Oxford.

McHale, J. (2007) *Healthcare Law: Text and Materials*, 2nd edn, Sweet and Maxwell, London.

Tingle, J. and Cribb, A. (2007) *Nursing Law and Ethics*, Blackwell Publishing, Oxford.

4 The ethics of prescribing

Learning outcomes

By the end of this chapter, the reader should be able to:

- describe three key ethical theories
- understand how ethical theory may be applied in prescribing practice
- consider ethics in relation to conscience, law and ethical codes
- reflect on unique ethical problems in prescribing.

Ethics, or moral philosophy as it is also known, is concerned with questioning and justifying what individuals do, and particularly what actions are thought right or wrong, or what sort of person one should try to be. Traditionally, this involved concerns about individuals' virtues but more recently focus has shifted to justifying individual acts. The aim in this chapter is to focus on ethical theories that have been influential in the healthcare setting – deontology, utilitarianism and the four principles of bioethics – and to consider how ethical decision making occurs in practice.

Deontology

Deontological ethical theories are concerned with 'duty' and with what acts are right. They put forward a number of specific acts which individuals are expected to follow regardless of the consequences of these actions. The most influential deontological theory was that of Immanuel Kant (1998) who argued that acts are right only if they are in accordance with the categorical imperative. There are two key statements of the categorical imperative: to act only in ways that can be accepted by everyone (universalised), and to treat individuals not as means to an end, but respect them as individuals. Deontological theories do not allow the consequences of a proposed act to have any influence. The prescriber, for example, who prescribes a medicine

The New Prescriber. Edited by J Lymn, D Bowskill, F Bath-Hextall, R Knaggs, © 2010 John Wiley & Sons.

to assist in suicide acts wrongly because to universalise such an act would threaten society. The prescriber who lies to a patient about a medicine's side effects to ensure they take it also acts wrongly according to the deontologist. Lying is not something that everyone would agree to if everyone were allowed to do it, and it does not respect the patient who is lied to.

Deontological, duty-based ethical theories have been criticised. Firstly, these duties are very demanding and, because every action must comply with the categorical imperative statements, they cannot be avoided. Secondly, it is not always obvious how to apply these rules in everyday situations.

Utilitarianism

In contrast to deontological theories based on duties, there are consequentialist theories that value the outcome or good of actions. The most influential of these, utilitarianism, involves a calculation of the overall measure of utility or good. The utilitarian must consider how a proposed act will affect everyone but, crucially, not allow anyone a greater weighting. Furthermore, the utilitarian can only be concerned with the single measure of utility and the best known, developed originally by Mill (1992), is happiness. The result is an ethical theory that is impartial in terms of individuals. One cannot give greater weighting to some (like family or friends) but not others and one cannot exclude particular acts (like lying or suicide) if they result in the greatest overall welfare.

Utilitarianism has been influential for political and policy-based decisions but has been criticised since it can justify in certain circumstances acts usually considered wrong, such as torture and killing. Taking a utilitarian approach, a prescriber might limit the prescribing of expensive medicines that only benefit a minority of patients when greater happiness could be gained from prescribing a different drug for a larger number of patients. Utilitarian justification cannot give any extra weighting to the suffering that would result from the minority denied a medicine.

Whilst utilitarian and deontological ethical theories have been influential within healthcare, a principle-based theory has been highly influential too.

Four principles of bioethics

Principlism is a form of ethical justification which recognises that certain principles should guide individuals in deciding upon what acts are right. For Beauchamp and Childress (2001), the question of what principles one should use can be answered using four principles: autonomy, beneficence (going good), non-maleficence (avoiding harm) and justice. Whilst acknowledging that these were not the only principles that should guide individuals in life more generally, they were argued to be sufficient to allow ethical decisions within healthcare to be made (along with several more specific rules).

Autonomy involves 'self-rule' and freedom from controlling influences and may be applied not only and obviously to patients but also to relatives, carers and healthcare professionals such as prescribers. For prescribers, this principle would require consideration of patients' decisions and wishes, but also the prescriber's autonomy, including concerns about not being coerced into prescribing. Beneficence and non-maleficence seem similar and that to not harm is to do good. Non-maleficence is considered the more demanding principle and not harming takes precedence over helping. For prescribers, this might involve consideration of not harming patients in prescribing and always prescribing to help them. This can be difficult for prescribers when, for example, the prescribed drug is known to have harmful side effects. The principle of justice involves the notion of the fair and equitable distribution of treatment according to needs – prescribers considering this principle would need to appreciate conflicting demands upon who would benefit most from medicines and how to allocate scarce resources in healthcare systems.

It is obvious that these four principles may conflict at times. For example, a patient's autonomous wish for an unproven or expensive medicine cannot always be respected, since this may deprive other patients of treatment (a justice concern) or harm the patient (non-maleficence). Whereas Kantian deontological duties require all categorical imperatives to be observed and utilitarian theory involves only one consistent calculation, the four principles accept that all four cannot necessarily be applied in all situations and that a process of deciding which to use or what weighting to give each must be used.

The answer to how to decide which principles to apply involves what is termed a process of reflective equilibrium, following the liberal theory of Rawls (1979). This requires individuals to engage in a process of specifying and balancing the respective principles – choosing which might apply, together with their relative importance, in a given situation, all whilst considering these in relation to their own intuition. If the choice of one principle cannot be accommodated with one's own intuition, then one must return to the problem and reconsider the available principles again.

 Stop and think

If there are several conflicting theories, which one should the new prescriber use in practice?
   Can you be utilitarian when you want a patient to take a beneficial medicine that they do not want, but a deontologist when you want to give a patient a medicine usually denied on cost grounds?

Making ethical decisions

To answer these questions, it is helpful to consider reasoning that is either 'top down' or 'bottom up'. The difference between these approaches is that 'top down' reasoning works from an ethical theory and seeks to apply it consistently to all cases. 'Bottom up' reasoning starts from a problem and applies theories to solve it. The bottom-up approach is not the intended use of individual theories but the approach is argued to be helpful in the practical aspect of resolving ethical problems. This approach also allows the practitioner to apply ethical theories alongside other factors, such as laws, codes and also personal beliefs. Although this seems to be a convenient 'having your cake and eating it' approach, it is recognised that certain ethical problems can be considered in relation to different theories and so selecting them accordingly is relevant (Seedhouse, 1998).

It should also be added that there are several other ways of justifying decisions and a frequently used method involves arguing by analogy. Instead of applying theory, the individual attempts to compare a proposed act or decision with another situation, to either support or contrast it. An obvious example is that of postcode prescribing in which a concerned prescriber who wants to prescribe a medicine which is not permitted in their area could argue using not only principles of justice but also analogy and question why a medicine can be given in another area but not their own. However, these approaches are often claimed to carry less ethical justification since they rely upon comparisons with acts that may only be socially or historically justified, rather than based upon ethical argument.

There is another approach to making ethical decisions that prescribers might find useful. It recognises that ethical theories are rather abstract and perhaps hard to apply in practice. This involves the development of several practical *models* of decision making (Cooper, 2007; Wingfield and Badcott, 2007). These may be contrasted with the three key ethical theories described so far in this chapter, in that they provide a series of steps or stages which individuals should work through to arrive at an ethical decision. Unfortunately, none of them does away with the fundamental need to apply some form of ethical reasoning to the problem at hand, but for the prescriber, such models may help in the gathering of relevant information and balancing other demands. Several models have been developed but the British Medical Association (2004) approach illustrates a typical example in Box 4.1.

Whilst such models might seem unduly reductive and raise concerns as to whether all decision making can be reduced to such discrete and convenient stages, they are appealing in providing an *aide-mémoire* to allow the prescriber to gain confidence and perhaps conceptualise what is needed to resolve each ethical problem. However, it can be seen from the above example that individuals must be prepared to consider not only ethical argument but also relevant law and this is now considered in terms of additional influences upon decision making in prescribing.

Conscience, codes and law

An ethical decision in prescribing unfortunately does not involve considering ethical theory alone and it is usually accepted that the prescriber must also consider their own personal beliefs and conscience, as well as relevant laws and professional codes of ethics. In relation to personal beliefs, it is recognised that all individuals will have such thoughts, perhaps about issues that they have considered over time, or they may be one's first thoughts about a new situation and these may be referred to as one's intuition or even one's conscience.

Box 4.1 British Medical Association Stages of Ethical Decision Making

1. Recognise ethical situation.
2. Break down dilemma into parts.
3. Seek information from patient and others.
4. Identify relevant legal and professional guidance.
5. If no solution found, apply critical ethical analysis.
6. Justify decisions with sound arguments.

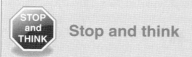

Stop and think

What sorts of beliefs or feelings might conflict with making an ethical decision?
   Should such beliefs and convictions be given any weight? Or should the three key ethical theories considered so far always be used instead?

Ethics and the individual

As noted, 'top down' approaches maintain that only one ethical theory applies and there can be no room for personal beliefs but others have recognised the appeal of such personal beliefs. Beauchamp and Childress, for example, believed that accommodating principles within one's own beliefs is a necessary process. Indeed, within healthcare, personal beliefs – be they religious or secular – are frequently (although not always) respected by the inclusion of conscience clauses in professional codes. However, there is a tension between accommodating personal beliefs and giving them primacy, since the latter introduces what is known as relativism. This is yet another ethical approach that, in various forms, maintains that different beliefs are possible amongst different individuals and, significantly, that these should all be valued. However, opponents have argued that this may mean that no agreement might be reached on anything, if individuals hold many different views. Applied to prescribing and healthcare, relativism and appeals to personal beliefs are therefore problematic because they may lead to different outcomes for different prescribers, and may be hard to justify to others. Despite such problems, appeals to conscience are often accepted in healthcare in relation to issues such as abortion, for example, and these are supported in ethical codes and also law (Royal Pharmaceutical Society, 2007). However, although these are distinct from more extreme views that all healthcare professionals must undertake tasks that are part of their professional role (Savulescu, 2006), caveats apply and conscientious objectors are usually required to provide details of where alternative services can be found. Hence, the prescriber who does not wish to prescribe contraception should indicate where such services are available, even if this is ethically problematic for them (Cooper, Bissell and Wingfield, 2008).

Ethics and professional codes

As well as personal beliefs, prescribers must also consider relevant ethical codes. The role of professional codes of ethics is to offer guidance to practitioners, and they often include principles similar to those described above, and may be identified in those issued by the Nursing and Midwifery Council (2008) and also the Royal Pharmaceutical Society (2007), for example. They have certain advantages over general ethical theories like utilitarianism and deontology in that they are usually specific to particular professions and hence offer potentially more specific advice related to practice. They also represent a formalisation of the standards of practice expected of a profession and may be used to measure standards of practice. They are therefore of importance in ethical justification in prescribing, but two problems should be mentioned: firstly, they appear not to be of relevance in ethical decision making in practice (Cooper, 2007; Holm, 1997) and, secondly, their contemporary and contextual nature means they are subject to revision and the criticism that they carry less ethical force than normative theories.

Ethics and the law

The relationship between ethics and law is also potentially problematic for the prescriber. As considered in Chapter 2, prescribing is circumscribed by laws that permit only certain individuals to issue prescriptions – furthermore, legal restrictions on which medicines may be prescribed and in what way are also in place and these carry potential penalties of prosecution if contravened. However, ethics can place conflicting demands upon prescribers; for example, should the supplementary prescriber who realises that a clinical management plan has not been signed by the doctor make the patient wait for an urgently needed medicine? In such cases, ethical considerations about the welfare of the patient come into conflict with legal rules. Many factors, including clinical judgement and the details of each situation, are important but these may be considered analogous to the scenario of stopping at a red light whilst driving a car, then seeing an ambulance behind that can only proceed if you drive through the red light to let it past. In such cases, ethical considerations are often thought to over-ride legal ones and for the prescriber, this is something that should be considered on occasion. However, when considering more extreme examples such as assisted euthanasia, for example, whilst one can develop strong ethical arguments – often utilitarian – to support prescribing medicines that will hasten death and prevent suffering, the courts may not be prepared to accept such ethical arguments, mainly due to the gravity of the situation in such cases. Hence, the balance between following laws and making an ethically informed decision is both difficult and dependent upon the exact nature of the problem.

 Stop and think

What ethical problems might you as a new prescriber encounter that are different from your previous clinical practice?

Example of an ethical problem in prescribing

Distributive justice – who should get what medicine?

Although all services and treatments within the NHS in the UK are limited by costs and time, this is particularly evident in relation to medicines due to the economic impact they have upon the NHS overall. Hence, as well as considering the necessary clinical and therapeutic aspects of prescribing, all prescribers must be aware of the impact that their prescribing has upon overall costs. The availability of primary care prescribing analyses and cost (PACT) data about prescribing has led to an increased understanding of costs but in relation to ethics, there may be situations where budgetary restrictions and local formularies prevent some medicines being available. For example, the well documented cases of 'postcode prescribing' arise due to different trusts taking different decisions about what medicines may be prescribed and these may lead to ethical concerns. Such decisions are often considered utilitarian, since they are intended to maximise the overall benefits for all patients, rather than provide help to specific individuals. Elsewhere, some doctors have circumvented financial issues such as NHS prescription charges by writing private prescriptions for cheaper medicines, helping patients to afford medicines and save money.

Summary

- The new prescriber has been introduced to several important ethical theories for healthcare – utilitarian, deontological and the four principles approaches.
- Such theories offer often conflicting justification for ethical decisions in healthcare but the use of 'bottom-up' approaches together with practical decision-making models can be helpful in applying theory and reaching ethical decisions.
- The influence of conscience, ethical codes and law may also be relevant and should be considered before making final ethical decisions.
- Ethical decision making remains variable and potentially difficult and this chapter offers a starting point for prescribers to develop the skills and confidence to make ethical decisions in their work.
- New prescribers are encouraged to explore ethics texts and although some are difficult for beginners (Kant, 1998), many are commendably approachable (Singer, 1993).

 Activity

Answer true or false to each of the following.
1. Prescribers must never act in an ethically justifiable way that is contrary to the law.
2. Duty based deontological justification involves considering the overall consequences of a proposed action.
3. 'Top down' ethical reasoning involves applying a particular ethical theory consistently to different problems.
4. If a prescriber conscientiously objects to prescribing a certain medicine, they may still have to appropriately refer the patient to an alternative prescriber.
5. If using the four principles of bioethics, only one principle can be considered at a time when making an ethical decision.

References

Beauchamp, T. and Childress, J. (2001) *Principles of Biomedical Ethics*, Oxford University Press, Oxford.

British Medical Association (2004) *Medical Ethics Today. The BMA's Handbook of Ethics and Law*, 2nd edn, BMJ Publishing, London.

Cooper, R.J. (2007) Ethical Problems and their Resolution by Community Pharmacists: a Qualitative Study, PhD thesis, University of Nottingham.

Cooper, R.J., Bissell, P. and Wingfield, J. (2008) Ethical decision-making, passivity and pharmacy. *J Med Ethics*, **34**, 441–445.

Holm, S. (1997) *Ethical Problems in Clinical Practice: The Ethical Reasoning of Health Care Professionals*, Manchester University Press, Manchester.

Kant, I. (1998) *Groundwork of the Metaphysics of Morals*, Cambridge University Press, Cambridge.

Mill, J.S. (1992) *On Liberty and Utilitarianism*, David Campbell, London.

Nursing and Midwifery Council (2008) *The Code Standards of Conduct, Performance and Ethics for Nurses and Midwives*, Nursing and Midwifery Council, London.

Rawls, J.A. (1979) *Theory of Justice*, Harvard University Press, Cambridge, MA.

Royal Pharmaceutical Society of Great Britain (2007) *Code of Ethics for Pharmacists and Pharmacy Technicians*, Royal Pharmaceutical Society of Great Britain, London.

Savulescu, J. (2006) Conscientious objection in medicine. *BMJ*, **332**, 294–297.

Seedhouse, D. (1998) *Ethics:The Heart of Healthcare*, Wiley, New York.

Singer, P. (1993) *Practical Ethics*, Cambridge University Press, Cambridge.

Wingfield, J. and Badcott, D. (2007) *Pharmacy Ethics and Decision Making*, Pharmaceutical Press, London.

Further reading

Hawley, G. (ed.) (2007) *Ethics in Clinical Practice: An Interprofessional Approach*, Pearson Education, Harlow.

Norman, R. (1998) *The Moral Philosophers: An Introduction to Ethics*, Oxford University Press, Oxford.

Seedhouse, D. (1988) *Ethics: The Heart of Health Care*, John Wiley, Chichester.

5 Prescribing in practice

Learning outcomes

By the end of the chapter the reader should be able to:

- understand the difference between independent and supplementary prescribing and know when to use them in practice
- understand the requirements of a clinical management plan
- identify approaches to the integration of prescribing into clinical practice
- identify factors which promote, hinder or prevent prescribing in teams and consider strategies to manage and reduce barriers.

This chapter spans the process of prescribing from education to the integration of prescribing in clinical practice. As a new prescriber, you may need to revisit the definitions and questions raised here from time to time. The transition to prescriber takes time and achieving a licence to prescribe is similar to passing a driving test, in that learning really begins after qualification.

Independent and supplementary prescribing

These two types of prescribing form the legal framework for medical and non-medical prescribing. They originate from the second Crown Report (DH, 1999) in which Dr June Crown proposed two types of prescriber, independent and dependent. The term 'dependent' was quickly replaced by the term 'supplementary prescriber' and introduced as a type of prescribing in 2003 (DH, 2003). Understanding the difference between the types and knowing how and when to use them in practice is the foundation of safe and accountable prescribing.

Independent prescribing

Prescribing by a practitioner responsible and accountable for the assessments of patients with undiagnosed or diagnosed conditions and for decisions about the clinical management required, including prescribing.

DH, 2006: p. 7.

The New Prescriber. Edited by J Lymn, D Bowskill, F Bath-Hextall, R Knaggs, © 2010 John Wiley & Sons.

Supplementary prescribing

A voluntary partnership between an independent prescriber (a doctor or dentist) and a supplementary prescriber to implement an agreed patient specific Clinical Management Plan with the patient's agreement.

DH, 2005: p. 8.

 Stop and think

Look carefully at the descriptions of independent and supplementary prescribing. Can you identify the difference between them?

The key difference between the two types of prescribing is the accountability and responsibility for diagnosis. Under independent prescribing, it is the independent prescriber (doctor, dentist, nurse, pharmacist or optometrist) who is responsible for the diagnosis and prescribing of treatment. Under supplementary prescribing, it is also the independent prescriber who makes the diagnosis but this must be a doctor or dentist (DH, 2005).

Supplementary prescribing and the clinical management plan (CMP)

Under supplementary prescribing arrangements, the supplementary prescriber will manage the care of the patient by prescribing drugs identified in a patient-specific clinical management plan. Two blank template clinical management plans have been developed by the Department of Health. Template 1 is designed for teams who have contemporaneous access to patient records and template 2 for teams who do not. Template 2 includes two additional boxes for the prescriber to record the medication and past medical history of the patient. The template chosen for use should reflect the supplementary prescriber's access to patient records. The templates are available to download from the Department of Health website. Search using the phrase 'template clinical management plan'.

What information must a clinical management plan include?

A patient-specific CMP must be prepared and agreed by the doctor, supplementary prescriber and patient before supplementary prescribing can begin. The Department of Health lists the information which must be included in a clinical management plan. This list can be seen in Box 5.1.

> **Box 5.1   The Clinical Management Plan Must Include**
>
> 1. The name of the patient to whom the plan relates.
> 2. The illness or conditions which may be treated by the supplementary prescriber.
> 3. The date on which the plan is to take effect and when it is to be reviewed by the doctor/dentist who is party to the plan.
> 4. Reference to the class or description of medicines or types of appliances which may be prescribed or administered under the plan.
> 5. Any restrictions or limitations of strength or dose of any medicine which may be prescribed or administered under the plan, and any period of administration or use of any medicine or appliance which may be prescribed or administered under the plan.
> 6. Reference to published national or local guidelines. However, these must clearly identify the range of medicinal products to be used in treatment of the patient and the CMP should draw attention to the relevant part of the guideline. The guidelines also need to be easily accessible.
> 7. Relevant warnings about known sensitivities of the patient to or known difficulties that the patient may have with particular medicines.
> 8. Arrangements for the notification of suspected or known reactions of clinical significance to any medicines which may be prescribed or administered under the plan, and suspected or known clinically significant reactions to any other medicine taken at the same time as any medicine prescribed or administered under the plan. Incidents occurring with the appliance which might lead or have led to the death or serious deterioration of state of health of a patient.
> 9. The circumstances in which the supplementary prescriber should refer to or seek the advice of the doctor/dentist who is party to the plan.
>
> www.dh.gov 2007. DH, 2005: p. 55.

Prescribers writing patient specific clinical management plans often seek clarification of points 3 and 6 in Box 5.1. It is useful here to explain these points in some detail.

Point 3 states that dates must be included in the plan. The date on which the plan comes into effect is easy to determine. The prescribers date and sign the CMP when it is written and an agreement for supplementary prescribing is reached. The review date, however, should be carefully considered. The patient will have in place a care or treatment plan which includes the evaluation and review of care needs. This plan will continue to be used alongside the CMP used for supplementary prescribing. The review of the clinical management plan should consider:

● if the aim of treatment remains valid
● if the drugs identified in the plan are suitable for the treatment aim
● if the drugs identified in the plan are appropriate for the patient
● whether there are new allergies or sensitivities
● the current health of the patient
● any recent changes to the patient's medical and medication history
● if the independent prescriber, supplementary prescriber and patient are happy to continue with supplementary prescribing arrangements
● guidelines, protocols or standards referred to in the plan are up to date.

Department of Health guidance (2005: p. 55) states that the plan must include:

'the date on which the plan is to take effect and when it is to be reviewed by the doctor or dentist who is party to the plan'. Prescribers sometimes use the terms 'annually' or '6 monthly' as a review date. The use of the word 'date' in this context suggests that a date, in day, month and year form is required. This is considered best practice; it takes no longer to write and provides clear information for those who are using the plan. Patient and prescribers should be involved in the review of the CMP. Where this is not possible it is advised that the independent prescriber should review the patient and discuss the patient's future management with the supplementary prescriber. Agreement should be recorded and a new date agreed for the plan to remain valid.

DH, 2005: p. 65.

Point 6 states that 'CMPs will often be based on national and local guidelines'. In the CMP it is not acceptable to write 'NICE guidelines' or 'practice protocol'. Guidelines, standards and protocols should be identified with their full title and date of development. Wherever possible, the chapter, sections or pages referred to when developing the clinical management plan should be specified.

Disease-specific CMPs have in the past been written and used as templates in some areas of clinical practice. Prescribers must, however, be warned. The Medicine and Healthcare products Regulatory Body (MHRA) were quoted by the NMC as saying: 'if an independent prescriber agrees in advance that the supplementary prescriber can prescribe for a patient by virtue of them being on an agreed practice register and using the same CMP for all patients incorporating these into the patient computer records, this is illegal practice and does not meet clear legislation requirements' (NMC, 2006: p. 22).

When the patient-specific CMP is prepared, agreed and in place, the supplementary prescriber can prescribe drugs within the boundaries agreed in the plan. This agreement is a voluntary partnership and supplementary prescribers must remember that all partners can end the agreement at any time.

Should I use independent or supplementary prescribing?

Supplementary prescribing is the only option for non-medical prescribers wishing to prescribe some controlled drugs. As outlined in Chapter 3, controlled drugs can be prescribed by nurse and pharmacist non-medical prescribers under supplementary prescribing. Nurses are allowed to independently prescribe a small number of controlled drugs. The independent prescribing of controlled drugs is restricted by the form of medicine and the clinical condition for which they may be prescribed. See the British National Formulary for details.

Aside from these restrictions, the framework of independent and supplementary prescribing presents non-medical prescribers with a choice: choosing to prescribe independently when the prescriber is competent to diagnose, manage and prescribe treatment, or choosing supplementary prescribing when the non-medical prescriber does not wish to or is not competent to take responsibility for the diagnosis.

It is important that non-medical prescribers always prescribe within the legal framework of independent and supplementary prescribing. In clinical practice, new prescribers can find it difficult to decide which type of prescribing is the most appropriate. The flow diagram in Figure 5.1 takes you through a patient consultation. Each box poses a question and is

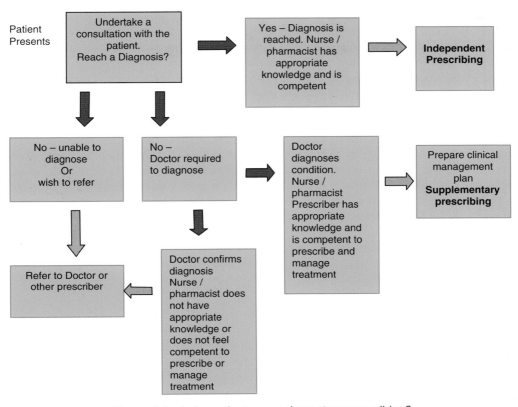

Figure 5.1   Independent or supplementary prescribing?

a decision point which directs the prescriber towards either independent or supplementary prescribing.

Prescribing in practice

In order to integrate prescribing skills and knowledge, non-medical prescribers need first to visualise how they will prescribe for patients in their clinical area. Forward thinking will enable the new non-medical prescriber to prepare themselves and the practice area for when prescribing begins.

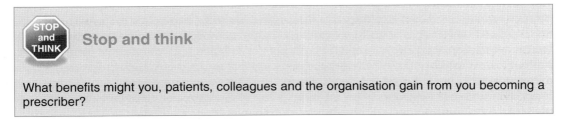

Stop and think

What benefits might you, patients, colleagues and the organisation gain from you becoming a prescriber?

Prescribing education takes a generic approach and will guide non-medical prescribers to develop a broad prescribing knowledge. As the pharmacology chapters in this book show, learning is based around body systems. This might mean revisiting topics you have not considered for a long time and will certainly involve learning about new ones. Non-medical prescribers working in narrow fields of specialist practice sometimes question why such broad knowledge is necessary. Advancements in medicine and pharmacology mean that patients who present for healthcare are often living with chronic disease and co-morbidities (Taylor and Field, 2007). Drugs are used to prevent, treat and manage the symptoms of disease and as a prescriber you must be aware of how these drugs might interact with or affect the drugs you prescribe. This broad prescribing knowledge is necessary to inform your prescribing practice and help you not only to decide when to refer but also to understand why. There is a lot to learn and a balance must be reached. You will need to think about how you can make sense of this new knowledge in the context of prescribing in your clinical area. Personal prescribing formularies are a really useful way of doing this.

Personal prescribing formularies

Personal prescribing formularies work by encouraging you to think about the drugs you will be prescribing in practice. This focus is a really useful way to build your confidence in prescribing (Bradley, Hyman and Nolan, 2007). Start your formulary by listing the drugs you are most likely to prescribe. The list provides a starting point from which you can begin to apply principles of pharmacology, consultation, law, accountability and ethics to your own prescribing practice.

As a new non-medical prescriber, it is easy to assume that the doctors and healthcare professionals with whom you work have a good knowledge of independent and supplementary prescribing. However, for most this is not the case and it is suggested in the prescribing literature that a lack of knowledge and misunderstandings about non-medical prescribing are common in healthcare teams (Bradley and Nolan, 2007). Your team needs to know and understand the general principles of independent and supplementary prescribing. In order to help the team make sense of these principles and to help you integrate prescribing into your team, you will find it useful to define your prescribing role.

Defining your prescribing role

Defining your role requires you to think about yourself as a prescriber in your clinical area. Prescribing education encourages you to focus on the expertise you have but at the same time provides you with an insight into what you do not know and even what you didn't realise you needed to know. For some prescribing students this can mean that whilst they entered prescribing with the belief that they had the knowledge and competence to diagnose a condition, further knowledge is actually required to achieve competence. When the Department of Health opened up the British National Formulary for independent nurse and pharmacist prescribing in May 2006, it did so by laying the responsibility for clinical competence directly with the prescriber. It may therefore be that at first you limit your prescribing whilst undertaking further education or developing clinical skills. Nurse prescribers describe three approaches to the integration of prescribing in nursing practice (Bowskill, 2009).

Approach 1

The prescriber takes an 'as prescribing opportunities present' approach. A full consultation is undertaken and should a prescription be necessary and the prescriber feels competent and confident, an independent prescribing prescription is written. If the prescriber is not competent or lacks confidence, the patient or client is referred to another prescriber to prescribe or alternatively supplementary prescribing is set up. This approach is most frequently described by those who prescribe in a specialist area where the condition(s) and range of drugs prescribed are limited.

Approach 2

The prescriber identifies in advance of starting to prescribe a range of conditions, clinics or patient groups. The prescriber will feel competent and confident with the condition(s) and treatments for this group of patients and will, following a full consultation, prescribe independently, refer and/or set up supplementary prescribing. The prescriber will go on to introduce prescribing into other areas of their role as confidence increases. This approach is most frequently described by general prescribers who treat a wide range of conditions for patients or clients of all ages.

Approach 3

The prescriber takes a patient-specific approach. Prescribers start by prescribing for patients they know well and slowly build a small group of patients for whom they regularly prescribe. As with the other groups, following a full consultation the prescriber will choose to prescribe independently, refer and/or set up supplementary prescribing. Knowing the patient and their past medical and medication history is important to these prescribers as their patients often have co-morbidities and multiple drug therapies. For these prescribers this approach offers a way to manage the risk of prescribing for patients with complex conditions. As confidence, knowledge and prescribing experience grow the number of patients prescribed for increases. The approach is most commonly described by those caring for patients with complex conditions.

These three approaches provide a useful starting point for new prescribers who are feeling unsure about where to start prescribing in practice. Having defined your prescribing role and decided how you will approach prescribing in practice, the next step is to consider how non-medical prescribing will be integrated into the team.

Prescribing in teams

Start by looking at the team(s) you will prescribe in.

 Stop and think

- Who needs to be informed that you are a prescriber? Make a list. Think about the whole prescribing process: who is involved – pharmacist, administering nurses, receptionist, line manager, lead pharmacist, prescribing lead and so on.

- Do your prescribing colleagues expect you to prescribe as they do? Are there areas of potential conflict between you and medical or non-prescribers in the team?
- What systems are in place for you to access and record information about the consultation and the items prescribed? Can you access these systems and if not, who do you need to contact in order to facilitate access?

Prescribing cannot occur in isolation – to do so could put patient safety directly at risk. You must be aware of, and communicate with, others who prescribe, supply or administer medicines to the patient at all times. The prescribers identified on your list are the people you should talk to first. Explain the difference between independent and supplementary prescribing, define your role and explain what you can prescribe from the BNF. Where appropriate, be clear about restrictions to independent prescribing, prescribing off or outside the product label and prescribing unlicensed products.

Support from the team is very important to new prescribers. The prescribing literatures suggest that those working in supportive teams are most likely to be prescribing for patients (Latter *et al.*, 2005). Non-medical prescribers can, however, face negativity about their prescribing role. Bradley and Nolan (2007) found that colleagues who are not prescribers are not always enthusiastic about new prescribing roles. Take time to explain to the team how prescribing integrates within your role, explain your prescribing boundaries, how you will use prescribing and how your prescribing can benefit patients and the team.

Nurse and pharmacist prescribers have identified situations where other prescribers in the team have a preference for a particular product and the new prescriber is expected to conform. You must remember that you are accountable for your prescribing decisions whether you choose to prescribe or not. Facing these 'conflicts' in prescribing situations can be daunting for new prescribers. Defining your role and providing information about prescribing to the team in advance of qualification can offer a valuable opportunity for you to outline your professional accountability and detail how you will proceed in these situations before they arise.

Communicating prescribing decisions within the team

Record keeping and communication are fundamentally important to safe and effective prescribing. Prescribers have a responsibility to inform and record their prescribing activity and you must act within your employer's prescribing policy. Chapter 6 explores the issue of record keeping and prescribing policies. In the modern healthcare arena there are many prescribers. Communicating and recording prescribing activity must be a priority.

Organisations and employers

Prescribing is part of the clinical governance framework of the organisation and each employer will consider the clinical risk of prescribing. It is here that we identify differences between employers in terms of what they will allow their non-medical prescribers to do. The law, as set out in Chapter 3, details the legal boundaries of prescribing for all healthcare professionals. Within frameworks of clinical governance, healthcare employers sometimes place restrictions on non-medical prescribing. You should access your employer's prescribing policy for guidance. Non-medical prescribers are often employed in roles which require prescribing across primary and secondary care services. These prescribing situations present a series of questions about the provision of FP10 prescription pads, access to patient records, record keeping and financial responsibility for prescribed items. If you are going to be prescribing in such a situation when qualified, you must talk to managers to address these questions before you begin to prescribe.

The most obvious restriction to prescribing is one which applies to all prescribers and is an accepted part of modern healthcare – the local prescribing formulary. Here the prescriber has an obligation to prescribe items included within the formulary, so get to know what is on the formulary. You also have an obligation from a public health perspective to prescribe within local antimicrobial guidelines. Make sure you always work with the most up-to-date guidelines and recommendations.

Integrating prescribing into your clinical practice is something which you alone can do. There is an awful lot to think about before you can use prescribing in your practice. Refer back to the questions raised in this chapter as you learn to prescribe and prepare your team and your employer to accept you as a prescriber. There is nothing worse than successfully passing the course and not being able to prescribe because there is something stopping you which you could have prepared for in advance.

Summary

- There are two types of prescribing – independent and supplementary.
- It is important that prescribers always prescribe within the legal framework of independent and supplementary prescribing.
- Doctors are always independent prescribers. Following the successful completion of prescribing education, nurses, pharmacists and optometrists become independent and supplementary prescribers. Allied health professionals become supplementary prescribers.
- Under supplementary prescribing the independent prescriber must be a doctor or dentist.
- A patient-specific clinical management plan must be prepared and an agreement signed by the independent prescriber (a doctor), the patient and supplementary prescriber before the supplementary prescriber can prescribe.
- Prescribing cannot occur in isolation; to do so would put patient safety directly at risk.
- As a prescriber you must be aware of and communicate with others who prescribe, supply and administer medicines to the patient or client at all times.

Activity

1. What is the key difference between independent and supplementary prescribing?
2. Using the BNF, under what type of prescribing (independent or supplementary) can a nurse prescriber prescribe morphine sulphate to be taken orally for symptom management in palliative care?
3. Under what type of prescribing can a physiotherapist prescribe non-steroidal anti-inflammatory drugs?
4. Can a pharmacist prescriber be the independent prescriber named on a clinical management plan?

Useful websites

The Department of Health website holds all government documents related to prescribing and medicines management. It also has a useful 'Frequently Asked Questions' section for non-medical prescribers. www.dh.gov.uk.

References

Bowskill, D. (2009) The Integration of Nurse Prescribing: Case Studies in Primary and Secondary Care, DHSci thesis, University of Nottingham, School of Nursing, Midwifery and Physiotherapy.

Bradley, E. and Nolan, P. (2007) Impact of nurse prescribing: a qualitative study. *J Adv Nurs*, **59**(2), 120–128.

Bradley, E., Hyman, B. and Nolan, P. (2007) Nurse prescribing: reflections on safety in practice. *Soc Sci Med*, **65**, 599–609.

Department of Health (1999) *Review of Prescribing, Supply and Administration of Medicines. Final Report*, Department of Health, London.

Department of Health (2003) *Supplementary Prescribing by Nurses and Pharmacists Within the NHS in England. A Guide for Implementation*, Department of Health, London.

Department of Health (2005) *Supplementary Prescribing by Nurses, Pharmacists, Chiropodists/Podiatrists, Physiotherapists and Radiographers within the NHS in England. A Guide for Implementation*, Stationery Office, London.

Department of Health (2006) *Improving Patients' Access to Medicines: A Guide to Implementing Nurse and Pharmacist Independent Nurse and Pharmacist Independent Prescribing within the NHS in England*, Department of Health, London.

Latter, S., Maben, J., Courtenay, M., *et al.* (2004) *An Evaluation of Extended Formulary Independent Nurse Prescribing. Final Report*, University of Southampton, Southampton.

Nursing and Midwifery Council (2006) Prescribing practice. Clinical management plans. *NMC News*, **8**, 16.

Taylor, S. and Field, D. (2007) *Sociology of Health and Health Care*, 4th edn, Blackwells, Oxford.

Further reading

Department of Health (2006) *Medicines Matters. A Guide to Mechanisms for the Prescribing, Supply and Administration of Medicines*, Stationery Office, London.

National Prescribing Centre (2003) *Maintaining Competency in Prescribing: An Outline Framework to Help Pharmacist Supplementary Prescribers*, National Prescribing Centre, Liverpool.

National Prescribing Centre (2003) *Maintaining Competency in Prescribing: An Outline Framework to Help Nurse Supplementary Prescribers*, National Prescribing Centre, Liverpool.

National Prescribing Centre (2004) *Maintaining Competency in Prescribing: An Outline Framework to Help Allied Health Professional Supplementary Prescribers*, National Prescribing Centre, Liverpool.

Nursing and Midwifery Council (2006) *Standards of Proficiency for Nurse and Midwife Prescribers*, Nursing and Midwifery Council, London.

Section 1

6 Record keeping

Learning outcomes

By the end of the chapter the reader should be able to:

- discuss the importance of record keeping from professional, legal and employer accountability perspectives
- consider the form and content of record keeping in the context of prescribing
- review the expectations of patients, public and professional bodies of the prescribing record
- identify local prescribing policies and work to the standards for prescribing records included within them.

The importance of record keeping

You are probably already very familiar with the principles of effective record keeping. However, this is an opportunity to rehearse your knowledge and practice of these principles and to consider how they might be exercised in terms of professional, legal and employer accountability, within the context of non-medical prescribing.

Records Management: NHS Code of Practice (DH, 2006a: p. 5) reminds us of the value of keeping accurate and up-to-date records, since this information may be needed:

- 'to support patient care and continuity of care
- to support day-to-day business which underpins the delivery of care
- to support evidence-based clinical practice
- to support sound administrative and managerial decision making, as part of the knowledge base for NHS services
- to meet legal requirements, including requests from patients under subject access provisions of the Data Protection Act or the Freedom of Information Act
- to assist clinical and other types of audits

The New Prescriber. Edited by J Lymn, D Bowskill, F Bath-Hextall, R Knaggs, © 2010 John Wiley & Sons.

Section 1

- to support improvements in clinical effectiveness through research and also to support archival functions by taking account of the historical importance of material and the needs of future research, or
- to support patient choice and control over treatment and services designed around patients'.

 Stop and think

Take a few minutes to consider which of the elements above might be particularly relevant to your prescribing practice. What influenced your choices?

Supporting patient care and ensuring continuity of care are probably the two most significant reasons for making records related to prescribing. As an independent prescriber, you will take time to assess each patient, establish a diagnosis, discuss possible treatment options and determine appropriate therapeutic interventions, including prescribing medicines. Your records should support your decision making and can assist you and other colleagues in future evaluation and care of patients. You may refer to therapeutic guidelines published by specialist groups such as the British Dermatology Association or the British Society of Haematology or national recommendations such as those from the National Institute for Health and Clinical Excellence, all of which draw on clinical evidence in their formulation.

As a supplementary prescriber, you will be working closely with a doctor or dentist, who is the independent prescriber, to provide ongoing management for patients who typically have long-term medical conditions. The doctor or dentist makes the initial diagnosis, decides on the medicines to be prescribed and must review these patients within a predetermined and agreed timescale. Your records will provide essential information of patients' progress, problems such as drug interactions or side effects and solutions achieved through medicines adjustments. The clinical management plan, which determines the drugs you may prescribe for an individual patient, is likely to refer to evidence-based, nationally or locally recognised guidelines.

There is little point in prescribing drugs if patients are not willing or able to take them. In your initial and ongoing assessments, you should aim to establish a relationship with patients that enables them to be as involved as they wish to be in choosing treatment. Patients may have very particular reasons for selecting one medicine over another: keeping a record of their reasoning and decisions can help you demonstrate that you are working towards 'medicines concordance' (Cline, Granby and Picton, 2007) and supporting patient choice and control over their treatment. This is a very different strategy from that aimed at achieving medicines compliance. Dean *et al.* (2002: p. 1377) suspect that 'prescribing, as understood by doctors, is primarily the naming of a drug, and that all subsidiary information and acts are seen as secondary'. Consequently, it is not common to find reasons for prescribing a drug, details of side effects experienced or explanations of adjustments to doses, timing, formulation and so on documented in a patient's records. Non-medical prescribers have the opportunity to establish different priorities within their record keeping, which may in turn influence prescribing records in the future.

If you are planning to prescribe using FP10 prescription forms, you are advised to keep a record of the serial numbers of the first and last sheets in every prescription pad issued to you (DH, 2006b). At the end of each working day you might also note the serial number of the next available form in the pad. These strategies can alert you to missing forms or pads, either of which should be reported following the processes set out in your employer's local non-medical prescribing policy. Similarly, if you are working in an outpatient department you may be required to sign out and sign in your outpatient prescription pad at the beginning and end of your clinic. This is a risk management strategy, instigated to reduce the possibility of these pads being misappropriated or misused. These are examples of record keeping that support the day-to-day business which underpins prescribing practice.

You may have identified other elements from the list of reasons for record keeping which you feel are relevant to your own prescribing practice. Some of these, such as legal reasons for keeping prescribing records, will be discussed in this chapter, but others may not be. Do take the opportunity to discuss your thoughts with colleagues; it can help to shape your thinking about effective record keeping.

Types of prescribing record

When you think about prescribing records, you probably have in mind your entries into the patient's health record detailing initial assessment, progress and problems and the document on which you write your patient-specific direction. These are certainly the records that support direct patient care, but there are other types of record that support prescribing and therefore contribute indirectly to the safe management and continuity of care of patients.

 Stop and think

Make a list of all the records that you can think of that are associated with non-medical prescribing. Here are some questions to prompt your thinking.

- Where could notes about the patient be made?
- What types of prescription form are there?
- What personal records might you hold related to non-medical prescribing?
- What non-patient records might the organisation hold that support safe and effective prescribing practice?

Compare your answer with the information contained in Table 6.1, which provides a review of possible prescribing records. This is not a definitive summary, but it offers insight into the range of records associated with non-medical prescribing. Remember, there are variations in the types of prescribing record that you will use, influenced by whether you are employed within primary care, secondary care or the independent sector, and by employer guidance and your regulatory body's requirements.

You can see in Table 6.1 that prescribing records are considered from three perspectives:

Table 6.1 Types of prescribing record.

Patient	Personal	Employer
Health record: • GP patient health record • NHS hospital patient health record • Non-medical prescriber patient record • Independent sector patient record • Clinical management plan • Patient-held record: for example, NPSA Yellow Book for anticoagulation monitoring	**Qualification record:** • Confirmation from Higher Education institution • Certificate from HEI • Confirmation of registration as an independent/supplementary prescriber from regulatory body	**Qualification record:** • Confirmation of registration with regulatory body • Confirmation of additional registration as non-medical prescriber • Notification of prescriber details to the NHS Business Services Authority
Prescription forms: • FP10 prescriptions • FP10SS prescriptions • Hospital inpatient prescription record[a] • Internal hospital prescription forms (typically used for outpatient prescribing)	**Professional record:** • Portfolio (professional, multi-purpose) • Significant events analyses • Reflective accounts • Case studies • Supervision records • Evidence of up-to-date prescribing knowledge and competence • Indemnity insurance	**Prescribing related records:** • Database of non-medical prescribers • Specimen signatures of non-medical prescribers • Prescription pad serial numbers • Documentation for distribution and return of prescription pads • Non-medical prescribing policies and procedures
Incident forms: • Yellow Card scheme for reporting adverse drug reactions • Employer incident forms for reporting prescribing-related incidents	**Audit information:** • Prescription form serial numbers • Appropriateness of prescribing • Patient satisfaction • Cost data, for example ePACT, ePFIP	**Audit information:** • Cost data (ePACT for PCT contract prescribers; ePFIP for GP Contract prescribers) • Prescribing monitoring analysis as part of overall prescribing audit cycle

[a]May go under a variety of names: for example, medicines administration record, drug prescription and administration record, ward drug chart.

Section 1

1. those that relate directly to patients
2. those that relate to professional regulation and personal development
3. those that the employer is required to develop and maintain.

The Department of Health (2005, 2006b) provides specific guidance about non-medical prescribers' record keeping. The key principles are that records should be:

- accurate
- legible
- unambiguous
- contemporaneous
- completed within 48 hours of writing the prescription
- relevant
- sufficient to enable all professionals involved in the patient's treatment to provide safe and effective care
- dated, timed and signed

and with respect to the prescription should include:

- the date the prescription was written
- the name of the prescriber, profession and whether acting as an independent or supplementary prescriber
- the name of the medicines prescribed, together with the dose, frequency, route, formulation and duration of treatment.

So for example you would write:
Paracetamol oral suspension 120 mg/5 ml to be taken every 4 hours by mouth as required for pain, maximum of 20 ml in any 24 hours.
There is no single template or method for writing records, particularly because there is a wide range of patient health records currently in use. However, there are well tried and tested practices and approaches to recording your diagnostic assessment and treatment recommendations, which are covered elsewhere in this book, as are the specifics of completing a prescription form (see Chapter 3) or creating a clinical management plan (see Chapter 5).

Once you successfully complete your non-medical prescribing course, your education institution will inform your regulatory body, who will send you the necessary paperwork to record your qualification on their register. You should keep all your personal records related to non-medical prescribing safe, as you will need to present them to new employers if you move employing organisation. Similarly, you need to be able to demonstrate that you are maintaining and developing your prescribing knowledge and skills, so do include relevant learning in your professional portfolio.

Your employer has a whole range of responsibilities associated with record keeping for non-medical prescribing. These include the maintenance of a register of prescribers, along with their specimen signatures, so that if queries arise from dispensing pharmacists regarding an individual's prescribing status this can be easily confirmed. There must be a robust process in place for ordering, distributing and receiving returned prescribing pads and for reporting missing prescription pads or single prescription forms. The employer must also audit aspects of

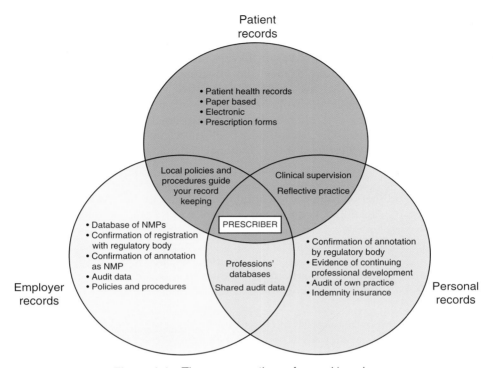

Figure 6.1 Three perspectives of record keeping.

non-medical prescribing and may need to report audit findings as part of internal and external quality assurance checks. For primary care organisations, information regarding medicines prescribed and costing is available electronically from the NHS Business Services Authority.

Now have a look at Figure 6.1, which illustrates the relationships amongst patient records, personal records and employer records. You, the non-medical prescriber, sit at the centre of the process of record keeping and make a fundamental contribution to each of these record types.

There are clear distinctions and overlaps amongst the three perspectives discussed. In some instances the overlapping areas suggest a cyclical relationship. For example, you may choose to share a patient's prescribing record during a clinical supervision session. This gives you the opportunity to explore your decision-making processes with a knowledgeable colleague which may, in turn, influence your prescribing practice and the records that you keep in the future.

Accountability and record keeping

Chapter 2 provides a comprehensive overview of the nature of accountability and its application to non-medical prescribing. We now encourage you to think specifically about your accountability for record keeping, with reference to the expectations and requirements of your patients, your professional body and your employer.

Patients

As well as being healthcare professionals, we are also likely to be patients too at some time during our lives. What expectations do you have with regard to your own personal health records? You probably expect them to meet the principles for record keeping set out above. In addition, you might hope that they contain information you have shared with healthcare professionals, because you believe it to be relevant to your management, and that this information will be acknowledged by other healthcare professionals who may be responsible for your treatment in the future. The frustration of self-knowledge not being valued by health professionals is graphically illustrated in the National Patient Safety Agency report (2006: p. 52) on anticoagulant therapy:

> One participant said that consultants often did not understand the drugs he was on, even when he offered explanations. As an example, there had been a lack of recognition that phenindione was an anticoagulant, confusing it with phenytoin ... He recounted that on one occasion, he allowed a procedure to continue, although he knew it was inappropriate: 'They cut into my groin and the blood came shooting out and I said, "Well, I did tell you". Of course, the crash team and everybody else panicked and said, "Why did you do that?". I said, "Because I got fed up of telling you that I'm on phenindione".'

Clearly, one of the important aspects of effective record keeping is to listen carefully to what patients tell you, clarify what they say if you are unsure and then document this in their health records. The effects that drugs exert on the body are influenced by individual physiological functioning, so if patients report particular responses or side effects these should be noted for future reference and their treatment regimens adjusted if necessary.

Professional body

The professional bodies which regulate all those professional groups named in supplementary and independent prescribing legislation require their registrants to work to codes of conduct, performance and ethics. Whilst each code is profession specific, there is acknowledgement by the regulating bodies that healthcare professionals have a shared set of values, which find their expression in these codes.

 Stop and think

Have a look at your own professional body's code and see what it says about record keeping. You may also note that there are linked standards relating to confidentiality and working with colleagues.

Some of the record-keeping standards expressed in codes of conduct replicate the guidance given in the non-medical prescribing guidance (DH, 2005; DH, 2006b). For example, the

Nursing and Midwifery Council code (NMC, 2008) requires registrants to keep clear, legible and accurate records, complete them in a timely way and ensure that they are dated and timed. It also states that nurses and midwives:

- must not tamper with original records in any way
- must ensure any entries made in electronic records are clearly attributable
- must ensure all records are kept securely.

In addition to standards expressed in codes of conduct, performance and ethics, professional bodies also provide specific guidance on record keeping. For example 'Guidance on Recording Interventions' (Royal Pharmaceutical Society of Great Britain, 2006) includes a helpful section on the factors that pharmacists should consider when determining whether it is necessary to record particular interventions and suggests where records should be made if there is no access to the patient's medical record. It is worth noting that professional bodies do not always provide consistent advice: for example, the NMC (2007) states that records must not include abbreviations, whereas the RPSGB (2006) says that established abbreviations that are common to all healthcare professionals are acceptable. You should follow the guidance set out by your own professional body, since this is the body to which you are accountable.

Remember, record keeping:

- is an integral part of professional practice
- is a tool that supports patients' treatment and care processes
- is not an optional extra to be omitted if you are short of time
- is a reflection of your standards of practice

and good record keeping:

- is the mark of a skilled and safe practitioner.

Employer

As discussed in Chapters 2 and 3, your contract of employment implies that you will work to the policies and procedures of your employer. Your employer is responsible for translating legal statutes and national guidance into policies and procedures that will enable you to practise safely and legally whilst in their employ. This is a positive aspect of policies and procedures, designed to protect both you and the organisation. However, policies and procedures may be used in other ways to restrict or control your practice, perhaps for financial reasons, which you may find professionally challenging. For example, if you are a non-medical prescriber based in secondary care, you may not be allowed to prescribe on FP10 prescribing forms. This is not necessarily discriminating against non-medical prescribers and may well apply to doctors/dentists within the organisation too. This restriction ensures that all drugs prescribed within the organisation can only be dispensed by the hospital pharmacy, thus making it easier for the hospital to manage its annual pharmacy budget.

Table 6.2 Local policies and procedures directly relevant to non-medical prescribers.

Policy/procedure	Focus of policy/procedure
Medicines Code of Practice	Overarching policy that sets out the organisation's approach to prescribing, supply and administration of medicines.
Non-medical prescribing policy	This may be an annex to the Medicines Code of Practice. Sets out the principles for non-medical prescribing. Is likely to set out the expectation with respect to record keeping.
Non-medical prescribing procedures	Linked to the non-medical prescribing policy. Determines precise steps related to non-medical prescribing processes, for example: ● confirming your qualification and signature with your employer ● ordering prescription forms ● verifying the medicines that you will be prescribing.

Stop and think

Identify the policies and procedures in your organisation that have direct relevance to your role as a prescriber.

You are likely to have identified some or all of those set out in Table 6.2. As well as these, you need to be familiar with the policies that relate to record keeping, which might include: patient records, confidentiality, data protection, incident reporting and personal development review. Take time to read through all the relevant policies and to note any requirements that they put on you in your role as a non-medical prescriber. It isn't possible here to look at these areas in detail but, for example, in reading through your policy on incident reporting you might identify a specific template for reporting medicines-related incidents, which supplements the standard incident forms.

Returning to your employer's policy for non-medical prescribing, are there any particular points to note regarding record keeping? Does it stipulate which forms are to be used for prescribing? Does it refer you to your own regulatory body's guidance for record keeping? Whatever requirements are expressed, ensure that you incorporate these into your prescribing practice.

Conclusion

Your records relating to non-medical prescribing serve a number of purposes for you. Your registration with your professional body confirms that you have the legal right to practise in your particular sphere and as a non-medical prescriber. Your employer may also provide additional confirmation of your non-medical prescribing role. Your professional portfolio demonstrates that your prescribing knowledge and skills are up to date and that you are continuously seeking ways to maintain and develop your practice. Your entries into the patient's health record and

Section 1

on prescribing forms demonstrate your patient assessment and therapeutic decision-making processes and provide an essential source of evidence if ever a clinical negligence claim is made against you.

Ultimately your records lie at the heart of your non-medical prescribing practice. They are integral to your non-medical prescribing role and their quality is a hallmark of the standard to which you practise this role.

Summary

- The Department of Health and the professions regulatory bodies provide explicit guidance regarding record keeping: be familiar with this guidance.
- Your employer should have specific guidance, usually in the form of policies and procedures, which will shape your non-medical prescribing records.
- Non-medical prescribing records fall into three categories: patient records, personal records, employer records. You contribute to all three types.
- You have the opportunity to develop patient records that support medicines concordance and so do much more than simply naming the medicines prescribed.
- Record keeping is an integral part of your professional practice and good record keeping marks you out as a skilled and safe practitioner.

 Activity

Answer true or false to each of the following.

1. Patients have a right to access their health records, as determined by the Data Protection Act.
2. Supplementary prescribers can prescribe medicines other than those named on the clinical management plan.
3. Medicines concordance involves the process whereby patients' behaviours are measured to determine the extent to which they are taking their medicines according to their prescriptions.
4. A prescription must include the prescriber's name, profession and whether acting as a supplementary or independent prescriber.
5. An instruction to administer or supply medicines will always be written on an FP10/FP10SS form.

Useful websites

The British Association of Dermatologists. www.bad.org.uk.

The British Society for Haematology. www.b-s-h.org.uk.

National Institute for Health and Clinical Excellence. www.nice.org.uk.

References

Cline, W., Granby, T. and Picton, C. (2007) *A Competency Framework for Shared Decision-Making with Patients. Achieving Concordance for Taking Medicines*, National Prescribing Centre, Liverpool.

Dean, B., Schachter, M., Vincent, C. and Barber, N. (2002) Causes of prescribing errors in hospital inpatients: a prospective study. *Lancet*, **359**, 1373–1378.

Department of Health (2005) *Supplementary Prescribing by Nurses, Pharmacists, Chiropodists/Podiatrists, Physiotherapists and Radiographers within the NHS in England*, Department of Health, London.

Department of Health (2006a) *Records Management: NHS Code of Practice*, www.dh.gov.uk/en/Publicationsandstatistics/Publications/PublicationsPolicyAndGuidance/DH_4131747?IdcService=GET_FILE&dID=27250&Rendition=Web.

Department of Health (2006b) *Improving Patients' Access to Medicines: A Guide to Implementing Nurse and Pharmacist Independent Prescribing within the NHS in England*, Department of Health, Leeds.

National Patient Safety Agency (2006) *Risk Assessment of Anticoagulant Therapy*, National Patient Safety Agency, London.

Nursing and Midwifery Council (2007) *A-Z advice sheet. NMC Record Keeping Guidance*, Nursing and Midwifery Council, London.

Nursing and Midwifery Council (2008) *The Code, Standards of Conduct, Performance and Ethics for Nurses and Midwives*, Nursing and Midwifery Council, London.

Royal Pharmaceutical Society of Great Britain (2006) *Guidance on Recording Interventions*, Pharmaceutical Press, London.

Further reading

Department of Health (2006) *Medicines Matters. A Guide to Mechanisms for the Prescribing, Supply and Administration of Medicines*, Department of Health, London.

7 Public health issues

Learning outcomes

By the end of this chapter the reader should be able to:

- understand what is meant by public health
- identify the professional groups which contribute to public health
- describe where to find evidence in relation to public health
- identify health-promoting settings
- describe the differences between evidence-based approaches in medicine and public health
- demonstrate an awareness of public health and how prescribers can contribute to key areas.

In the past, prescribers have made significant contributions to improving the public's health by prescribing medicines and providing health advice on a range of important areas including smoking, contraception and the safe use of medicines. Prescribers as a group have considerable 'reach' as they work in a number of settings including primary care, hospitals and workplaces. In the future, prescribers' public health roles are likely to increase as the government is keen to enlist the support of key professionals to tackle pressing public health priorities.

This chapter will discuss the meaning of public health and some of the different influences on health. It will also consider evidence-based approaches and priority topics and explore how prescribers can increase their role in public health.

What is public health?

There are a plethora of definitions of public health. However, the definition that is accepted by the Faculty of Public Health and is widely used within the NHS is:

> The science and art of preventing disease, prolonging life and promoting health through organised efforts of society.
>
> Acheson, 1988

The New Prescriber. Edited by J Lymn, D Bowskill, F Bath-Hextall, R Knaggs, © 2010 John Wiley & Sons.

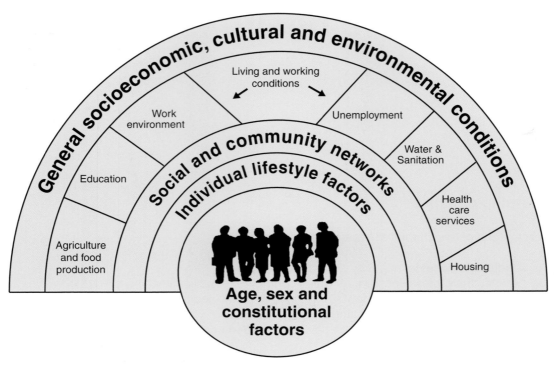

Figure 7.1 The main determinants of health (Dahlgren and Whitehead 1991) (with permission from the author).

This definition is broad and includes an emphasis on prevention, the collective responsibility for health and a focus on whole populations. Public health incorporates a range of disciplines and professions and individuals may work in or across different settings, including primary care, workplaces, schools and local communities.

For those wanting to promote health, it is crucial to understand the different types of influences on health. The main determinants of health have been classified by Dahlgren and Whitehead (1991) into five categories (Figure 7.1). These categories include both fixed factors (age, sex, hereditary factors) and potentially modifiable ones (e.g. individual lifestyle factors and working conditions). The diagram illustrates the range of different influences on health, and draws attention to areas that should be targeted in order to produce improved health outcomes.

Although public health activities are many and varied, the Faculty of Public Health has classified them into three key domains of public health practice (Table 7.1). These domains overlap and together they provide an insight into the real breadth and complexity of the public health function. Prescribers have important roles to play in all three of the domains.

In relation to health improvement, prescribers are already working on some public health priority topics and examples include providing support for smokers, reducing teenage pregnancy and tackling obesity. Health protection examples include working on strategies to control antimicrobial resistance and the supply of condoms, dental dams and advice.

Table 7.1   Three domains of public health activity.

Domain	Area of activity
Health improvement	Lifestyles Inequalities Education Housing Employment Family/community Surveillance and monitoring of specific diseases and risk factors
Improving services	Clinical effectiveness Efficiency Service planning Audit and evaluation Clinical governance Equity
Health protection	Disease and accident prevention Chemicals and poisons Radiation Emergency response Environmental health hazards

Contributions to public health

For prescribers to make an effective contribution to public health, they must be able to identify their own public health role as well as that of others. According to the Chief Medical Officer, there are three main groups in the public health workforce (DH, 2001).

1. Wider workforce – this includes individuals who have a role in health improvement but they may not have recognised this. They need to adopt a public health 'mindset'. This is the biggest group and includes nurses, teachers, social workers, local government workers, transport engineers, doctors and other healthcare professionals.
2. Public health practitioners – spend a major part or all of their time in public health practice. Examples include health visitors, environmental health officers and community development workers.
3. Public health consultants and specialists – who work at a strategic or senior management level.

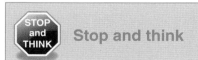 **Stop and think**

Which group reflects your public health role?

Although most prescribers will be part of the wider public health workforce, in each of these groups there will be individuals who will be integrating their prescribing skills and knowledge into their public health practice.

Effective approaches to promoting public health prescribing

In the past there has been a dearth of information about the effectiveness of public health interventions but public health theory provides a number of frameworks which can be used to guide action (Tones and Green, 2004; Davies and Macdowall, 2006; Pencheon *et al.*, 2006). There are, for example, theories to help identify relevant factors, theories to guide changing individual behaviour and theories to guide changing organisations and communities. In addition, the World Health Organization's Ottawa Charter provides clear direction for those wanting to develop effective interventions (World Health Organization, 1986).

More recently, there have been a growing number of articles and books that highlight opportunities for key people to promote health, especially in the priority areas identified in the government public health strategy for England, 'Choosing Health: Making Healthy Choices Easier' (DH, 2004). This strategy sets out proposals for action on a range of important areas, including obesity, smoking and sexual health. The role of the prescriber in tackling these public health challenges will be discussed in a later section.

As part of the government's Choosing Health initiative, a commitment was made to publish a strategy for pharmaceutical public health. 'Choosing Health Through Pharmacy' expanded the contribution that pharmacists can make to improving health in all sectors: community, hospital, industry and primary care (DH, 2005). Building on this, 'Pharmacy in England' sets out some of the major health and social challenges, identifies reforms that are needed and indicates how and where pharmacists could contribute (DH, 2008b). Although both these documents were produced for pharmacists, they are relevant to all prescribers. They contain key public health information, real-life case studies of innovative public health practice and priorities for action.

The government documents are good starting points for locating evidence-based priorities. Additionally, there are national organisations that support professionals who are seeking details about effective public health approaches (Box 7.1).

The NICE is an excellent source of guidance on the promotion of good health and the prevention of ill health. For example, it has published a reference guide for stop smoking services in primary care, pharmacies and other settings (NICE, 2008). Another relevant production presented a set of generic principles that can be used for behaviour change at population, community and individual levels (NICE, 2007). As a prescriber, it is important to always work from the most up-to-date guidelines, so always check the date that they were produced.

Two other national organisations are PharmacyHealthLink and the Royal Pharmaceutical Society of Great Britain (RPSGB). Together they have commissioned a series of evidence-based research reviews in order to promote effective pharmacy-based health improvement initiatives. The most recent systematic review covers evidence published in peer-reviewed journals between 2004 and 2007, on the contribution of community pharmacy to improving the public's health (Anderson, Blenkinsopp and Armstrong, 2008). This work strengthens the evidence base for key public health priorities including smoking cessation, diabetes, coronary heart disease and hypertension.

At a primary care trust level, effectiveness information can be found in the annual reports of the director of public health and in multi-agency health strategies. These documents should

---

Box 7.1 Key Organisations

The faculty of public health

A faculty of the Royal College of Physicians. It promotes, for the public benefit, the advancement of knowledge in the field of public health and seeks to develop public health with a view to maintaining the highest possible standards of professional competence and practice. The site has a wide range of resources and links to other organisations involved in public health.
www.fphm.org.uk/about_faculty/default.asp

Health protection agency

This is a special health authority that deals with infectious diseases, radiation, chemicals and poisons and provides emergency responses. In relation to infectious diseases, it collects, collates, analyses and interprets information to identify outbreaks and monitor patterns in the prevalence of infectious diseases and the performance of vaccine programmes.
www.hpa.org.uk/webw/HPAweb&Page&HPAwebHome/Page/1153496333353?p=1153496333353

National Institute for Health and Clinical Excellence (NICE)

An independent organisation responsible for providing national guidance on promoting good health and preventing and treating ill health. Guidance is produced in three areas: public health, health technologies and clinical practice.
www.nice.org.uk/

Pharmacy health link

A national charity which works with the government, pharmacists, health professionals and the public. Seeks to broaden the role that pharmacists and their staff can play in helping the public achieve good health. Provides research-based guidance, runs training events, conferences and other events. The site has briefing cards on key topics (including physical activity, alcohol, smoking and weight management).
www.pharmacyhealthlink.org.uk/

UK Public Health Association (UKPHA)

A multidisciplinary independent voluntary organisation which brings together individuals and organisations from all sectors who share a common commitment to promoting the public's health.
www.ukpha.org.uk/default.asp?action=category&ID=1

---

be used to guide prescribing in a public health context. They can usually be found on primary care trust websites.

Gold standards: health-promoting settings

The World Health Organization's Ottawa Charter for Health Promotion is a seminal document of the new public health (World Health Organization, 1986). The Charter was influential in guiding the development of the 'settings approach' which is an important cornerstone for successful public health. Prescribers need to know about the settings approach as the concept is fundamental to contemporary practice in public health, and prescribers will work in different settings.

Internationally, examples of a wide range of health-promoting settings can now be found including:

- health-promoting schools
- health-promoting workplaces
- health-promoting prisons
- health-promoting hospitals.

For some of these, for example health-promoting schools and health-promoting hospitals, a considerable amount of academic literature has been produced, including theoretical papers, descriptive studies and evaluations. However, for others, including the health-promoting general practice (Watson, 2008) and the health-promoting pharmacy, little has been written.

The settings approach moves public health interventions away from merely focusing on individuals who are ill and towards organisations, systems and the environment that can be used to prevent ill health and promote health. In a health-promoting school, for example, there are many aspects that can be health inhibiting or health promoting. The most notable are the curriculum, the physical environment, relationships within the school and with the community, and the general ethos of the school. In a health-promoting school, the health of pupils and staff would be promoted.

The pharmacy setting provides many opportunities for promoting health. However, it is essential to differentiate between a health-promoting pharmacy and health promotion in the pharmacy. Health promotion in the pharmacy may merely involve certain aspects of health promotion carried out as part of the normal dealings with customers. In contrast, the health-promoting pharmacy enables a more comprehensive and co-ordinated approach. A health-promoting pharmacy will have a positive ethos, have appropriate care for clients and staff and a strong sense of community.

Baric (1994) suggests that to become recognised as a health-promoting setting, the staff must commit to fulfil three conditions (see Figure 7.2).

Evidence-based approaches in medicine and public health

Having described some of the effective approaches available to prescribers for working on public health, including gold standards, it is important to briefly discuss some of the differences between evidence-based approaches in medicine and in public health.

There are four main differences: quantity of evidence; time from intervention to outcome; type of evidence; and the decision-making process (Brownson *et al.*, 2003).

Quantity of evidence

In general, fewer resources have been devoted to the evaluation of public health interventions compared to medical interventions. As a result there are fewer studies of public health effectiveness to be found. One important exception is for the topic of smoking, as here considerable research has been undertaken.

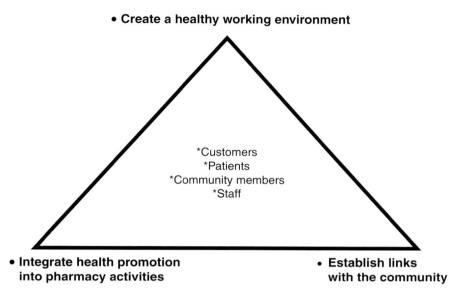

Figure 7.2   Three criteria for a health-promoting pharmacy.

Time taken

The time from intervention to outcome is a significant difference between studies in medicine and in public health. For public health initiatives there may be very long-term goals and therefore the time taken is generally longer than that for medicine. For example, certain community campaigns to reduce coronary heart disease are likely to take decades.

Type of evidence

For many healthcare studies randomised controlled trials are often the appropriate study design and will provide the most valid and reliable evaluation evidence. This may also be the case for some public health interventions, particularly those that are covering a single topic in one tightly controlled setting such as a clinic or a school. However, for many public health interventions, for example those operating in a number of different settings, a combination of quantitative and qualitative designs may be needed which may or may not include a randomised controlled trial (Watson, Woods and Kendrick, 2002).

Decision-making process

In medicine a decision is often made by a single person, whereas in public health it may be made by a group of individuals who have very different values, beliefs and levels of public health knowledge. For example, a local accident prevention group may include a health visitor, doctor, road safety officer, social worker and voluntary group members. The different members may have very different ideas of what counts as a successful outcome and what counts as evidence.

Key priority areas for public health

The government's public health strategy Choosing Health proposes action in six initial key priority areas (see Box 7.2) (DH, 2004).

Box 7.2 Choosing Health priorities

1. Tackling health inequalities.
2. Reducing the numbers of people who smoke.
3. Tackling obesity.
4. Improving sexual health.
5. Improving mental health.
6. Reducing harm and encouraging sensible drinking.

 Stop and think

As a prescriber, will you be caring for patients/clients in these priority areas?

Below we will look at these priorities, particularly in relation to how prescribers can contribute.

● In this country smoking prevention is one of the public health success stories but smoking is still the UK's single greatest cause of preventable illness and early death (DH, 2004). It causes a wide range of illnesses, including cancer, heart disease and respiratory disease. Prescribers can contribute through participating in NHS stop smoking services, providing opportunistic advice, prescribing products to support quitting, and participating in no smoking campaigns.
● Obesity is a growing public health challenge that is now receiving more resources (DH, 2008a). Being obese or overweight increases the risk of contracting important diseases such as heart disease, cancer and diabetes. There is no single way to promote healthy eating – a variety of strategies will be needed, utilising the knowledge and skills from a range of disciplines. Action will be needed in a range of different settings including schools, primary care, workplace and hospitals. Examples of activities that prescribers may be involved in include weight management clinics, lifestyle checks and advice, making healthy options more available, education campaigns and prescribing obesity drugs.
● The sexual health priority aims to reduce the incidence of chlamydia, the most common sexually transmitted infection, HIV, cervical cancer and unintended pregnancies. Prescribers can support this priority by raising awareness of safer sex messages, providing advice and contraception (including condoms and emergency hormonal contraception) and participating in local and national campaigns. A recent example of a campaign in

which prescribers are participating is one that aims to protect against the virus that causes most types of cervical cancer. The vaccination programme is targeting girls in secondary schools and is supported by mass media initiatives.

● Although drinking alcohol is an integral part of many societies, excessive consumption causes major public health problems (BMA Board of Science, 2008). Alcohol misuse contributes to a range of negative health consequences including alcohol poisoning, cancer, cardiovascular disease and injuries resulting from accidents. The British Medical Association report 'Alcohol Misuse: Tackling the UK Epidemic' describes a wide range of public health measures that are needed to tackle this key public health area (BMA Board of Science, 2008). Measures needed include fiscal, reducing availability and actions in a range of settings including primary and secondary care. Prescribers can contribute to this key area by providing brief interventions, supervising medicines to treat alcohol withdrawal and providing advice aimed at raising awareness of the health consequences of excess alcohol (DH, 2008b).

● A considerable number of people have mental health problems (DH, 2004). Stress-related conditions are the most common reported cause of absence from work, and up to one in four consultations with a general practitioner is thought to concern mental health issues (DH, 2004). Prescribers can support this key area by helping individuals with mental health problems to take their medicines correctly, referring individuals to appropriate agencies, helplines, websites and support groups, and by contributing to the development of health-promoting settings such as the workplace.

● The final key area is one that is linked to all the others and that is tackling health inequalities. Although on average people are living healthier and longer lives, life expectancy and health are not shared equally across the population (DH, 2004). There are large differences in health between certain groups both within communities and across the country. People in higher socio-economic groups tend to live longer, be ill less often and suffer fewer long-standing illnesses than those in lower socio-economic groups. Many prescribers will be in good positions to understand the needs of, and be able to reach, disadvantaged and vulnerable individuals and families. Prescribers can support this priority by working in areas of greatest need, targeted working with high-risk groups and on key topics. They can also direct individuals to services that offer translation, support families with young children and assist with housing.

Further health challenges

The Department of Health outlines further health challenges that are relevant to prescribers in 'Pharmacy in England' (DH, 2008b).

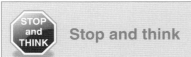 **Stop and think**

How can you contribute to public health challenges?

To gain a better understanding of how you can contribute to some of the pressing public health challenges, go to the Department of Health website www.dh.gov.uk/en/ Publicationsandstatistics/Publications/PublicationsPolicyAndGuidance/DH_083815 and download a copy of 'Pharmacy in England: Building on Strengths – Delivering the Future'. Select one of the health challenges in Annex 1 and think of all the ways in which you can contribute to tackling this challenge.

Long-term conditions

Of all medicines prescribed, about two-thirds are for people with long-term conditions, including arthritis, asthma, diabetes, heart disease and stroke (DH, 2008b). Prescribers can support this health challenge by participating in health campaigns, providing support to patients in the effective use of medicines and developing concordance programmes and carrying out reviews.

Healthcare-associated infections

Healthcare-associated infections can add significant time to a patient's stay in hospital and are costly to the NHS. Some infections have occurred due to the overprescription of general antibiotics. However, public health campaigns are now under way that not only focus on cleanliness and washing hands, but also encourage prudent prescribing of antibiotics. It is important that prescribers are up to date with the latest local antimicrobial guidelines, and that they participate in increasing public awareness on antibiotic resistance and infection control matters.

Medication errors

Medication errors are an important but sometimes under-recognised cause of avoidable harm to patients. Mistakes can occur at any stage from prescribing and dispensing, through to administration and monitoring (DH, 2008b). Prescribers can help to tackle this challenge by working with patients to ensure they have a better understanding of medicines, by clearly documenting medication allergies, providing opportunistic advice when appropriate and carrying out reviews.

Summary

- Public health is concerned with preventing disease, prolonging life and promoting health.
- There are three main groups in the public health workforce: public health consultants and specialists; public health practitioners; and the wider workforce.
- Public health encompasses a wide range of activities in different settings. Prescribers in all sectors have important roles to play.
- Key priorities for public health have been set by the government.
- Evidence-based guidance is now available to enable prescribers to make positive contributions to all domains of public health.
- There are a number of effective approaches, but the health-promoting setting is considered the gold standard.

Section 1

Activity

1. What are the three domains of public health?
2. In which Canadian city was the Wold Health Organization's Charter for Health Promotion launched?
3. What is the name of the latest public health strategy for England?
4. What are the three criteria for a health-promoting pharmacy?

References

Acheson, D. (1988) *Public Health in England*, HMSO, London.

Anderson, C., Blenkinsopp, A. and Armstrong, M. (2008) *The Contribution of Community Pharmacy to Improving the Public's Health: Literature Review Update 2004-7. Management Summary*, PharmacyHealthLink, London

Baric, L. (1994) *Health Promotion and Health Education in Practice. Module 2. The Organisational Model*, Barns Publications, Altrincham.

British Medical Association Board of Science (2008) *Alcohol Misuse: Tackling the UK Epidemic*, British Medical Association, London.

Brownson, R., Baker, E., Leet, T. and Gillespie, K. (2003) *Evidence-Based Public Health*, Oxford University Press, Oxford.

Dahlgren, G. and Whitehead, M. (1991) *Policies and Strategies to Promote Social Equity in Health*, Institute of Future Studies, Stockholm.

Davies, M. and Macdowall, W. (eds) (2006) *Health Promotion Theory*, Open University Press, Maidenhead.

Department of Health (2001) *The Report of the Chief Medical Officer's Project to Strengthen the Public Health Function*, The Stationery Office, London.

Department of Health (2004) *Choosing Health: Making Healthy Choices Easier*, Department of Health, London.

Department of Health (2005) *Choosing Health through Pharmacy. A Programme for Pharmaceutical Public Health 2005-2015*, Department of Health. London.

Department of Health (2008a) *Healthy Weight, Healthy Lives: A Cross Government Strategy for England*, Department of Health, London.

Department of Health (2008b) *Pharmacy in England. Building on Strengths – Delivering the Future*, The Stationery Office, London.

National Institute for Health and Clinical Excellence (2007) *Behaviour Change at Population, Community and Individual Levels. NICE Public Health Guidance 6*, National Institute for Health and Clinical Excellence, London.

National Institute for Health and Clinical Excellence (2008) *Smoking Cessation Services in Primary Care, Pharmacies, Local Authorities and Workplaces, Particularly for Manual Working Groups, Pregnant Women and Hard to Reach Communities. NICE Public Health Guidance 10*, National Institute for Health and Clinical Excellence, London.

Pencheon, D., Guest, C., Mezler, D. and Gray, M. (eds) (2006) *Oxford Handbook of Public Health Practice*, Oxford University Press, Oxford.

Tones, K. and Green, J. (2004) *Health Promotion. Planning and Strategies*, Sage, London.

Watson, M. (2008) Going for gold: the health promoting general practice. *Qual Primary Care*, **16**(3), 177–185.

Watson, M., Woods, A. and Kendrick, D. (2002) Randomised controlled trials in primary care. *Community Practitioner*, **75**(4), 131–134.

World Health Organization (1986) *Ottawa Charter for Health Promotion*, World Health Organization, Copenhagen.

Section 1

Section 1: The patient activity answers: Chapters 1–7

Chapter 1: The consultation

1. It is important to prepare for a consultation by studying the information you have available. This should include referral letters, past medical history, medicine history, near-patient test results and any record of allergies.

2. Presenting complaint:
   History of the presenting complaint
   Past medical and surgical history
   Family history
   Medications, drug history and allergies
   Personal and social history
   Systems review.

3. False; the purpose of the physical examination and near-patient tests is to supplement your findings from the history and to support or refute your diagnostic hypothesis.

4. Any of the following:
   Unexplained weight loss
   Night sweats
   Unexplained chronic pain
   Pain that keeps the patient awake at night.

5. Ascertain the patient's name, DOB, address, hospital or NHS number.
   Check weights were appropriate particularly when prescribing for children.
   Check for allergies.
   Check there are no interactions with other medicines the patient is taking.
   Ensure the patient has no other medical condition that might be exacerbated by the medication.
   Inform the patient of mild and more serious side effects of the medication.

Chapter 2: Accountability

Answer true or false.

1. False; they act to protect the patient/society.

2. False; you are legally and professionally liable for acts and omissions under the law of negligence and your code of practice.

The New Prescriber. Edited by J Lymn, D Bowskill, F Bath-Hextall, R Knaggs, © 2010 John Wiley & Sons.

3. False; practitioners are expected to maintain their level of competence in meeting the standards of care required of the reasonable prescriber.

4. This is broadly true though under Bolam a practitioner only has to accept your actions as being reasonable. Do note that since the case of Bolitho you do need to be able to provide evidence for your acts to the court.

5. True; this could be yrue if your prescribing amounts to gross negligence.

6. False; a tort is a civil wrong actionable in the civil courts.

7. False; practitioners do cause harm to their patients, for example giving injections and so on. These harms are balanced against the benefits of the treatment.

Chapter 3: Legal aspects of prescribing

1. False

2. True

3. False

4. False

5. True

6. False

7. True

8. False

9. False

Chapter 4: Ethics of prescribing

1. False

2. False

3. True

4. True

5. False

Chapter 5: Prescribing in practice

1. The key difference between the two types of prescribing lies in the accountability for diagnosis. Under independent prescribing, the independent prescriber (doctor, dentist, nurse, pharmacist or optometrist) is responsible for the diagnosis and prescribing of treatment. Under supplementary prescribing, the independent prescriber who takes responsibility for the diagnosis must be a doctor or dentist.

2. Morphine sulphate can be prescribed under independent prescribing in oral form for use in palliative care.

3. Supplementary prescribing with a patient-specific clinical management plan. AHPs are supplementary prescribers.

4. No, under arrangements for supplementary prescribing the independent prescriber must be a doctor or a dentist.

Chapter 6: Record keeping

1. True

2. False

3. False

4. True

5. False

Chapter 7: Public health issues

1. Health improvement,
   Improving services,
   Health protection.

2. Ottawa

3. Choosing Health, Making Healthy Choices Easier.

4. Create a healthy working environment,
   Establish links with the community,
   Integrate health promotion into pharmacy activities.

Section 1: The patient glossary

Act: Primary legislation that is considered as a Bill and debated by both Houses.

Administrative law: Statutory law delegating power to public bodies and setting out their accountability for quality; the body itself may be fined or contractors may be fined with the money passing to the public body.

Black triangle: Symbol in the BNF denoting newly licensed medicines that are monitored intensively by MHRA.

Civil law: Law expressing duties owed by citizens to one another, particularly duty of care.

Clinical management plan: A written patient-specific agreement between independent and supplementary prescribers, which details the condition(s) to be managed and the medicines that may be prescribed.

Clinical negligence: The branch of law dealing with the duty of care between health professionals and their users and alleged failures in care. If proven to cause harm, compensation may be ordered.

Conscience clauses: Part of many codes of ethics in healthcare that respect the personal (including religious) beliefs of individuals, and broadly exempt individuals from undertaking acts that conflict with their conscience.

Controlled drug: Any dangerous or otherwise harmful substance included in the Misuse of Drugs Act 1971 or subsequent Misuse of Drugs Regulations.

Criminal law: Statutory law with criminal sanctions, such as fines going to the Treasury and prison, generally enforced by the police service.

Deontology: Ethical theories that claim individuals have certain duties, which must be followed at all times, irrespective of the outcome.

Determinants of health: The range of personal, social, economic and environmental factors that determine the health of individuals or communities.

Distributive justice: A concern, usually ethical, about how resources and money should be allocated amongst individuals and in society in the fairest way.

Duty of care: An obligation to provide care to a reasonable standard; the duty relates to both acts and omissions.

ECT: Electroconvulsive therapy. A treatment for depression which involves the passing of an electric current across the brain to induce an epileptic-type seizure.

The New Prescriber. Edited by J Lymn, D Bowskill, F Bath-Hextall, R Knaggs, © 2010 John Wiley & Sons.

Ethics: Ethics, or moral philosophy as it is often also called, involves questioning and justifying what individuals do, and particularly what actions are thought right or wrong, or what sort of person one should try to be.

Four principles of bioethics: Influential ethical theory which argues that four key principles – autonomy, beneficence, non-maleficence and justice – can be applied to decide the ethical problems that arise in healthcare.

Independent prescribing: Prescribing by a practitioner responsible and accountable for the assessments of patients with undiagnosed or diagnosed conditions and for decisions about the clinical management required, including prescribing.

Medicinal purpose: Marketed for the purpose of treating or preventing disease or related purposes.

Medicines compliance: A measure of patient behaviour: the extent to which patients take medicines according to the prescribed instructions.

Medicines concordance: A two-way consultation process: shared decision making about medicines between a healthcare professional and a patient, based on partnership, where the patient's expertise and beliefs are fully valued.

Negligence: Negligence is a tort involving a civil action for compensation arising from a breach of the duty of care which has caused damage.

Non-medical prescriber: A prescriber who is not a doctor.

Off-label, off-licence, outwith the licence: Using a licensed medicinal products in circumstances not covered by the licence.

Patient Group Direction: A written instruction for the supply and/or administration of a medicine(s) in an identified clinical situation, signed by a doctor or dentist and a pharmacist. It applies to groups of patients who may not be individually identified before presenting for treatment.

Patient-specific direction: The traditional written instruction, from a doctor, dentist, nurse or pharmacist independent prescriber, for medicines to be supplied or administered to a named patient.

Professional law: Statutory law with professional sanctions, such as being struck off a professional register.

Public health: 'The science and art of preventing disease, prolonging life and promoting health through organised efforts of society' (Acheson, 1988).

Regulations: Secondary or subordinate legislation that implements the details of an Act; usually 'laid before' Parliament only.

Statute: Instruments of legislation passed by Parliament, i.e. Acts, Regulations and Orders.

Statutory law: Law that has been made by Parliament.

Statutory administrative law: Statutory law delegating power to public bodies and setting out their accountability for quality; the body itself may be fined or contractors may be fined with the money passing to the public body.

Statutory criminal law: Statutory law with criminal sanctions, such as fines going to the Treasury and prison, generally enforced by the police service.

Statutory professional law: Statutory law with professional sanctions, such as being struck off a professional register.

Supplementary prescribing: A voluntary partnership between an independent prescriber (a doctor or dentist) and a supplementary prescriber to implement an agreed patient-specific clinical management plan with the patient's agreement.

Tort: A tort is a civil wrong.

Unlicensed: Using a product or substance which does not have a licence for a medicinal purpose.

Utilitarianism: Ethical theory which deems acts right only if they lead to the greatest overall happiness (or welfare in some versions) for the greatest number of individuals.

Vicarious liability: The liability held by employers for the actions of their employees, specifically in relation to costs for harm caused to patients.

Written directions: The form of instruction for prescribing medicines to hospital inpatients (bed chart, ward chart, etc.).

Yellow Card scheme: MHRA-administered scheme for reporting and monitoring the occurrence of ADRs.

Section 2

Evidence–Based Practice

Section introduction

This section of the book should be regarded as a brief introduction to evidence-based practice and does not attempt to replace the vast number of highly detailed texts available on the subject. We hope that by the end of this section of the book you will have a better understanding about how evidence-based practice has developed over the years. We hope that as you wind your way through the different chapters, you will acquire new skills to take back into practice; for example, framing a question that emerges from clinical practice, searching effectively for evidence, critically appraising the research evidence you have found and finally gaining a better understanding about how to implement research evidence into practice.

8 What is evidence-based practice?

Learning outcomes

By the end of this chapter the reader should be able to:

- have a better understanding of evidence-based practice – what it is and why it is important in prescribing
- identify the key milestones in evidence-based practice
- define the term 'evidence-based practice'
- identify the five steps involved in evidence-based practice
- understand the main components to framing a question (step 1 in evidence-based practice).

Evidence-based practice – what is it and why is it important for prescribers?

The way the healthcare professions have approached training, until recently, has been based on an apprentice type system that might have involved anecdotal evidence and others' personal experience which could have been unreliable and biased. Remember, experience is made up of personal values as well as social and cultural influences which could unknowingly influence our opinions. Nowadays most of us recognise that professional practice should be based on sound evidence in addition to personal expertise, that is acquired with time and experience; in reality this is not so easy. As a practitioner/prescriber you are probably only too aware of how difficult it is to keep up with new emerging evidence, not to mention how time consuming it can all be. In fact, studies done in the USA and The Netherlands suggest that around 30–40% of patients are not receiving the most appropriate care according to present evidence, and 20–25% of care provided is not needed and could be potentially harmful (Grol, 2001; Schuster, McGlynn and Brook, 1998).

So what is evidence-based practice? Evidence-based practice (EBP) is a somewhat recent development and has emerged partly due to difficulties in keeping up to date with the

The New Prescriber. Edited by J Lymn, D Bowskill, F Bath-Hextall, R Knaggs, © 2010 John Wiley & Sons.

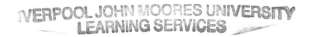

tremendous amount of new information. Just think, more than 50 new trials and 2000 new research articles are published per day! EBP is also a product of our time, since without the availability of technologies such as electronic databases and internet searching, the process of searching for evidence would take an extraordinary amount of time and could be out of date almost immediately.

As prescribers, it is essential to keep up to date with new emerging evidence and Chapter 9 will help you understand how to go about finding this. It is also important to remember that you will be targeted by pharmaceutical companies who will try and convince you that their product is the best thing since sliced bread. Be careful; remember that a study all wrapped up in a glossy cover doesn't mean that it is a good study! The following chapters will arm you with the necessary skills to practise and develop EBP in your clinical area. A cautionary note, however; it's all well and good to be aware of the evidence but it's another thing to be able to translate that evidence into practice. This process can be difficult and challenging and is addressed in Chapter 13.

The emergence of evidence-based practice has to be one of the success stories of the 1990s. In the space of ten years the movement has had a significant impact on health care and policy.

Trinder, 2001

Practice application

All healthcare professions need to understand the principles of evidence-based practice (EBP), recognise evidence-based practice in action, implement evidence-based policies, and have a critical attitude to their own practice and to evidence. Without these skills, professionals and organisations will find it difficult to provide best practice.

Dawes *et al.*, 2005

Stop and think

When you last made a clinical decision, was it based on recent and appropriate evidence?

Key milestones in evidence-based practice – a little bit of history

The move towards EBP began more than 30 years ago and for medicine, it was largely due to Archibald (Archie) Cochrane.

1972

Professor Archie Cochrane gives a lecture at Edinburgh University drawing attention to the lack of precise evidence for the effectiveness or otherwise of medical treatment in the UK health service. The publication of the monograph 'Effectiveness and Efficiency: Random Reflections on Health Services' (Cochrane, 1972) commands international attention, and becomes a best seller which will underpin the development of EBP ideals in healthcare professions.

Archie Cochrane also suggests that the results of research would be more likely to influence clinical practice if they could be systematically reviewed and if well-founded findings could be aggregated.

1977

A Canadian survey suggests that doctors are failing to keep up to date with current research (Sackett *et al.*, 1977). These findings prompt McMaster University in Canada to develop and introduce both undergraduate and Master's level curricula encouraging medical students to keep up to date with medical research in order to inform their clinical decision making.

1980s

Archie Cochrane's ideas are taken up by Ian Chalmers who begins reviewing care during pregnancy and childbirth.

1987

Archie Cochrane refers to Ian Chalmers' review as 'a milestone in the history of randomised controlled trials and in the evaluation of care'.

1988

The Cochrane Collaboration is formed in order to prepare, maintain and disseminate reviews of the effects of healthcare based on randomised controlled trials.

1992

The term evidence-based medicine (EBM) appears for the first time in medical literature (Evidence-Based Medicine Working Group, 1992). The Cochrane Centre in Oxford is established.

Evidence-based medicine develops rapidly and key concepts are developed in other disciplines and professions under the generic title of evidence-based practice, for example evidence-based dentistry, nursing, public health, physiotherapy and so on.

1994

The NHS Centre for Reviews and Dissemination (CRD) is established in the UK. The CRD undertakes systematic reviews evaluating the research evidence on health and public health questions of national and international importance. The CRD also produces the Database of Abstracts of Reviews of Effects (DARE), the NHS Economic Evaluation Database (NHS EED)

Section 2

and the Health Technology Assessment (HTA) database. These databases are used by health professionals, policy makers and researchers around the world.

1996

The Centre for Evidence-Based Nursing is established in the UK, to further evidence-based nursing through education, research and development.

1996

The Joanna Briggs Institute (JBI) in Australia is founded to address the needs of the nursing profession for EBP.

2000

The Campbell Collaboration is established in the USA. It produces, maintains and disseminates systematic reviews of research evidence on the effectiveness of social interventions. The Collaboration is closely associated with the Cochrane Collaboration.

Since the 1990s EBP has made a significant impact on healthcare and policy and has rapidly developed globally.

Definitions of evidence-based practice

The term EBP has become widespread and in the literature you will find numerous definitions. The most quoted definition, written by Sackett and colleagues, was originally confined to the description of evidence-based medicine.

> Evidence-based medicine is the conscientious, explicit, and judicious use of current best evidence in making decisions about the care of individual patients, based on skills which allow the doctor to evaluate both personal experience and external evidence in a systematic and objective manner.
>
> Sackett *et al.*, 1996

However, since that first description of EBM, many healthcare professions have adopted the evidence-based approach to practice.

Here are a few more definitions

Evidence-Based Practice

> Evidence-based practice (EBP) is an approach to health care wherein health professionals use the best evidence possible, i.e. the most appropriate information available, to make clinical decisions for individual patients. EBP values, enhances and builds on clinical expertise, knowledge of disease mechanisms, and pathophysiology. It involves complex and conscientious decision making based not only on the available evidence but also on patient characteristics, situations, and preferences. It recognizes that health care is individualized and ever changing and involves uncertainties and probabilities. Ultimately

EBP is the formalization of the care process that the best clinicians have practiced for generations.

McKibbon, 1998

Evidence based practice provides a framework and process for the systematic incorporation of research evidence and patient preference into clinical decision making at the level of the individual practitioner and the healthcare organisation.

Newman and Papadopoulos, 2000

Evidence-Based Clinical Practice

Evidence-based clinical practice is an approach to decision-making in which the clinician uses the best evidence available, in consultation with the patient, to decide the option which suits the patient best.

Gray, 1997

Evidence-Based Healthcare

Evidence-Based Health Care extends the application of the principles of Evidence-Based Medicine (see above) to all professions associated with health care, including purchasing and management.

Centre for Evidence-Based Medicine glossary

As you can see from the definitions above, best research evidence (BRE) is just one source of evidence. We must not forget other sources of evidence including clinical expertise (CE) derived from experience and, of course, the patient preference (PP) (Figure 8.1). You might want to think of this in the form of the following equation:

$$CE + PP + BRE = EBP$$

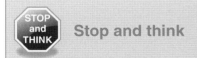 **Stop and think**

Think back to when you last saw a client. Did you consider all three components of evidence-based practice?

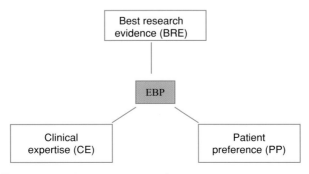

Figure 8.1   Main components for evidence-based practice.

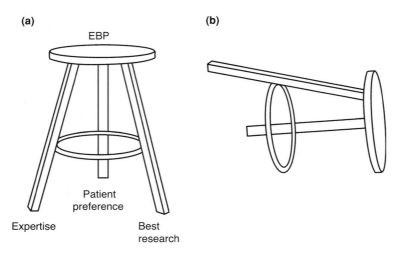

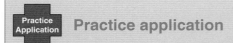

Figure 8.2 (a) The stool illustrating three key components of EBP. (b) One of the key components (legs) is missing!

A useful way to think about EBP is to consider a stool. The seat of the stool could represent EBP but remember, for the stool to be functional, it requires three legs, and the legs are best research evidence, clinical expertise and patient preference (Figure 8.2a). For the stool to remain upright then all three legs need to be used (Figure 8.2b).

Practice Application **Practice application**

If you apply the principles of EBP to buying a family car, you might want to consider the following:

- the needs of the family (patient preference)
- your driving experience (clinical expertise)
- research to find a car for the job (best research evidence).

You might also need to consider your budget! (cost implications).

After all, as a parent of four children, you would be foolish to buy this car (Figure 8.3) for the school run!

So far we have looked at a number of definitions for EBP, how EBP developed and the main components of EBP. Now we are going to move on to look at the five key steps involved in EBP and in this chapter, we will look in detail at the first.

The five steps involved in evidence-based practice

The evidence-based approach to decision making can be broken down into five key steps.

1. Asking the question.
2. Finding the evidence that best answers the question (Chapter 9).

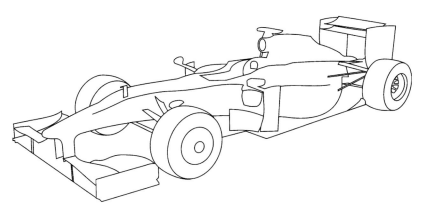

Figure 8.3   Formula 1 car.

3. Appraising the evidence for its validity, impact and applicability (Chapter 11).
4. Acting on the evidence – that is, implementing the evidence in practice (Chapter 13).
5. Evaluation and reflection.

Of course, going through the above five steps is time consuming and not always possible so there have been a number of developments that have made this whole process more manageable, for example the creation of systematic reviews of the effects of healthcare, the creation of evidence-based journals of secondary publication and evidence-based summary services such as Clinical Evidence.

Let's now look at step 1 in EBP. Have you ever asked yourself the question: 'Is this the best treatment for this person?'.

Step 1: Asking the question

Take yourself back into your practice area and try to think of a relevant, answerable question (Figure 8.4). It is crucial that you take your time over this step, as it will save you time in the long run. Asking a question forces you to clarify the problem in your own mind and also helps you to define the kind of evidence that you will need to answer the question.

Try and use a structured approach to framing your question. It has been proposed that a well-built question contains three or four components (Richardson, 1995; Sackett *et al.*, 1997; Flemming, 1998). To help with remembering the four components you could use the mnemonic **PICO** which stands for **P**articipants, **I**ntervention, **C**omparison and **O**utcome.

1. The patient or the problem (**P**).
2. The intervention (or exposure) you are considering (**I**).
3. The comparison (if this is relevant) – what is the treatment compared to? (**C**)
4. The outcome – what are you trying to achieve? You may need to think about a time point here, if relevant (**O**).

Of course, questions can be classified in a number of different ways and it does depend on the focus. Questions might be around diagnosis, prognosis, patient/client prospective or intervention.

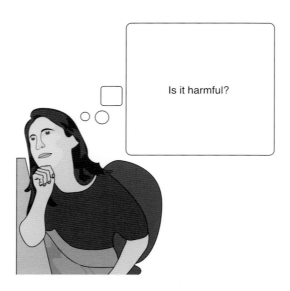

Figure 8.4 Step 1 – Asking the question.

Different questions will lead to you looking for different types of evidence Go to Chapter 9 to look at different types of evidence.

Here are a couple of examples of well-formulated questions. Notice that they follow the PICO format. Both of these examples are taken from Cochrane systematic reviews and concentrate on questions of intervention.

The first question below looks at topical treatments for cutaneous warts (Gibbs and Harvey, 2006).

P – population/patient

People with *clinically* observed viral warts.

I – intervention

All *local* treatments aimed at eradicating viral warts. Local treatments are defined here as all topical, intralesional and surgical treatments, including cryotherapy but not including systemic or psychological treatments.

C – comparison

Local treatments versus placebo or local treatment versus other local treatment.

O – outcome

Primary outcomes
(1) Clinical cure at the end of the treatment period. (Clinical cure is defined as complete disappearance of elevated/warty skin.)
(2) Participant satisfaction/dissatisfaction.
(3) Quality of life measures.

Secondary outcome

(1) Adverse events such as blistering, pain and scarring.

This second question looks at interventions for basal cell carcinoma (BCC) (Bath-Hextall *et al.*, 2007).

P – population/patient

All adults who have one or more *histologically* proven, primary basal cell carcinoma, who were eligible for randomisation to active treatment, placebo/open or other treatment. Excluded: studies solely of participants with Gorlin syndrome (or basal cell naevus syndrome), organoid naevi or other genetic syndromes. Persistent (where a number of treatments have been tried with no success) or recurrent tumours.

I – intervention

Treatments for BCC including:
- **Surgical**
  - (i) excisional – margin of clinically normal tissue specified or unspecified
  - (ii) Mohs micrographic surgery.
- **Destructive**
  - (i) curettage and cautery/electrodesiccation – any margin – any number of cycles
  - (ii) cryosurgery – any number of cycles
  - (iii) photodynamic therapy
  - (iv) laser surgery
  - (v) radiotherapy.
- **Other techniques**
  - (i) topical therapy, for example imiquimod, 5-fluorouracil
  - (ii) intralesional interferon
  - (iii) chemotherapy.

C – comparison

Treatment versus placebo or treatment versus other treatment.

O – outcome

Primary outcome

Recurrence at 3–5 years, measured clinically (to reflect what actually happens in clinical practice).

Secondary outcome

Early treatment failure within 6 months, measured *histologically*.

Adverse effects

- (i) Aesthetic appearance to participants: atrophy, scarring, changes in pigmentation at 6 months, 1 year and 5 years.
- (ii) Aesthetic appearance to observer: atrophy, scarring, changes in pigmentation at 6 months, 1 year and 5 years.
- (iii) Discomfort to participants in terms of pain during treatment and thereafter.

Section 2

If you are interested in qualitative questions about health issues, please refer to the Joanna Briggs Institute website, listed at the end of this chapter.

Stop and think

Think back to problems you have encountered. Try and frame the question around the following headings: **P**roblem, **I**ntervention, **C**omparison, **O**utcome.

Summary

- Evidence-based practice began more than 30 years ago and has been one of the success stories of recent times.
- One of the key players in the evidence-based medicine movement was Archie Cochrane.
- Evidence-based practice can be thought of as a product of our technological age.
- There are a number of key milestones in evidence-based practice.
- Many definitions of evidence-based practice exist but all versions include best research evidence, clinical expertise and patient preference.
- There are five major steps involved in evidence-based practice: asking the question, finding the evidence, appraising the evidence, acting on the evidence, and evaluation and reflection.
- Framing a question involves three or four components: the problem, the intervention, a comparison and an outcome. Questions can be classified in a number of different ways including diagnosis and prognosis, interventions, patient/client perspective, and efficiency and effectiveness.

Activity

1. List the five steps involved in evidence-based practice.
2. List the main components in evidence-based practice – remember the stool!
3. When did the term 'evidence-based medicine' first appear in the literature?

Useful websites

The Cochrane Collaboration. www.cochrane.org

Centre for Evidence Based Medicine Glossary. www:cebm.jr2.ox.ac.uk/docs/glossary

Centre for Reviews and Dissemination, University of York. www.york.ac.uk/inst/crd/

Joanna Briggs Institute for Evidence-based Nursing and Midwifery, Australia. www.joannabriggs.edu.au

Campbell Collaboration. www.campbellcollaboration.org

(Critical Appraisal Skills Programme) (CASP) – aims to enable individuals to develop the skills to find and make sense of research evidence, helping them to put knowledge into practice. www.phru.nhs.uk/Pages/PHD/CASP

(Centre for Evidence-Based Medicine) (CEBM). www.cebm.net

(Centre for Evidence-Based Mental Health) (CEBMH). http://cebmh.warne.ox.ac.uk/cebmh

(Centre for Evidence-Based Nursing) (CEBN), Department of Health Sciences, University of York. www.york.ac.uk/healthsciences/centres/evidence/cebn.htm

Reusable learning objects
Asking the question

www.nottingham.ac.uk/nursing/sonet/rlos/ebp/systematic_reviews/index.html

References

Bath-Hextall, F.J., Perkins, W., Bong, J. and Williams, H.C. (2007) Interventions for basal cell carcinoma of the skin. *Cochrane Database Syst Rev*, 1, CD003412).

Cochrane, A. (1972) Effectiveness and efficiency: random reflections on health services, in *The Nuffield Provincial Hospitals Trust*, Burges & Son, Abingdon, pp. 19–20.

Dawes, M., Summerskill, W. and Glasziou, P., *et al.* (2005) Sicily statement on evidence-based practice. *BMC Med Educ*, **5**, 1.

Evidence-Based Medicine Working Group (1992) Evidence-based medicine. A new approach to teaching the practice of medicine. *JAMA*, **268**, 2420–2425

Flemming, K. (1998) Asking answerable questions. *Evidence-Based Nurs*, **1**(2), 36–37.

Gibbs, S. and Harvey, I. (2006) Topical treatments for cutaneous warts. *Cochrane Database Syst Rev*, **3**, CD001781).

Gray, J.A.M. (1997) *Evidence-based Health Care: How to Make Health Policy and Management Decisions*, Churchill Livingstone, Edinburgh.

Grol, R. (2001) Successes and failures in the implementation of evidence-based guidelines for clinical practice. *Med Care*, **39**(suppl 2), 46–54.

McKibbon, K.A. (1998) Evidence based practice. *Bull Med Library Assoc*, **86**(3), 396–401.

Newman, M. and Papadopoulos, I. (2000) Developing organizational systems and culture to support evidence based practice: the experience of the evidence based ward project. *Evidence-Based Nurs*, **3**, 103–105.

Section 2

Richardson, W., Wilson, M., Nishikawa, J. and Hayward, R.S. (1995) The well-built clinical question: a key to evidence-based decisions [editorial]. *ACP J Club*, **123**, A12–A13.

Sackett, D.L., Rosenberg, W., Taylor, D.W., *et al.* (1977) Clinical determinants of the decision to treat primary hypertension. *Clin Res*, **24**, 648.

Sackett, D.L., Rosenberg, W.M., Gray, J.A., *et al.* (1996) Evidence based medicine: what it is and what it isn't. *BMJ*, **312**(7023), 71–72.

Schuster, M., McGlynn, E. and Brook, R. (1998) How good is the quality of health care in the United States? *Milbank Q*, **76**, 517–563.

Trinder, L. (2000) The context of evidence-based practice, in *Evidence Based Practice: A Critical Appraisal* (eds L. Trinder and S. Reynolds), Blackwell Science, Oxford, pp. 1–16.

Further reading

Sackett, D. (2000) *Evidence-based Medicine: How to Practice and Teach EBM,* 2nd edn, Churchill Livingstone, London.

Sackett, D.L. and Wennberg, J.E. (1997) Choosing the best research design for the question. *BMJ*, **315**, 1636.

Straus, S.E., Richardson, W.S., Glasziou, P. and Haynes, R.B. (eds) (2005) *Evidence-Based Medicine. How to Practice and Teach EBM*, 3rd edn, Elsevier Churchill, Edinburgh.

9 How do we find the evidence?

Learning outcomes

By the end of this chapter the reader should be able to:

- use the Cochrane Library to find the answer to a question by using one search term
- construct a simple search strategy combining several disease terms with boolean operators
- search for randomised controlled trials (RCTs)
- construct a more complex search strategy
- search a variety of databases.

Finding the evidence is the second step in the evidence-based practice approach to decision making.

Step 2: Finding the evidence that best answers the question

It is easy enough to find information on the internet by 'Googling' any word. The real difficulty is in deciding if the information found has answered the question and that the answer is true, reliable and free of bias (see Chapters 10 and 11).

The first step towards finding the evidence is to be very clear about the question you are asking. Remember, we covered **Step 1 'Asking the question'** in Chapter 8.

Let's take one of the questions that we looked at in that chapter – topical treatments for cutaneous warts.

The next step then is to find the evidence – so where is the best place to look for a reliable answer to this question? Traditionally, in the pre-internet world, the first port of call would have been a library to find a textbook on skin conditions and treatment for warts. This may have been good reliable evidence based on the experience of many practitioners in the field

The New Prescriber. Edited by J Lymn, D Bowskill, F Bath-Hextall, R Knaggs, © 2010 John Wiley & Sons.

or it may have been one person's opinion. It would inevitably have been information that was quite dated and was unlikely to have been sourced internationally.

Now with access to the internet there is far more information available, which is more up to date. BUT! There is a jungle of information out there so if you Google 'treatment common wart', how do you know that you can trust the lotions and potions suggested? The answer is: you need to search websites that you can trust.

Guidelines

You could search the National Library for Health site and if you click on 'guidance' you will find a link to the National Library of Guidelines. If you then click this link it will take you to the National Library of Guidelines Specialist Library and then all you do is enter the term 'warts' in the search box and this will reveal 'Guidelines for the management of cutaneous warts'. Guidelines will have gathered information from different sources. A word of caution: do please check the date of any guidelines that you find because they can rapidly go out of date.

However, if there are no guidelines on your subject of interest, then the next step is to look for systematic reviews.

Systematic reviews (secondary research)

The best place to find systematic reviews is the Cochrane Library. Systematic reviews are the most reliable source of evidence for the effectiveness of an intervention (see Chapter 11). However, be careful not to confuse a *systematic review* with a *literature review*. A systematic review is not simply a narrative written by one person expressing their opinion. It is a structured body of work usually conducted by a group of people where a clear research question has been posed. A plan (known as the protocol) has been written to set out how the systematic review is to be conducted. These reviews are usually updated every 2 years. More about systematic reviews in Chapters 10 and 11.

The first step in finding out about a treatment for warts is to conduct a basic search in the Cochrane Library.

The Cochrane Library

Figure 9.1 shows a screen shot of the front page of the Cochrane Library.

The simplest search is to go to the Search Box indicated and type in the free text term 'warts' and click 'go'. As you can see, the first systematic review that is displayed in the Cochrane Library is 'Topical treatments for cutaneous warts'. So if you read through this, you will find the answer to the question we asked about the best way to treat warts. Remember always to check the date of the systematic review to see how up to date the information is.

The above example was very easy because the search term 'warts' was in the title of the review.

Basic searching strategies

If you look at the search strategy used within this review 'Topical treatments for cutaneous warts' to find the primary research (in this case the randomised controlled trials RCTs), you will see the authors did not just search for the word 'warts' but they used all the names for warts that they could think of and combined them using Boolean operators (Box 9.1). Here all

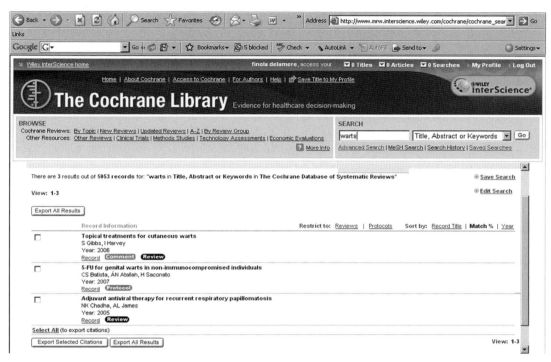

Figure 9.1   Cochrane Library page. The Cochrane Library: Copyright © Cochrane Collaboration, reproduced with permission.

the disease terms were combined together with the Boolean operator 'OR'. They then searched for all the terms that might be used to describe clinical trials: these were also combined with the Boolean operator 'OR'. The findings from the two groups were then combined with the Boolean operator 'AND' – so that all the papers found are on the subject of warts and clinical trials. In this example the authors have looked for any treatment for warts so they do not need to have a third group of search terms.

If the authors wanted to only find topical treatments they would have had to search on all the terms for topical ointments that they could think of, combined all these with 'OR' and then added them to the other two groups so that they had disease terms AND clinical trials

---

Box 9.1   Boolean Operators Explained

Search for fruits: apples, pears, bananas, tomatoes
Search for vegetables: turnips, onions, potatoes, tomatoes
A combination of FRUITS **AND** VEGETABLES would only include 'tomatoes' as they are in the FRUIT list AND the VEGETABLE list.
A combination of FRUITS **OR** VEGETABLES would be the sum of the 2 groups as each group contains:
  apples OR pears OR bananas OR tomatoes
  OR turnips OR onions OR potatoes.
Tomatoes would only be included once as they are duplicated in the two lists.

Section 2

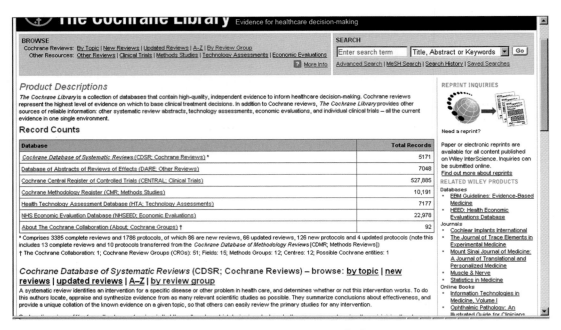

Figure 9.2 Search results. The Cochrane Library: Copyright © Cochrane Collaboration, reproduced with permission.

terms AND topical treatment terms. This is an example of a pragmatic approach to searching: they have been as inclusive as possible to try to find all the records.

The Cochrane Library is composed of several databases, not just the one that contains the systematic reviews (known as CDSR). As you can see in the screen shot in Figure 9.2, there is a database known as CENTRAL. This contains records for over half a million clinical trials. If our simple search for 'warts' had not yielded a systematic review because a systematic review had not been done on this subject, then we would have had to see if we could answer our question by looking at the evidence from clinical trials. As you will see in CENTRAL, the term 'warts' is in the title, abstract or keywords of over 400 records (Cochrane Library, Issue 1, 2008). You will note that the other databases also have records on 'warts'.

BUT! If we had only searched on the word 'warts' we may have missed lots of RCTs that would have helped us answer our question. So in this instance we should search on all the disease terms and combine them together as explained above. Don't be worried about using the 'advanced search' in the Cochrane Library just because it is called 'advanced'. It is actually more useful because it is more flexible than the one-line search box. Now go to 'advanced search' as shown in screen shot Figure 9.3 and type the following into each of the boxes and select 'search all text' and also select 'OR':

Warts

Verruca

Papilloma virus

Mosaic warts

Section 2

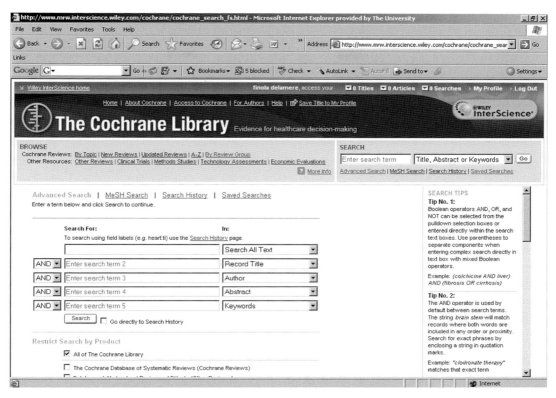

Figure 9.3   Advanced search. The Cochrane Library: Copyright © Cochrane Collaboration, reproduced with permission.

Now tick the box and 'go directly to search history' and click 'search'. If you scroll further down the screen you will see that you can also limit your search to a specific date range.

Screen shot Figure 9.4 shows the search history page with the sum of the disease terms combined with 'OR'. If you double-click on the line indicated, this will take you to the following screen where the numbers of records in each of these databases is indicated in brackets. Screen shot Figure 9.5 indicates the number of records with the 'warts' disease terms that are in the systematic reviews database and the clinical trials databases.

The clinical trials database in the Cochrane Library is the biggest source of RCTs and controlled clinical trials in the world. So the hard work has been done for you because many databases and journals have been searched for clinical trials and even records that have never been on databases before have been gathered together in one place. But the database can never be completely up to date so it is important to search other databases. For further information on what a RCT is, see Chapters 10 and 11.

Other databases

If you look at a systematic review of interventions you will see the authors will have searched for RCTs (primary research) in several different databases.

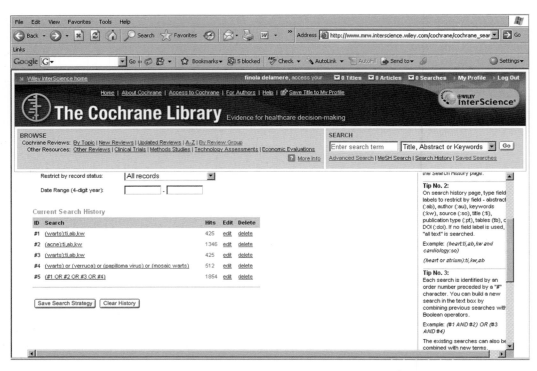

Figure 9.4 Advanced search continued. The Cochrane Library: Copyright © Cochrane Collaboration, reproduced with permission.

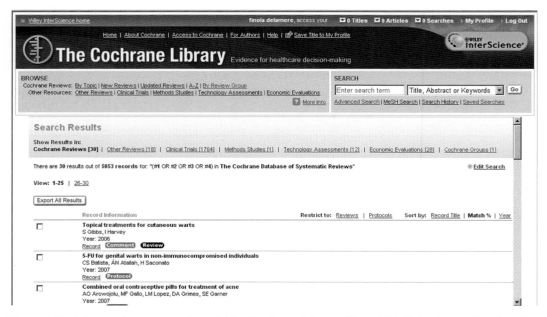

Figure 9.5 Advanced search continued. The Cochrane Library: Copyright © Cochrane Collaboration, reproduced with permission.

The aim is to maximise the chances of finding as many reports of trials as possible. Each database has its own characteristics and although you may use similar search terms for diseases or interventions or clinical trials, they will be indexed and displayed differently in each database. So a systematic review should have each search strategy for each database clearly displayed with the date that the search was conducted. This is because new records are constantly added to new databases and methods of indexing are constantly being developed.

By the time this book is published the optimal search for RCTs will have been updated. See the Cochrane Handbook for the latest search strategy.

The second database to search would be PubMed or MEDLINE. PubMed is a service of the US National Library of Medicine that includes over 17 million citations from MEDLINE and other life science journals for biomedical articles back to the 1950s. These databases have different platforms by which they are accessed and therefore are searched differently. These databases contain many types of records so that in a search for RCTs for a disease, the search strategy would need to combine disease terms AND intervention terms AND clinical trial terms. You can find the latest advice on search filters in Chapter 6.4.11 in the Cochrane Handbook.

Databases all have their own formats so that although search strategies may use the same terms, they all need to be in the format that can be 'read' by that database. The PubMed format to search for RCTs is shown in Box 9.2 and the MEDLINE (OVID) format is shown in Box 9.3.

You will see in the search strategies in Boxes 9.2 and 9.3 that records are indexed with Medical Subject Headings (MeSH). MeSH headings are also used in the Cochrane Library as many of the clinical trials come from MEDLINE. It is advisable to combine free text terms

---

Box 9.2 Search Strategy for Locating RCTs in PubMed

#1	randomised controlled trial [pt]
#2	controlled clinical trial [pt]
#3	randomised [tiab]
#4	placebo [tiab]
#5	clinical trials as topic [mesh: noexp]
#6	randomly [tiab]
#7	trial [ti]
#8	#1 or #2 or #3 or #4 or #5 or #6 or #7
#9	humans [mh]
#10	#8 and #9

The Cochrane Library: Copyright © Cochrane Collaboration, reproduced with permission.

PubMed search syntax

[pt] denotes a Publication Type term
[tiab] denotes a word in the title or abstract
[sh] denotes a subheading
[mh] denotes a Medical Subject Heading (MeSH) term ('exploded')
[mesh: noexp] denotes a Medical Subject Heading (MeSH) term (not 'exploded')
[ti] denotes a word in the title

Box 9.3 **Search Strategy for Locating RCTs in MEDLINE (OVID)**

1	randomised controlled trial.pt.
2	controlled clinical trial.pt.
3	randomised.ab.
4	placebo.ab.
5	clinical trials as topic.sh.
6	randomly.ab.
7	trial.ti.
8	1 or 2 or 3 or 4 or 5 or 6 or 7
9	humans.sh.
10	8 and 9

The Cochrane Library: Copyright © Cochrane Collaboration, reproduced with permission.

OVID search syntax

.pt. denotes a Publication Type term
.ab. denotes a word in the abstract
.fs. denotes a 'floating' subheading
.sh. denotes a Medical Subject Heading (MeSH) term
.ti. denotes a word in the title

---

and MeSH terms in a search strategy to maximise the records found. In fact, MeSH terms can sometimes give clues about other free text terms to use in a search.

A simple example in the Cochrane Library

Go to MeSH search and type in 'atopic eczema'. You will see that this is not a term that is indexed, but a list of possible MeSH descriptors is given. One of these is atopic dermatitis. This would then give a clue that in the free text search, 'atopic eczema' and 'atopic dermatitis' need to be used as disease search terms.

Other places to find randomised controlled trials

There are other good-quality databases that should be searched when looking for primary research.

- EMBASE, which is a biomedical and pharmacological database, gives you access to the most up-to-date information about medical and drug-related subjects.
- LILACS (Latin American and Caribbean Health Sciences Literature) covers health sciences literature that has been published in countries of Latin America and the Caribbean.
- AMED (Allied and Complementary Medicine Database) is a unique bibliographic database produced by the Health Care Information Service of the British Library.
- PsycINFO database is the comprehensive international bibliographic database of psychology.
- CINAHL (Current Index to Nursing and Allied Health Literature).

Searching for observational studies

Observational studies (e.g. case–control studies, cohort studies) cannot be found in big databases by applying the equivalent of a clinical trial search filter because there is no simple way to label them. Searches have to include MeSH terms such as 'cohort studies', 'case–control studies', 'prospective studies', 'qualitative research', 'health surveys' and other terms such as 'observational research' that are not currently MeSH terms. Look at Chapter 10 for more information about observational studies.

Searching for adverse effects

Generally RCTs only report common side effects of interventions. To report rare and possibly serious adverse effects, the trials would require impractically large numbers of participants. Observational studies such as surveys done after the drug has been released for use may be designed to find adverse effects, as are reports to the Yellow Card scheme by the MHRA. The Adverse Effects Methods Group of the Cochrane Collaboration is developing a search strategy to search for side effects of interventions.

Summary

- The Cochrane Library is a source of systematic reviews as well as reports of clinical trials.
- Use of Boolean operators enables search terms to be combined.
- Each database can be searched with the same terms but these need to be in strategies compatible with their own format.

 Activity

1. List two Boolean operators.
2. Go to the National Library of Health and click on 'guidance'; now list the different types of guideline sites available.
3. List five databases that you could search for primary research.
4. To gain further understanding about how databases are all slightly different, go to the Cochrane Library and download the pdf of the review on basal cell carcinoma listed in the references.
   - Look at the section entitled: 'Search Methods for Identification of Studies'.
   - Type the basic disease terms into the Cochrane Library, MEDLINE and EMBASE. You could even print off the search histories for each database to compare how in each one the terms will look slightly different. This is because each database stores information in a different way.
   - Look at how many records each database generates using the same search terms. You will also see that some records are the same – this is because the databases are taking information from the same sources, usually journals. You will also see that some records are unique to each of these three databases.
   - Look at the date of the last search done in the review on 'Interventions for basal cell carcinoma'.
   - See if there are more RCTs have been published since that date.

Section 2

Useful websites

The Cochrane Library. www.thecochranelibrary.org

The (InterTASC Information Specialists' Sub-Group) (ISSG) at York University, a good source of information about the development of search filters for observational studies. www.york.ac.uk/inst/crd/intertasc/

The Joanna Briggs Institute. www.joannabriggs.edu.au

The National Library for Health. www.library.nhs.uk

The Adverse Effects Methods Group of the Cochrane Collaboration. www.mrw.interscience. wiley.com/cochrane/clabout/articles/CE000150/frame.html

Reusable learning objects

- Literature searching. www.nottingham.ac.uk/nursing/sonet/rlos/studyskills/lit_search/
- Searching for RCTs. www.nottingham.ac.uk/nursing/sonet/rlos/ebp/rctsearch/

Further reading

Bath-Hextall, F.J., Perkins, W., Bong, J. and Williams, H.C. (2007) Interventions for basal cell carcinoma of the skin. *Cochrane Database Syst Rev*, 1, CD003412.

Gibbs, S. and Harvey, I. (2006) Topical treatments for cutaneous warts. *Cochrane Database Syst Rev*, **3**, CD001781.

Higgins, J.P.T. and Green, S. (eds) (2008) *Cochrane Handbook for Systematic Reviews of Interventions* Version 5.0.0, updated February 2008. Cochrane Collaboration. Available from www.cochrane-handbook.org.

10 What are the different types of study design?

Learning outcomes

By the end of this chapter the reader should be able to:

- understand the meaning of quantitative and qualitative research
- understand the difference between primary and secondary research
- understand the different types of studies
- recognise the advantages and disadvantages of different types of study
- understand when to use different types of studies.

Research studies are often referred to as being either quantitative or qualitative in design. These terms refer to different research methodologies. Quantitative studies collect facts and use numbers to describe things whereas qualitative studies are very exploratory and focus on the perceptions and beliefs of individuals. Some research studies use a mixture of quantitative and qualitative methodologies and are referred to as mixed methods studies (see RLO 'Qualitative and Quantitative Research'). This chapter focuses mainly on quantitative research methods.

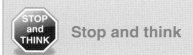 **Stop and think**

Do you know the difference between primary research and secondary research?

The New Prescriber. Edited by J Lymn, D Bowskill, F Bath-Hextall, R Knaggs, © 2010 John Wiley & Sons.

Differences between primary and secondary research

Primary research: studies in which original data are collected to answer a specific research question. Randomised controlled trials, cohort studies, case–control studies and surveys are all examples of primary research studies.

Secondary research: uses information from existing studies, that is, publications, or expert opinion to answer a specific research question. Systematic reviews, meta-analysis (quantitative data), metasynthesis (qualitative or narrative data) and guidelines are types of secondary research studies.

This chapter focuses on primary research designs. Details of secondary research designs are described in Chapter 11.

Randomised controlled trials

What are they and why they are done?

Randomised controlled trials (RCTs) are experimental studies in which an intervention of some kind is evaluated. In many cases the intervention of interest is a new treatment but other interventions such as an initiative to manage patients in a different way or an educational programme to help patients cope with their illness may be assessed.

The most common design is one in which participants are randomly allocated to one of two or more groups. In the simple case where there are two groups, one group receives the intervention and the other group acts as a control. The control group may receive the care they would usually receive, that is, the care they would get if the RCT did not exist, or no active intervention. Both groups are then followed up over time and at the end of this period, specific outcome measures that were identified when the study was designed are recorded. These outcome measures are then compared between the two groups.

 Stop and think

Why is a control group needed?

If there is no control group, it is difficult to know whether any changes that have occurred in the intervention group are due to the intervention received or whether they could have occurred because of other reasons.

In studies where there are more than two groups, two or more interventions are compared to a control group.

Randomised controlled trials are regarded as being the gold standard in study design because they are less prone to bias than other study designs. Further information on bias is given in Chapter 11.

The most common types of randomised controlled trials are described in this section.

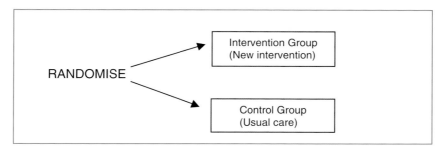

Figure 10.1 Two-group parallel trial.

Parallel group trials

In the previous section, a two-group parallel group trial was described. These trials occur when participants are randomly allocated to one of the two groups (Figure 10.1). These groups are studied concurrently and the outcome measures are compared at the end of the follow-up period. In this design all participants receive only one of the interventions (either the new (experimental) intervention or the control (usual care) intervention). Parallel group trials with more than two groups are less common than the two-group design but the same principle applies – participants are randomly allocated to one of the intervention groups.

Cross-over trials

Cross-over trials differ from parallel group trials because all participants receive both interventions (or all, if there are more than two interventions). In this case, randomisation is used to determine the order in which the interventions are received (Figure 10.2). Half of the participants receive intervention A in the first part (period 1) of the trial and the remaining half receive intervention B. In the second part of the trial (period 2), the participants receive the intervention they did not receive in the first part of the trial. In these trials, participants act as their own control and within-participant differences are compared rather than between participants. This means that they require smaller sample sizes than parallel group trials. Cross-over trials are not as common as parallel trials even though they have the advantage of requiring a smaller sample size. This is because the cross-over design is often not appropriate.

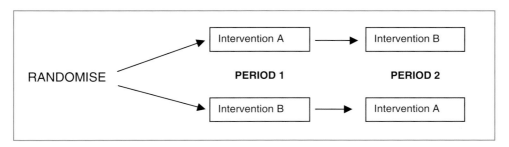

Figure 10.2 Two-period cross-over trial.

Stop and think

Would a cross-over design be an appropriate way to compare the efficacy of surgery and radiotherapy in the treatment of people with basal cell carcinoma?

No, a cross-over design is only appropriate for interventions that do not bring about a permanent effect. A fair comparison of two interventions can only be made if the participant's condition at the beginning of the second period of the study is the same as it was when they entered the first period of the study. Sometimes a 'wash-out' period, during which the participants receive no intervention, is needed to allow the effects of the intervention received in the first period of the study to wear off before the start of the second period. The length of the 'wash-out' period depends on how long it takes for the effect of the intervention received in the first period to disappear. Just remember that interventions that do not have a reversible effect are inappropriate for a cross-over trial.

Stop and think

In what other situations would it be inappropriate to use a cross-over design?

The type of condition being studied and the duration of follow-up period both need to be considered. Participants with progressive disorders are not suitable for inclusion in cross-over trials because their condition is not stable over time. If their condition is deteriorating over time then they will be less well when they enter the second period of the study than when they entered the first period and therefore may not be able to benefit from the intervention as well as they would have done if they had received it in the first period. The duration of follow-up is also important because all patients receive both interventions and if the follow-up period is too long, a considerable number of participants may drop out before the trial is completed.

Cluster randomised controlled trials

In the above two types of trials, participants are randomly allocated to treatment groups (parallel group trials) or treatment sequences (cross-over trials). In some trials participants are nested within some sort of unit, for example hospital wards, general practices, schools. Participants within the same unit are likely to be more similar to each other than to those in another unit. Patients within one general practice, for example are more likely to be similar to each other than to those in another general practice because they are treated by the same clinicians and are managed according to the same policies of the practice. In this situation, it is not appropriate to randomly allocate individual participants to treatment groups but it is better to randomly allocate the units, for example general practices. In this case, all participants within the same unit receive the same intervention. This reduces the risk of contamination which could arise if health professionals administering the treatments are asked to give different treatments to different patients within the same unit. One of the disadvantages of this type of trial, however, is that a larger sample size is required because the greater similarity between patients within the same unit must be allowed for.

Why is randomisation important?

The main reason for randomisation is to reduce bias. If participants have been randomly allocated to treatment groups and differences between the participants in the treatment groups are observed, these differences will have arisen by chance. Other non-randomised methods of allocation such as alternate or systematic allocation can introduce selection bias.

The concealment of treatment allocation is also an important feature of a RCT. Even if patients have been randomly allocated to a treatment group, it is possible that knowledge of the group to which a patient was randomised will create bias. Further details of selection bias and the biases that can be introduced through lack of treatment concealment are given in Chapter 11.

Types of randomisation

Simple randomisation

This is the simplest form of randomisation. Each participant has an equal chance of being allocated to the intervention groups. This method of randomisation is equivalent to tossing a coin and entering people to the active intervention group if the outcome is 'heads' or to the control group if the outcome is 'tails' (Figure 10.3).

A word of caution: simple randomisation may create large differences in treatment group sizes in small studies.

Block randomisation

This is similar to simple randomisation but participants are allocated in blocks so imbalances between treatment groups can be restricted to a certain size. If a block size of six is used in a trial in which there are two intervention groups, this means that within each block, three participants will be allocated to the active intervention group and three to the control group. In some studies the block size is fixed but the disadvantage of this is that it may become possible to predict which intervention group the next participant will be allocated to (even if the treatment allocation is concealed). To overcome this, you can vary the block size so it is much more difficult to predict the group to which the next participant will be allocated.

Stratified randomisation

This method aims to produce intervention groups that are similar with respect to one or more key variables that are known to affect the outcome measure. Separate randomisation lists are prepared (one for each stratum) and block randomisation is used to randomly allocate participants to an intervention group. Sometimes this method is not suitable because not enough is known about which variables influence the outcome. Stratified randomisation is often used in multicentre trials. Remember that the variables to stratify by should be chosen at the design stage of the study and the number of these variables should be kept to a minimum (usually no more than 2–3).

Section 2

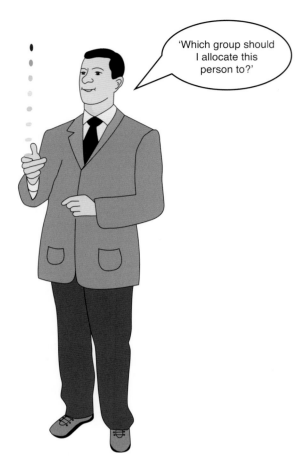

Figure 10.3   Tossing a coin.

Alternative methods of allocation

Minimisation is an example of an alternative method of allocation. Although participants are not randomly allocated to an intervention group, this is still a valid approach to use. It aims to produce intervention groups that are closely balanced for a number of key prognostic factors. Minimisation works well even in small studies but it is complicated to perform.

Box 10.1 gives a summary of some of the advantages and disadvantages of RCTs.

Box 10.1   Advantages and Disadvantages of RCTs

Advantages

- Less prone to bias than other study designs.
- Randomisation tends to balance prognostic factors across study groups.
- Usually easier to blind participants and study personnel than in other study designs.

● Assumptions of statistical tests tend to be met.

Disadvantages

● Can be very expensive in terms of cost and time.
● Participants may not comply or they may withdraw from the study.
● Strict eligibility criteria can lead to limited generalisability of findings.
● May not be ethical to randomise participants to intervention groups, for example if a potentially effective treatment is withheld from some participants or if some participants are exposed to a substance known to be harmful.

Observational studies

Although RCTs are regarded as the gold standard for primary research studies, sometimes it is not possible or appropriate to use such a design. In some cases it may be unethical to randomise participants to certain groups – for example, to randomise participants to an intervention such as smoking that is known to be harmful. Other factors may make a RCT design unfeasible, such as the need for a very large sample size (e.g. for rare conditions) or a long period of follow-up before an effect can be observed,. In these situations it may be more appropriate to use other research designs such as observational studies. Cohort, case–control studies and cross-sectional surveys are all examples of observational studies. We will now look at each of these in turn.

Cohort studies

These are similar to RCTs in that a cohort of participants is followed up over time to see what happens to them but participants are not randomly allocated to an 'intervention group'. Usually the aim is to see if participants develop a certain outcome. At the start of the study, all participants are free of the outcome of interest and they are followed up over time to see whether they develop it (Figure 10.4). No intervention is given to participants. Information on the exposure to one or more prespecified factors is collected over time. At the end of the follow-up period the frequency of the occurrence of the outcome is compared between participants in the exposed and non-exposed groups (control).

This type of study design can be very efficient because the development of more than one outcome can be studied at the same time. The results of cohort studies are presented as relative risks and these are explained in more detail in Chapter 12. The relative risk is the ratio of the incidence of the outcome in the exposed group relative to the non-exposed group.

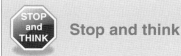 **Stop and think**

What types of outcomes would it be inappropriate to study using a cohort study design?

Section 2

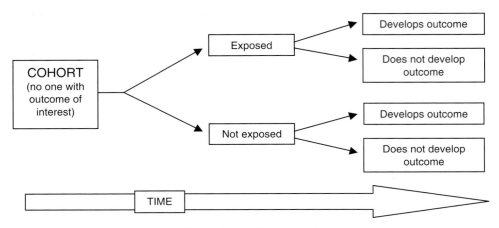

Figure 10.4   Cohort study.

Outcomes which take a long time to develop would need a long period of follow-up. This of course increases the cost of the study and the chance of people being lost to follow-up. Reasons for loss to follow-up include the failure of participants who move away to inform the research team of their new contact details; the participant's decision to withdraw from the study; the participant's death. Losses to follow-up can lead to biased results so it is very important that a real effort is made to keep these to a minimum.

It is also not helpful to use cohort studies when the outcome of interest is rare. This is because a very large cohort of people would need to be studied in order to get enough people with the outcome of interest. This would obviously be very costly and time consuming and it would be more appropriate to use an alternative study design.

Retrospective cohort studies are based on cohorts that were formed in the past and rely on baseline and outcome data that were collected in the past. They have the same sort of benefits as a prospective cohort study but are restricted by the quality of the data recorded since the data were not collected specifically for the current study.

Box 10.2 summarises some of the advantages and disadvantages of cohort studies

---

Box 10.2   Advantages and Disadvantages of Cohort Studies

Advantages

- Several different outcomes can be studied at the same time.
- The incidence of the outcome in the exposed and non-exposed groups can be determined.
- Can establish time sequence of events.
- Easier to administer and cheaper than RCTs.

Disadvantages

- Large sample sizes are required if outcome of interest is rare.
- Can be expensive and time consuming.
- Long periods of follow-up would be needed for outcomes that take a long time to develop.
- Loss of people to follow-up may lead to biased results.

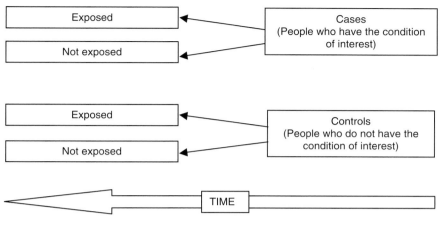

Figure 10.5   Case–control study.

Case–control studies

In case-control studies two groups of participants are identified at the start of the study. One group consists of participants who have a prespecified outcome (cases) and the other group are participants who do not have the outcome (controls). Information on the past exposure to certain factors is collected from both groups and this is then compared between the groups (Figure 10.5).

Case-control studies are more useful than cohort studies when diseases are rare or in situations in which there is a long period of time between exposure and outcome. This is because the status of participants (whether or not they have the outcome of interest) is known at the start of the study and there is no need to wait to see who develops it. This means that case-control studies tend to be of shorter duration and require fewer participants than cohort studies. This also tends to make them less expensive to carry out.

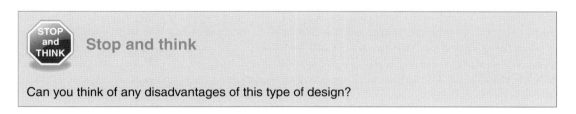

In these studies, participants are asked to look back over time and recount their behaviour and experiences. Data collected in this way are likely to be less accurate than data collected prospectively. This is because it is harder to remember events that occurred in the past than it is to describe current events. It is also possible that participants in the group with the outcome of interest (cases) may recall things differently from those in the control group. This is referred to as recall bias. Further details of recall bias and other biases that arise in case-control studies can be found in Chapter 11.

Other disadvantages of case-control studies include the fact that it is often quite difficult to select an appropriate control group and confounding can be a problem. Chapter 11 explains

---

Box 10.3 Advantages and Disadvantages of Case–Control Studies

Advantages

- Good for studies of rare diseases or for situations in which there is a long period between exposure and outcome.
- Can be carried out more quickly and less expensively than other study designs.
- Often do not require as many participants as cross-sectional designs.
- Loss to follow-up is not a problem.

Disadvantages

- Selection of control group may be difficult.
- Retrospective collection of data may mean data are less accurate.
- May be difficult to interpret the results since confounding could be present.
- Cannot calculate incidence of outcome of interest.

---

this more fully. It is also not possible to estimate the incidence of the outcome of interest in the exposed and non-exposed groups. The results of case–control studies are presented as odds ratios and these are explained in more detail in Chapter 12. The odds ratio is a good approximation to the relative risk when diseases are rare.

Nested case–control studies are case–control studies in which the cases and controls have been drawn from participants who were enrolled in a prospective cohort study. These are not subject to recall bias since data were collected prospectively and selection bias should not be a problem since cases and controls are drawn from the same cohort. Box 10.3 summarises some of the advantages and disadvantages of case–control studies.

Cross-sectional surveys

Cohort and case–control studies are both examples of longitudinal studies. These look for associations between outcomes of interest and events and exposures that have occurred over time. Cross-sectional surveys are studies that look at one point in time and describe what is happening at that time. All measurements (exposures and outcomes) are taken at the same time. These studies can be used to estimate the prevalence of conditions but are not good for determining causality. Box 10.4 summarises some of the advantages and disadvantages of cross-sectional surveys.

Box 10.4 Advantages and Disadvantages of Cross-Sectional Surveys

Advantages

- Usually cheap and quick to conduct.
- Good for providing descriptive information and prevalence estimates.
- Ethically safe.

> **Disadvantages**
>
> ● Can examine associations but cannot establish causality.
> ● Non-response may lead to biased results.
> ● Cannot estimate incidence of conditions.

Which type of design should be used?

There is no simple answer to this question because it very much depends on what your research question is. Sometimes it is clear that there is only one possible design that can be used but in other cases more than one type of design could be considered. Randomised controlled trials are regarded as being the gold standard study design to use in primary research studies but they are not always feasible or appropriate. If more than one study design would be suitable to answer your research question then the design which gives the strongest level of evidence should be used provided it is feasible and is within cost and time restraints. Chapter 11 gives further details of the hierarchy of evidence.

Summary

● Research studies may be quantitative or qualitative in design.
● Primary research uses original data whereas secondary research uses information from existing studies.
● There are lots of different study designs but randomised controlled trials are regarded as being the gold standard in study design.
● Randomised controlled studies are less prone to bias than other study designs.
● Different research questions require different study designs.
● There are advantages and disadvantages for all study designs.

Section 2

> ✎ **Activity**
>
> Look up the following references and decide which type of study design they are.
>
> 1.
>   A. Katz, K.A., Marcil, I. and Stern, R.S. (2002) Incidence and risk factors associated with a second squamous cell carcinoma or basal cell carcinoma in psoralen + ultraviolet a light-treated psoriasis patients. *J Invest Dermatol*, **118**,1038–1043.
>   B. Thissen, M., Nieman, F., Ideler, A., Berretty, P. and Neumann, H. (2000) Cosmetic results of cryosurgery versus surgical excision for primary uncomplicated basal cell carcinomas of the head and neck. *Dermatol Surg*, **26**, 759–764.
>   C. Moffatt, C.J., Franks, P.J., Doherty, D.C., Smithdale, R. and Martin, R. (2006) Sociodemographic factors in chronic leg ulceration. *Br J Dermatol*, **155**, 307–312.
> 2. List three different types of randomisation.

Useful websites

Understanding medical research. www.patientinform.com/understanding-medical-research/

Methodological research issues. www.ingentaconnect.com/content/routledg/psyres/2007/00000017/00000001/art00005;jsessionid=4qae1fc06fqs1.alexandr

Reusable learning objects

● Qualitative and quantitative research.
www.nottingham.ac.uk/nursing/sonet/rlos/ebp/qvq/index.html

Further reading

Altman, D.G. (1991) Designing research, in *Practical Statistics for Medical Research* (ed. D.G. Altman), Chapman and Hall, London.

Bland, J.M. and Kerry, S.M. (1997) Trials randomised in clusters. *BMJ*, **315**, 600.

Grimes, D.A. and Schulz, K.F. (2002) An overview of clinical research: the lay of the land. *Lancet*, **359**, 57-61.

Grimes, D.A. and Schulz, K.F. (2002) Descriptive studies: what they can and cannot do. *Lancet*, **359**, 145-149.

Grimes, D.A. and Schulz, K.F. (2002) Cohort studies: marching towards outcomes. *Lancet*, **359**, 341-345.

Hulley, S.B., Cummings, S.R., Browner, W.S., *et al.* (2006) *Designing Clinical Research*, Lippincott Williams and Wilkins, Philadelphia.

Petrie, A. and Sabin, C. (2000) *Medical Statistics at a Glance*, Blackwell Science, Oxford.

Schulz, K.F. and Grimes, D.A. (2002) Case–control studies: research in reverse. *Lancet*, **359**, 431-434.

Schulz, K.F. and Grimes, D.A. (2002) Generation of allocation sequences in randomised trials: chance, not choice. *Lancet*, **359**, 515-519.

11 Appraising the evidence

Learning outcomes

By the end of this chapter the reader should be able to:

- understand different levels of evidence
- understand the need to critically review research studies
- understand the meaning of bias
- understand the key types of bias for systematic reviews, randomised controlled studies (RCTs) and observational studies
- know where to find critical appraisal tools for different types of studies, reviews and guidelines.

In Chapter 10 we covered different types of study design. In this chapter we see how some studies give better evidence than others and we look at the various levels of hierarchy that have been developed. Table 11.1 gives details of a simple classification of strengths of evidence. You will see from the table that more bias is introduced as we go down the table and therefore we will be less confident that the research findings are a true reflection of what has happened. Although RCTs are considered to be the gold standard study design for primary research, well-conducted systematic reviews of RCTs are regarded as being the type of study that provides the strongest evidence. Other classifications are essentially the same but give greater detail on the hierarchy of non-randomised studies or with regard to different question types, for example therapy or prevention, prognosis, diagnosis, economic and decision analyses. Listed at the end of the chapter are a number of useful websites which have further information on hierarchy of evidence.

Step 3: Appraising the evidence

A word of warning. If you are using guidelines which, let's face it, are a very convenient source of information, just remember that they are *guidelines* and you should treat them very

Table 11.1 Classification of strengths of evidence (taken from Bandolier, 1995; 12,1).

Type	Strength of evidence	
I	Strong evidence from at least one systematic review of multiple well-designed RCTs.	INCREASING BIAS
II	Strong evidence from at least one well-designed RCT of appropriate size.	
III	Evidence from well-designed trials without randomisation, single group pre/post, cohort, time series or matched case–control studies.	
IV	Evidence from well-designed non-experimental studies from more than one centre or research group.	
V	Opinions of respected authorities, based on clinical evidence, descriptive studies or reports of expert committees.	

much like any other source of evidence. This means that you should appraise them in just the same way as any other evidence. Appraisal of guidelines is not covered in the section but the Evidence-based Medicine Toolkit covers appraisal of guidelines in detail. Also look at AGREE, which is an international collaboration of researchers and policy makers who are looking to improve the quality and effectiveness of clinical practice guidelines. AGREE have developed an appraisal instrument to assess the quality of clinical guidelines and the link to their website is given at the end of this chapter.

The need to critically review research studies

In the previous chapter we saw that evidence can come from many different types of studies. Unfortunately, not all studies are done well and therefore we need a way to appraise them. So whatever the evidence, you will need to decide if you can trust the results and then if you can, decide what they mean and whether they are relevant to your practice. Have a look at the RLO 'Why critique research?'.

Systematic reviews

A systematic review is a secondary source of evidence because it evaluates and summarises the relevant primary sources (RCTs and other research). If you cannot remember the difference between primary and secondary research, refer back to Chapter 10.

The key thing about systematic reviews is that they should be conducted according to an explicit methodology and should be reproducible.

Is a systematic review the same as a literature review?
The first thing to clarify is the difference between a literature review and a systematic review.

 Stop and think

Do you know the difference between a systematic review and a literature review?

Table 11.2 Differences between literature reviews and systematic reviews.

	Literature review	Systematic review (conducted according to an explicit methodology and reproducible)
Framing the question	Often a broad question	Well-structured question
Identifying relevant literature	Not usually specified, often not reproducible	Clear and reproducible search strategy
Assessing the quality of the literature	Variable	Rigorous critical appraisal
Summarising the evidence	Often a qualitative summary	May be qualitative or quantitative depending on the question[a]
Interpreting and exploring clinical relevance of findings	May be biased	Usually evidence based

[a]Quantitative summary that includes a statistical synthesis is a meta- analysis or metasynthesis in the case of qualitative systematic reviews.

Table 11.2 summarises the main differences. Take care – literature reviews of healthcare interventions rarely use methods designed to reduce the risk of bias. The fact that literature reviews are often written by experts in the field just compounds the risk of bias.

Why do we need systematic reviews?

All of us are inundated with unmanageable amounts of information on healthcare. One of the main aids for practitioners, researchers and policy makers is the systematic review which is regarded as the highest level of evidence for medical decision making. Systematic reviews can support individual patient decisions, help in the preparation of guidelines and treatment protocols and in the development and planning of new trials.

But please be careful: systematic reviews of low methodological quality or those which are out of date can be misleading.

Different kinds of systematic reviews

Quantitative systematic reviews

These reviews use a characteristic set of methods for analysing data, called meta-analysis. However, it may not always be possible to conduct a meta-analysis (Chapter 12), especially if the studies identified have different protocols or are of very different design.

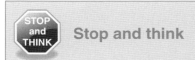 **Stop and think**

Where can you find systematic reviews?

Section 2

The best place to find systematic reviews is the Cochrane Library. Remember, we covered this in Chapter 9.

Qualitative systematic reviews

These reviews involve interview, focus groups, ethnographic data and phenomenological data and are not covered in this book. If you would like to look at some qualitative systematic reviews then visit the Joanna Briggs Institute (JBI); the website is given at the end of this chapter.

So how can you judge if a systematic review is of good methodological quality?

Well, if you go to the (Critical Appraisal Skills Programme) (CASP) website, click on appraisal tools and then click on systematic reviews, you will find 10 questions to help you make sense of systematic reviews. You can also look at the QUOROM (**Qu**ality **O**f **R**eporting **O**f **M**eta-analyses) guidelines. First published in 1999, these provide guidance to ensure the proper reporting of systematic reviews. Just remember to check that the reviewers have critically appraised the individual studies included in the review.

Quality assessment of studies

A few terms that you will have to get to grips with are as follows.

Validity

The validity of an individual study is the extent to which its design and conduct (how it is carried out) are likely to prevent systematic errors or bias (Moher *et al.*, 1995). Studies designed to avoid bias (defined further on) should be more likely to give results that are closer to the truth. Studies with varying degrees of validity can produce 'false-positive' results if the less thorough studies are biased towards overestimating treatment effectiveness. Studies with varying degrees of validity can also produce 'false-negative' results if less thorough studies are biased towards underestimating an intervention's effect (Detsky *et al.*, 1992).

Precision

A common mistake is to confuse validity with precision. Precision is a measure of the likelihood of chance effects leading to random errors. It is reflected in the confidence interval (CI) around the estimate of effect from each study and the weight given to the results of each study when an overall estimate of effect or weighted average is derived. We will look at this in more detail in Chapter 12. For now, you just have to be aware not to confuse it with validity.

Before we go any further, we need to look at the definition of 'bias'.

Definition of bias

Any process at any stage of inference tending to produce results that differ systematically from the true values.

Murphy, 1976

Just remember that biases can lead to an underestimation or overestimation of the true intervention effect. Biases can vary in magnitude: some can be small and insignificant compared with the observed effect whilst others can be much larger, so much so that an apparent finding may be entirely due to bias.

Cast your mind back to Chapter 10, in which we talked about randomised controlled trials (RCTs) as being the 'gold standard' in study design because they are less prone to bias than other study designs. Remember, this is only true if they are done properly!

Randomised controlled trials (RCTs)

The four key bias types that may impact on the internal validity of a study are selection bias, performance bias, detection bias and attrition bias. We shall look at each of these in turn.

Selection bias

Selection bias is about researchers consciously allocating participants to a particular group. One of the most important factors that may lead to bias and distort treatment comparisons is that which can result from the way in which comparison groups are assembled (Kunz and Ixman, 1998). What we are trying to do when we conduct a randomised controlled study is to achieve an equal distribution of known and unknown confounders (prognostic factors) between the two groups. If there are imbalances of these confounders between the groups, it becomes very difficult for differences in outcome to be confidently attributed to the intervention. It is therefore very important to ensure that randomisation is done appropriately.

Randomisation consists of two parts. The first part is the generation of the randomisation sequence and the second part is concealment of allocation. Generating the randomisation sequence is about ensuring that the allocation of patients to the groups is independent of the characteristics of the patient, so all patients have the same chance of being assigned to either group. Concealment of allocation is about ensuring that neither the trial subjects nor the investigators are able to influence the group into which each person is put. Clearly, selecting patients alternatively from a list or by the day of the week is not going to ensure allocation concealment; we sometimes call this quasi-randomisation. A really good way of generating allocation sequences and ensuring concealment of allocation is to use telephone or internet randomisation.

 Stop and think

When you last read a RCT paper, did it clearly state how the randomisation process was done?

Performance bias

Performance bias is about differences in care received by the participants in the comparison groups other than the intervention under investigation. Some studies have shown that if you unintentionally give the intervention to the control group or even if you give unintended additional care to either comparison group then this can affect the study results (CCSG, 1978; Sackett, 1979). One way of getting around this is to 'blind' those people receiving and giving the care – in this way you can protect against unintended differences in care and placebo

Section 2

effects. Remember that blinding is not always possible and will very much depend on what is being studied. However, where possible, every effort should be made to achieve blinding.

Detection bias

Detection bias arises when there are differences in how outcomes of the intervention are assessed for each of the participant groups. For example, if as an outcome assessor you are unaware of which group the participants are in, you are more likely to treat each group the same. Blinding the outcome assessor is one way to ensure that you treat each group in the same way. Blinding is particularly important in studies with subjective outcome measures such as pain (Schulz *et al.*, 1995).

Attrition bias

Attrition bias relates to the differences in terms of losses of subjects between groups. If a number of patients cannot be included in the analysis then that number should be reported together with the reasons why those patients were not included. All randomised patients should be included in the analysis and they should be kept in the original group to which they were assigned even if they did not fully comply with the intervention, changed over to the other group during the study or dropped out of the study before its completion. The analysis should be done according to the (intention-to-treat) principle (ITT) which requires data for all patients. Remember, the study should always tell you how many people dropped out of the study and for what reason.

If you look in the Cochrane Handbook you will find a more in-depth explanation of the above four key biases (Higgins and Green, 2008). You might also find it helpful to look at the CONSORT statement (link provided under Useful Websites) which was developed to increase the quality of trials and their reporting. The CONSORT statement has a checklist of items that should be recorded when reporting randomised controlled trials.

Other types of bias

Watch out for other types of bias: carry-over in cross-over trials and recruitment bias in cluster randomised trials.

 Stop and think

Find a RCT that you are familiar with and then go to the CONSORT checklist using the web link provided at the end of this chapter and look at the quality of your RCT. Was it of good methodological quality?

Sources of bias in studies of diagnostic accuracy

Just like randomised controlled studies, diagnostic test studies should be appraised. They have a number of unique features in terms of design and therefore the criteria to assess the quality of these studies differ from studies of therapeutic interventions. You might find the QUADAS tool useful when assessing studies of diagnostic accuracy. The QUADAS tool is an evidence-based quality assessment tool for use in systematic reviews of diagnostic accuracy studies. Another checklist that might be helpful is the STARD statement (STAndards for the Reporting of Diagnostic accuracy studies) which hopes to improve the accuracy and completeness of reporting of studies of diagnostic accuracy.

Sources of bias in observational studies

Observational studies are prone to a variety of biases and it is important to assess the potential for bias when appraising these studies. In the past this has been difficult because many observational studies have not been reported very well. Checklists for appraising observational studies can be found at the CASP website. You can also look at recent guidelines on how to report observational studies (STROBE statement).

Many biases can occur in observational studies and details of the key types of bias are given below.

Selection bias

Selection bias occurs when there are differences between the groups of participants being compared. In case–control studies, the cases and controls should be as similar as possible with the exception of the disease of interest (Grimes and Schulz, 2002). Selection bias can occur if the cases are not representative of the defined population or if the controls are not representative of the population from which the cases were selected (Bailey, Vardulaki and Chandramohan, 2005).

 Stop and think

How would you choose a control group?

Selecting an appropriate control group is often quite difficult in case–control studies. Ideally, controls should be selected from the same source as the cases but this needs to be done with care to prevent a biased sample. Hospital, community or neighbourhood controls may be selected. Table 11.3 summarises some of the advantages and disadvantages of each type of control group. You might find it helpful to look at a couple of articles (Schulz and Grimes, 2002; Grimes and Schulz, 2005) for further information on the selection of controls for case–control studies. In cohort studies the exposed and unexposed groups should be as similar as possible with the exception of the exposure of interest (Grimes and Schulz, 2002). If exposure data are collected prospectively, that is, as the cohort of individuals is followed up, selection bias should not usually be a problem. However, if exposed and unexposed groups are identified at the beginning of the study, as is the case when occupational cohorts are studied, it is possible that these two groups will differ on factors other than the exposure of interest.

Section 2

Table 11.3 Advantages and disadvantages of different types of control groups.

	Advantages	Disadvantages
Hospital	Convenient	Results will be biased if controls are diagnosed with a condition that is related to the exposures of interest
Community	If randomly sampled controls should be representative of people at risk of developing the disease	May be less motivated to take part in a study (could be *non-response bias*)
Neighbourhood	Cases and controls should be from similar social backgrounds	Expensive and uses homes rather than people as a sampling unit

As described by Grimes and Schulz (2005) and Petrie and Sabin (2000).

 Stop and think

Would it make sense to use the general population as a control (unexposed) group if the exposed group were from an occupational group?

If an occupational group is compared to the general population then the results are likely to be biased because these groups differ according to their health status as well as to their exposure. The exposed group will tend to be healthier than the general population because it includes individuals who are fit enough to work whereas the general population includes those who are well enough to work and those who are not. This is known as the healthy worker effect. In these types of studies it is preferable to select an alternative control group such as a group of individuals who work for another company but who are not exposed to the exposure of interest.

Information bias

This type of bias arises when data on the outcome and/or exposure are collected, measured or classified differently in the groups being compared. It may also be referred to as measurement, classification or observation bias (Grimes and Schulz, 2002). There are several different ways in which biases can occur. Here are some of the most common ones.

● **Interviewer bias**

This happens when interviewers do not interview individuals in the groups being compared (cases and controls in case–control studies or exposed and unexposed groups in cohort studies) in the same way. If the interviewer is aware of the study hypothesis and knows the person is a case or a control, for example, they may either phrase questions differently or probe more deeply when interviewing cases. This type of bias can be reduced if the interviewer is unaware of the study hypothesis. The same structured interview schedule should be used to collect data from all participants.

- **Misclassification bias**

  This occurs if participants are incorrectly classified according to exposure (cohort studies) or disease status (case–control studies). If misclassification is more likely to occur in one group than the other then the results could be biased in either direction. If, however, misclassification is equally likely to occur in both groups then the results will be biased towards finding no association and real differences could be missed (Kahn and Sempos, 1989).

- **Surveillance bias**

  This type of bias can occur when participants in the groups being compared are not managed in the same way. If, for example, participants in the exposed group of a cohort study are followed up or undergo investigative procedures more often than those in the non-exposed group then the outcome of interest is more likely to be detected than in the non-exposed group. This may also be referred to as *ascertainment* or *detection* bias. This type of bias can be prevented if all participants are managed in the same way and assessors are unaware of the group to which each participant belongs.

- **Recall bias**

  This is a problem in case–control studies since participants are asked to recall events in the past. Cases may spend more time thinking about their behaviour in the past and whether this could have been linked to their diagnosis. This may lead to cases being able to report their past exposures more accurately and controls under-reporting their exposure. This type of bias can be reduced if study participants are unaware of the study hypothesis and if data from other sources such as routinely collected medical records are also collected.

- **Loss to follow-up bias**

  Cohort studies are prone to this type of bias since individuals are followed up over time. Losses to follow-up can occur when participants move away, die or no longer wish to take part in the study. Participants who are lost to follow-up may be different from those who continue in the study so it is important to keep these losses to a minimum. It is also possible that the reason for the loss to follow-up is related to the outcome of interest or the exposure variables and that loss to follow-up is greater in one group, for example the exposed group, than the other. Every effort to maintain contact with members of the cohort should therefore be made.

Confounding

The presence of confounding should also be considered when appraising studies. This occurs when the association between an outcome and an exposure variable is distorted by a third variable. Age, for example, could be a confounder in studies of myocardial infarction (MI) and oral contraceptive (OC) use. This is because the risk of having a MI and the use of OCs are both associated with age; that is, the risk of MI increases and the use of OCs decreases with increasing age. If the age distribution of women in the two groups being compared, for example cases and controls, is different, confounding will occur. For a factor to be classed as a confounder, it has to be associated with the outcome of interest and also the exposure of interest. Confounders can be controlled for at both the design and analysis stages of a study.

Stop and think

Find an observational study relating to your practice area that you have already read and then download the appropriate appraisal tool from the CASP website and appraise the study. Was the quality of the study as good as you thought the first time you read it?

There is a variety of appraisal tools available and these are listed at the end of the chapter. JBI critical appraisal tools are included in the MAStARI program and can be completed electronically for RCTs, case–control/cohort studies and descriptive/case series studies.

Critical appraisal of qualitative studies

The critical appraisal of quantitative studies has been established for quite some time but the development of tools to appraise qualitative studies is more recent. Although there is a recognised need for determining the quality of qualitative research papers, there has been much debate on how this should be done. Various tools for appraising qualitative studies have been proposed but these are varied and as yet there is no consensus on the items that should be included in a checklist (Greenhalgh and Taylor, 1997).

Summary

- A systematic review is not the same as a literature review.
- A systematic review can be qualitative or quantitative.
- A well-conducted systematic review of RCTs is regarded as the type of study that provides the strongest evidence.
- Biases can lead to underestimation or overestimation of the true intervention effect.
- There is a need to critically appraise all research studies.
- Critical appraisal tools are available to help with appraising many different study designs.

Activity

1. From the following list, identify adequate methods of sequence generation
      Computer-generated random numbers
      According to patient's date of birth
      Table of random numbers
      Tossing a coin
      Alternate patients

2. Which of the following methods below aim to prevent foreknowledge of allocation; that is, clear concealment of allocation sequence?
   The use of sealed envelopes
   The use of sealed opaque envelopes
   Central randomisation (i.e. away from the trial location)

Useful websites

Hierarchy of evidence including hierarchy of non-randomised studies. www.bmj.com/cgi/content/full/315/7102/243

CONSORT statement. www.consort-statement.org/consort-statement/

Hierarchy of evidence in ScHARR's guide to systematic reviews including details of the hierarchy of non-randomised studies, expert opinion and anecdotal evidence. www.shef.ac.uk/scharr/ir/units/systrev/hierarchy.htm

The (Joanna Briggs Institute) (JBI) gives details of the hierarchy of evidence it applies to conclusions drawn in JBI systematic reviews. www.joannabriggs.edu.au/pubs/approach.php

Oxford's (Centre for Evidence-Based Medicine) (CEBM) for hierarchy of evidence for different question types, for example therapy or prevention, prognosis, diagnosis, economic and decision analyses. www.cebm.net/index.aspx?o=1025

The (Critical Appraisal Skills Programme) (CASP) website. www.phru.nhs.uk/Pages/PHD/resources.htm

The CASP checklist for appraising qualitative studies. www.phru.nhs.uk/Doc_Links/Qualitative%20Appraisal%20Tool.pdf

QUOROM (**Qu**ality **Of R**eporting **Of M**eta-analyses) guidelines. These guidelines, first published in 1999, provide guidance to ensure the proper reporting of systematic reviews. www.greenjournal.org/misc/quorom.pdf

The STARD checklist. www.stard-statement.org/

Guidelines on how to report observational studies (STROBE statement). www.strobe-statement.org/

Greenhalgh's article on the interpretation of qualitative research papers. www.bmj.com/cgi/content/full/315/7110/740

Dixon-Wood's article on the problem of appraising qualitative research with suggested checklist. www.qshc.bmj.com/cgi/reprint/13/3/223

Joanna Briggs Institute for details of Qualitative Assessment and Review Instrument (JBI-QARI) designed to facilitate critical appraisal, data extraction and meta-aggregation of the findings of qualitative studies. www.joannabriggs.edu.au/services/sumari.php

Section 2

Appraisal of guidelines for research and evaluation. www.agreecollaboration.org/pdf/agreeinstrumentfinal.pdf

The development of QUADAS: a tool for the quality assessment of studies of diagnostic accuracy included in systematic reviews. www.biomedcentral.com/1471-2288/3/25

Reusable learning object

● Why critique research?
  www.nottingham.ac.uk/nmp/sonet/rlos/ebp/research_critique/index.html

References

Bailey, L., Vardulaki, K. and Chandramohan, D. (2005) *Introduction to Epidemiology*, Open University Press, Berkshire.

Bandolier (1995) 12, 1. www.medicine.ox.ac.uk/bandolier/band12/b12-1.html.

Canadian Cooperative Study Group (CCSG) (1978) The Canadian trial of aspirin and sulfinpyrazone in threatened stroke. *N Engl J Med*, **299**, 53–59.

Detsky, A.S., Naylor, C.D., O'Rourke, K., *et al.* (1992) Incorporating variations in the quality of individual randomized trials into meta-analysis. *J Clin Epidemiol*, **45**, 255–265.

Greenhalgh, T. and Taylor, R. (1997) How to read a paper: papers that go beyond numbers (qualitative research). *BMJ*, **315**, 740–743.

Grimes, D.A. and Schulz, K.F. (2002) Bias and causal associations in observational research. *Lancet*, **359**, 248–252.

Grimes, D.A. and Schulz, K.F. (2005) Compared to what? Finding controls for case–control studies. *Lancet*, **365**, 1429–1433.

Higgins, J.P.T. and Green, S. (eds) (2008) *Cochrane Handbook for Systematic Reviews of Interventions*. Version 5.0.1 [updated September 2008]. The Cochrane Collaboration. Available from www.cochrane-handbook.org.

Kahn, H.A. and Sempos, C.T. (1989) *Statistical Methods in Epidemiology*, Oxford University Press, New York.

Kunz, R. and Ixman, D. (1998) The unpredictability paradox: review of empirical comparisons of randomised and non-randomised clinical trials. *BMJ*, **317**, 1185–1190.

Moher, D., Jadad, A.R., Nichol, G., *et al.* (1995) Assessing the quality of randomised controlled trials: an annotated bibliography of scales and checklists. *Controlled Clin Trials*, **16**(1), 62–73.

Section 2

Murphy, E.A. (1976) *The Logic of Medicine*, Johns Hopkins University Press, Baltimore.

Petrie, A. and Sabin, C. (2000) *Medical Statistics at a Glance*, Blackwell Science, Oxford.

Sackett, D.L. (1979) Bias in analytic research. *J Chron Dis*, **32**(1-2), 51–63.

Schulz, K.F. and Grimes, D.A. (2002) Case-control studies: research in reverse. *Lancet*, **359**, 431–434.

Schulz, K.F., Chalmers, I., Hayes, R.J. and Altman, D.G. (1995) Empirical evidence of bias. Dimensions of methodological quality associated with estimates of treatment effects in controlled trials. *JAMA*, **273**, 408–412.

Further reading

Cook, D.J., Mulrow, C.D. and Haynes, R.B. (1997) Systematic reviews: synthesis of best evidence for clinical decisions. *Ann Intern Med*, **126**(5), 376–380.

Moher, D., Schulz, K.F. and Altman, D.G. (2001) The CONSORT statement: revised recommendations for improving the quality of reports of parallel-group randomised trials. *Lancet*, **357**(9263), 1191–1194.

Moher, D., Tetzlaff, J., Tricco, A.C., *et al.* (2007) Epidemiology and reporting characteristics of systematic reviews. *PLoS Med*, **4**(3), e78.

Pearson, A. (1998) Excellence in care: future dimensions for effective nursing. *NT Res*, **3**(1), 25–27.

Section 2

12 How do we interpret the evidence?

Learning outcomes

By the end of this chapter the reader should be able to:

- identify the two main types of data and give examples of each type
- define the four main measures of effect: odds ratio, relative risk, mean difference, numbers needed to treat/harm, and understand how to interpret them
- understand and interpret p values and confidence intervals
- describe what a meta-analysis is and understand how to interpret the results from a meta-analysis
- understand publication bias and interpret a funnel plot.

Evidence-based practice not only requires clinical expertise to determine which is the best course of action to take to treat a patient, but also requires being able to interpret the results of scientific studies and communicate the risks and benefits of each course of action to patients. Before we start to think about how we interpret the results of a study, we first need to think about the types of data that can be used.

How do we make sense of the results from scientific studies?

When we perform a scientific study, such as a randomised controlled trial, we collect observations on many different patients, such as their age, gender and previous history of diseases, using questionnaires, interviews or medical records. The individual observations are termed 'data' and we group these data together to form 'variables'. There are two main divisions of the type of data we can collect: these are termed 'categorical' and 'numerical' data. Categorical data relate to data where we want to know 'what type?' and numerical data relate to data where we want to know 'how much?'.

The New Prescriber. Edited by J Lymn, D Bowskill, F Bath-Hextall, R Knaggs, © 2010 John Wiley & Sons.

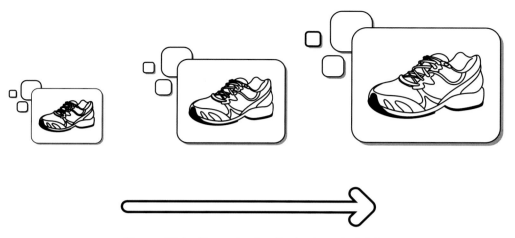

Figure 12.1   Example of ordinal categorical data.

Categorical data

Categorical data are any observations that can be grouped into distinct categories. For example, smoking status is a categorical variable as there are three distinct groups: the patient is a current smoker, an ex-smoker or they never smoked.

There are three subtypes of categorical data. termed 'binary', 'ordinal' and 'nominal'. Binary data can only take two distinct groups; for example, gender is binary as it can only be grouped as male or female.

Ordinal and nominal data have three or more distinct groups. Ordinal data have a natural order to their groupings, for example shoe size. There are many different shoe sizes, and as you go across the categories from size 3 to size 12, the shoe size also increases (Figure 12.1).

Nominal data have no natural order to their groupings, for example, method of drug administration. There are three main methods for administering drugs – intravenous, oral and transdermal – but there is no natural order to them (Figure 12.2).

Many patients are usually recruited into a scientific study so we end up with many individual observations for each variable. To make sense of the data, we present it in more manageable forms using either visual presentations, such as tallies, bar charts and graphs, or percentages or risks.

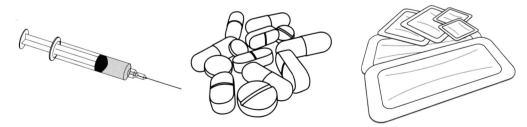

Figure 12.2   Example of nominal categorical data.

Section 2

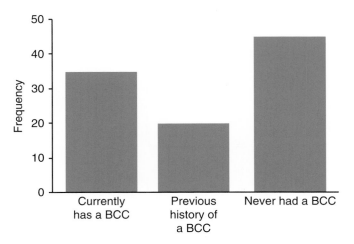

Figure 12.3   Example of a bar chart.

Figure 12.3 shows a visual presentation of BCC status from an observational study of 100 individuals at high risk of a basal cell carcinoma (BCC). We can see from this bar chart that 35 individuals currently have a BCC.

We can also present this as a percentage (or risk), where the risk is the probability that the event will happen. This is easily calculated by dividing the number of times the event occurs by the total number of people in the study. For example, the risk of having a BCC in the above example is:

$$35/100 = 0.35$$
$$= 35\%$$

Numerical data

Numerical data are any observations that can take a defined range of values. Numerical data are also called continuous data. Weight is numerical data as it can take integer and decimal values, for example 65.2 kg, and ranges from zero to infinity. Other examples include height, blood pressure or the number of GP visits in a year.

If numerical data are collected on numerous patients, we can make sense of these data by summarising them as a measure of location (for example, using a mean) and a measure of spread (for example, using a standard deviation) or using visual representations such as a histogram (Figure 12.4).

The data represented in Figure 12.4 are taken from a survey of 86 patients who had their temperatures taken on admission to hospital. From the figure we can see that the mean is 36.492°C, and the standard deviation is 0.604°C. Remember, you can distinguish between a bar chart and a histogram by seeing whether there are any gaps between the bars. A histogram should have no gaps as the numerical variable can take a defined range of values, whereas a bar chart can only take certain values which will be represented as distinct bars.

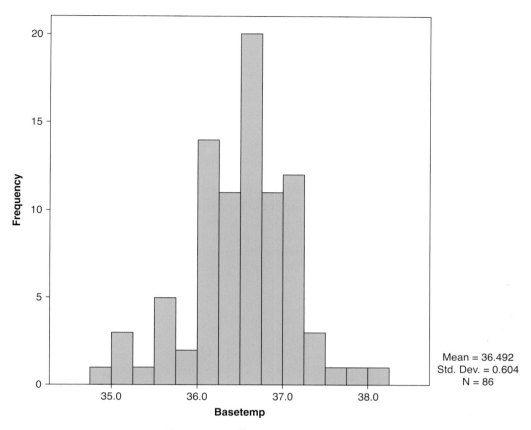

Mean = 36.492
Std. Dev. = 0.604
N = 86

Figure 12.4   Example of a histogram.

Other types of data

Categorical and numerical data are the most common types of data; however, other types of data exist, which include time-to-event (or survival) data. Time-to-event data are used when we are interested in the time taken for a binary outcome to occur, for example the time it takes for a disease to occur. This type of data is commonly used in cancer research. For example, a researcher could be interested in determining how long it takes for a skin cancer to appear once patients have stopped using a preventive treatment.

Measures of effect

When a scientific study is conducted, the researchers are usually interested in whether one treatment is better than another or a control treatment. This is usually achieved by splitting the patients recruited into two groups and exposing one of the groups to the new treatment (exposed group) and the other group to the conventional, control treatment or a placebo (un-exposed group). Researchers use measures of effect to describe how effective the treatments (or interventions) are as compared to each other in ways which can help people understand the relative benefit or harm. The type of measure of effect depends on the type of data that has been collected.

Odds ratio

The most commonly used measure of effect for categorical data is called the odds ratio which lets us describe the likely harm that a treatment or intervention might have caused. Before we can calculate the odds ratio, we need to determine what the term 'odds' means. The odds tell us how likely it is that the event will happen as compared to how likely it is that the event won't happen. The term is commonly used in gambling where, for example, the odds of a horse winning a race is 5 to 1. The odds of an event occurring is a more complicated term to understand compared to the term 'risk', and so usually isn't directly quoted to the general public; however, it is a very useful term for describing the likely harm or benefit a treatment will produce.

The odds is calculated by dividing the number of times an event happens by the number of times the event doesn't happen for each treatment group. For example, if one in every 25 patients suffers a side effect when taking the new treatment A (exposed group), then the odds of having a side effect is:

$$\frac{1}{(25-1)} = 0.04$$

For treatment B (unexposed group), if one in every 50 patients suffers a side effect when taking conventional treatment B, then the odds of having a side effect is:

$$\frac{1}{(50-1)} = 0.02$$

Once we have calculated the odds in each treatment group, we can then determine the odds ratio. The odds ratio is calculated by dividing the odds of the event in the new treatment group A by the odds of the event in the treatment B group:

$$\frac{0.04}{0.02} = 2$$

Therefore the odds ratio is 2. This means that patients in new treatment group A are twice (or 100%) as likely to have a side effect as patients on treatment B.

Here is another example. If a placebo-controlled trial found that four of 50 patients taking the new drug X died then the odds of dying in the exposed group is:

$$\frac{4}{(50-4)} = 0.087$$

Also, if six of the 50 patients on the placebo died then the odds of dying in the unexposed group is:

$$\frac{6}{(50-6)} = 0.136$$

Then the odds ratio would be calculated as:

$$\frac{0.087}{0.136} = 0.640$$

Therefore the odds ratio is 0.64. Since the odds ratio is less than one, this means that patients in the exposed group are less likely to die than patients on the placebo. This can be interpreted as the patients on drug X being 0.64 times as likely to die as the patients receiving placebo. However, this is not very intuitive so instead, researchers usually calculate by how much less likely they are to die by subtracting the odds ratio from 1.

$$1 - 0.640 = 0.360$$

This means that the patients on drug X are 36% less likely to die than the patients on the placebo. Remember, if the odds ratio is greater than 1 then the patients in the exposed (new treatment) group are more likely to have the event than the patients in the unexposed group. If the odds ratio is less than 1 then the patients in the exposed group are less likely to have the event than the patients in the unexposed group. An odds ratio of 1 means that there is no difference in the likelihood of the event in the two groups.

Relative risk

An easier measure of effect to understand is the relative risk (RR), also called the risk ratio. The relative risk tells us the likely harm or benefit a treatment might have caused. It can be estimated by dividing the risk of the event in the new treatment group (exposed group) by the risk of the event in the conventional or control group (unexposed group).

Using the side effect example above, if one in every 25 patients suffers a side effect when taking the new treatment A (exposed group), then the risk of having a side effect is:

$$\frac{1}{25} = 0.04$$

If one in every 50 patients suffers a side effect when taking treatment B, then the risk of having a side effect is:

$$\frac{1}{50} = 0.02$$

The relative risk is calculated by dividing the risk of the event in the new treatment group A by the risk of the event in the treatment B.

$$\frac{0.04}{0.02} = 2$$

Therefore the relative risk is 2. This means that patients in new treatment group A are twice (or 100%) as likely to have a side effect compared to patients on treatment B.

Using the second example from above, the risk of dying in the exposed drug X group is:

$$\frac{4}{50} = 0.08$$

The risk of dying in the placebo group is:

$$\frac{6}{50} = 0.12$$

The relative risk can thus be calculated as:

$$\frac{0.08}{0.12} = 0.667$$

Therefore, patients on drug X are 0.667 times as likely to die compared to patients receiving placebo. Since the relative risk is less than 1, we can calculate by how much less likely they are to die by subtract the relative risk from 1:

$$1 - 0.667 = 0.333$$

This means that the patients on drug X are 33% less likely to die than the patients on the placebo.

Remember, if the relative risk is greater than 1 then the patients in the exposed (new treatment) group have a greater risk of having the event than the patients in the unexposed group. If the relative risk is less than 1 then the patients in the exposed group are at a lower risk of having the event than the patients in the unexposed group. A relative risk of 1 means that there is no difference in the risk of the event in the two groups.

The relative risk and odds ratio will give the same result when there are few events in the exposed and unexposed groups. However, if the event is not rare (greater than 5–10%) then they will give very different values.

Risk reduction and number needed to treat

Although these measures of effect are only quoted in approximately 5% of scientific papers (Harris and Taylor, 2005), they are very easy to understand and are commonly used in clinical practice to answer the question 'How often does a treatment work?'. The risk reduction and number needed to treat are directly related to each other, since the number needed to treat is calculated using the risk reduction.

The risk reduction tells us the difference in the event rate between the two treatment groups. If a placebo-controlled trial found that one patient out of 50 had an adverse event on drug F and two patients out of 50 had an adverse event on placebo, then the risk of having an adverse event on drug F is:

$$\frac{1}{50} = 0.02 \qquad \text{(or 2\%)}$$

The risk of having a side effect when taking the placebo is:

$$\frac{2}{50} = 0.04 \quad (\text{or } 4\%)$$

The risk reduction is calculated by subtracting the risk of the event in the exposed group (drug F group) from the risk of the event in the unexposed group (placebo group).

$$0.04 - 0.02 = 0.02 \quad (\text{or } 4\% - 2\% = 2\%)$$

Therefore there is a 2% difference in the risk of having an adverse event between the two groups.

We can then use this value to calculate the number needed to treat (NNT) (Laupacis et al., 1988). The NNT tells you how many patients would need to be treated with the new treatment in order to prevent the event (bad outcome) occurring in one patient.

$$\text{NNT} = \frac{1}{0.02} = 50$$

Therefore 50 patients would need to be treated with drug F to prevent one patient having an adverse event.

Number needed to harm

The number needed to harm (NNH) is the converse of the NNT, and is used to assess how many patients need to be exposed to the treatment to cause harm to one patient who wouldn't have been harmed otherwise.

Suppose a trial finds that 14 out of 100 patients on drug G and only nine out of 100 patients on drug H have a recurrent skin cancer, then the risk of having a recurrent skin cancer on drug G is:

$$\frac{14}{100} = 0.14 \quad (\text{or } 14\%)$$

For drug H the risk of having a recurrent skin cancer is:

$$\frac{9}{100} = 0.09 \quad (\text{or } 9\%)$$

The risk reduction is calculated by subtracting the risk of the event in the treatment H group from the risk of the event in the treatment G group.

$$0.14 - 0.09 = 0.05 \quad (\text{or } 14\% - 9\% = 5\%)$$

Therefore there is a 5% difference in the risk of having a recurrent skin cancer between the two groups. We can then use this value to calculate the NNH.

$$\text{NNH} = \frac{1}{0.05} = 20$$

Section 2

This means that if 20 patients are exposed to treatment G, then one patient will be harmed by having a recurrent skin cancer that wouldn't have occurred if they were on treatment H.

Mean difference

The most commonly used measure of effect for numerical data is the mean difference (MD), calculated by subtracting means of the data in the two treatment groups. For example, the serum iron levels of patients on treatments Y and Z were measured in a trial to see if they differed.

- The mean serum iron level in the treatment Y group was 107 μg/dl.
- The mean serum iron level in the treatment Z group was 100 μg/dl.

Therefore the mean difference was:

$$107 - 100 = 7 \ \mu g/dl.$$

The value for the mean difference is positive; therefore we know that the patients on treatment Y (exposed group) have higher levels than the patients on treatment Z (non-exposed group). If the value was negative, then this would mean that the treatment Z group had higher levels than the treatment Y group.

A mean difference of 0 means there is no difference in the means of the variable between the two treatment groups. A positive value means the exposed group have a higher value. A negative value means the unexposed group have a higher value.

Statistical inference and *p* values

When researchers conduct scientific studies they identify a small group of individuals called a 'sample' and then relate those findings back to the population using statistical inference (Figure 12.5). We can use statistical inference to estimate a measure of effect, a measure of interval and hypothesis testing and p values to assess whether any findings we have seen are 'statistically significant'.

We have already talked about what measures of effect are and how to calculate them. We can directly use the value for the measure of effect from the sample to say what the true measure

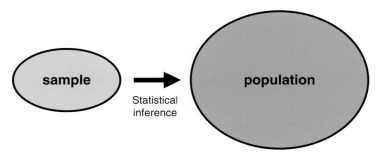

Figure 12.5 Statistical inference.

of effect would be in the whole population. However, we would also need to have a 'measure of interval' to allow us to say how confident we are about the reliability of the sample measure of effect value. The most commonly used measure of interval is the confidence interval (CI). We can determine how likely the confidence interval is to contain the population measure of effect value by setting a confidence interval level. The most commonly used is the 95% confidence interval which allows us to be 95% sure that the true population measure of effect lies within the range of values given. The 95% confidence interval gives us a range of values where the true population measure of effect is likely to lie. We can increase our confidence by increasing this to a 99% confidence interval, but this would widen the range of values within which the true population measure of effect value is likely to lie.

For example, suppose a placebo-controlled trial of a drug for the prevention of lung cancer found a relative risk of 0.60 and a 95% confidence interval of 0.40–0.80.

The relative risk is less than 1, therefore we need to subtract it from 1:

$$1 - 0.60 = 0.40$$

Thus, we know that on average, taking the drug reduces the patient's risk of lung cancer by 40%.

Next we can interpret the 95% confidence intervals. Since both of the confidence intervals are less than 1, we need to calculate by how much less likely they are to get lung cancer:

Lower confidence interval = 0.40: 1 - 0.40 = 0.60

Upper confidence interval = 0.80: 1 - 0.80 = 0.20

Since 0.20 is less than 0.60, we report the upper confidence interval first, and then the second. Thus, we are 95% sure that the true population relative risk is between a 20% reduction and a 60% reduction. Since both of the 95% confidence intervals are less than 1, it is likely that the finding of a lower risk of lung cancer is real.

Now let's look at an example using numerical data. Suppose the same placebo-controlled trial found a 10 mmHg lower systolic blood pressure in the drug group, with a 95% confidence interval of −24 to 2 mmHg. This means that on average, taking the drug lowers a patient's systolic blood pressure by 10 mmHg, and we are 95% sure that the true population mean difference would be between 24 mmHg lower in the drug group and 2 mmHg higher in the drug group. Therefore there is a chance that there is no difference between the blood pressures of the two groups since the 95% confidence intervals cross zero (no difference).

Confidence intervals are used to let us know a likely range of values for the population measure of effect; 95% confidence intervals are commonly used.

Stop and think

When you last read a paper, did you understand the significance of the *p* value?

Hypothesis testing and p *values*

When researchers conduct a scientific study, they wish to test a hypothesis, for example that a new treatment A is better than the conventional treatment B. The alternative to this is that there is no difference between new treatment A and conventional treatment B; this is called the null hypothesis. Researchers test whether the null hypothesis can be rejected or not using statistical tests based on interpreting p values. A p value is the probability that the finding we have seen in the scientific study is likely to have happened by chance, and ranges from 0 to 1. A p value of 0.05 means that there is a 5% chance that the finding from the study occurred by chance. A p value less than 0.05 is usually used to determine whether the finding is 'statistically significant', which means that it is unlikely that the finding occurred by chance and therefore is an important finding. The smaller the p value, the less likely it is that the finding has occurred by chance; therefore a p value less than 0.01 is usually reported as 'highly significant'.

Meta-analysis

A meta-analysis is 'a statistical analysis that combines or integrates the results of several independent clinical trials considered by the analyst to be combinable' (Huque, 1988). Meta-analyses can be used to calculate an 'average' measure of an effect by assembling the quantitative results from several studies together (Egger, Smith and Phillips, 1997). Each study in the meta-analysis has a measure of effect, such as an odds ratio, which tells the researcher whether there was, on average, an increase or decrease in the risk of getting the disease after being exposed to a treatment. The main aim of a meta-analysis is to improve the precision of these measures of effect by statistically combining the data from multiple studies and calculating a new single measure of effect, called the 'pooled result' or 'summary statistic'. The meta-analysis gives different 'weights' to each of the studies. Larger studies tend to give less spurious results and therefore are given relatively more weight in the meta-analysis than studies with smaller sample sizes.

Meta-analysis can be used when it makes sense to combine the results from different studies; therefore it assumes that the exposure and outcomes have been measured in similar ways in all of the studies and hence the studies are comparable. Also, since we are using the quantitative results from the studies, it is essential that all the studies present data for the outcomes. A meta-analysis which is based on only a couple of eligible studies should be interpreted carefully since excluding eligible studies may adversely affect the new single measure of effect from the meta-analysis.

A range of quantitative results may be used in the meta-analysis. Historically, p values from the studies were combined together to assess, overall, whether the exposure was significantly associated with the disease (Becker, 1994). A disadvantage with combining p values is that it only gives a feel for whether the result is significant. Raw data may be extracted from studies, for example the proportion of treated patients who develop the disease. Binary data are the most common form of data used in a meta-analysis and the most commonly used measures of effect are the odds ratio and the relative risk (risk ratio).

A meta-analysis is used to combine the quantitative results from several similar clinical studies to answer a specific research question. A meta-analysis produces a single pooled measure of effect by weighting the studies based on their relative sizes.

Section 2

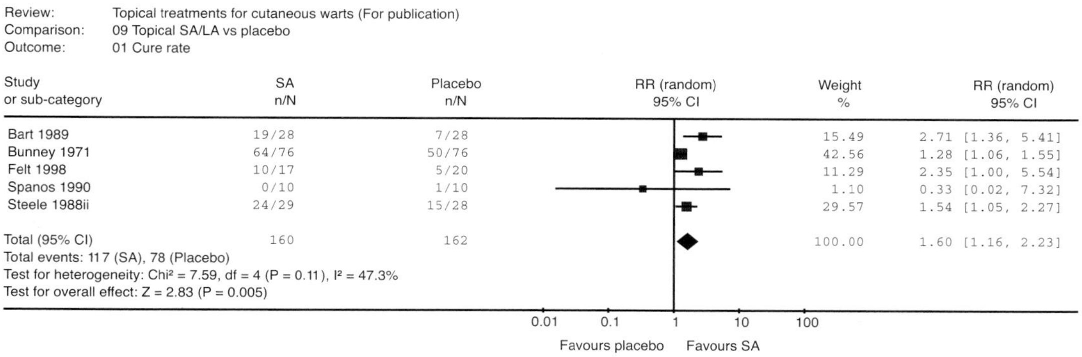

Review: Topical treatments for cutaneous warts (For publication)
Comparison: 09 Topical SA/LA vs placebo
Outcome: 01 Cure rate

Study or sub-category	SA n/N	Placebo n/N	RR (random) 95% CI	Weight %	RR (random) 95% CI
Bart 1989	19/28	7/28		15.49	2.71 [1.36, 5.41]
Bunney 1971	64/76	50/76		42.56	1.28 [1.06, 1.55]
Felt 1998	10/17	5/20		11.29	2.35 [1.00, 5.54]
Spanos 1990	0/10	1/10		1.10	0.33 [0.02, 7.32]
Steele 1988ii	24/29	15/28		29.57	1.54 [1.05, 2.27]
Total (95% CI)	160	162		100.00	1.60 [1.16, 2.23]

Total events: 117 (SA), 78 (Placebo)
Test for heterogeneity: Chi² = 7.59, df = 4 (P = 0.11), I² = 47.3%
Test for overall effect: Z = 2.83 (P = 0.005)

```
        0.01    0.1    1    10    100
     Favours placebo    Favours SA
```

Figure 12.6   Forest plot (from Gibbs and Harvey, 2006). Copyright Cochrane Collaboration, reproduced with permission.

Interpreting a meta-analysis

Once we have extracted the raw data from all the studies, we can present the results from each study, such as the relative risk and 95% confidence interval, visually, using a 'forest plot'.

An example arising from randomised controlled trials assessing the efficacy of a simple topical agent containing salicylic acid (SA) and lactic acid (LA) versus placebo for the treatment of warts (Gibbs and Harvey, 2006) is given in Figure 12.6. In this forest plot, the studies are represented in alphabetical order of author names from the top down, the squares representing the estimated relative risk for cure and the lines their associated 95% confidence intervals. The size of the study is represented by the size of the square where larger studies with more power have larger squares (in fact, the size of the square is proportional to the inverse of the variance of the log of relative risk). The diamond in the bottom line is the summary statistic, or pooled relative risk, and the width of the diamond is its 95% confidence interval.

We can see from this plot that patients on topical SA/LA are 1.60 times more likely to be cured than patients on placebo. The 95% confidence interval ranges from 1.16 to 2.23, and the p value is 0.005, which is statistically significant since it is less than 0.05 and therefore unlikely to be due to chance.

Figure 12.7 gives another example, this time looking at the effect of imiquimod on the risk of basal cell carcinomas, which is a non-melanoma skin cancer. We can see from this plot that patients on imiquimod are 0.25 times as likely (75% reduction in the risk) to suffer early treatment failure within 6 months of treatment than patients receiving vehicle alone. The 95% confidence interval ranges from 0.19 to 0.32 and the p value is less than 0.0001, which is highly statistically significant and therefore unlikely to be due to chance.

Forest plots are used to present the results from a meta-analysis. The centre of the diamond at the bottom of the plot represents the pooled measure of effect and the width of the diamond relates to the confidence intervals.

Assessing study heterogeneity

Once we have plotted the data visually using a forest plot, we then need to determine whether the results from each of the studies are similar. The degree to which the results from the studies vary is called 'heterogeneity'. We can only perform a meta-analysis when heterogeneity is not

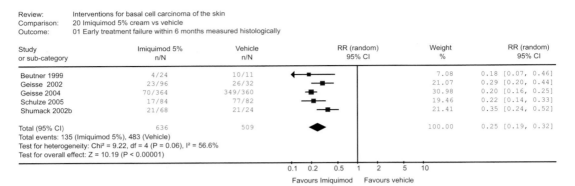

Figure 12.7 Forest plot (from Bath-Hextall *et al.,* 2007). Copyright Cochrane Collaboration, reproduced with permission.

a problem. The simplest way to assess the degree of heterogeneity is by visually looking at the forest plot and seeing whether the results from each study are similar. Figure 12.8 shows the forest plot from the meta-analysis assessing treatments for warts (Gibbs and Harvey, 2006).

To visually assess the presence of heterogeneity, we need to see whether the results from the individual studies lie within the 95% confidence intervals of the pooled result. We can do this by drawing imaginary lines from the 95% confidence intervals from the pooled result (Figure 12.8). From this forest plot, we can see that the trials vary slightly since not all the relative risks or 95% confidence intervals from the individual studies lie within the two red lines which relate to the 95% confidence intervals of the pooled result, thus indicating a slight degree of heterogeneity. If we compare this to the forest plot which is assessing the effect of imiquimod for basal cell carcinoma (Figure 12.9), these trials appear more similar to each other and hence a lot more homogeneous.

Alternatively, we can use a statistical test to assess the level of heterogeneity between the results of the studies, called I^2 (Higgins *et al.*, 2003). The value for I^2 can range from 0% to 100%. A value of 0% would indicate that there is no heterogeneity, a value of 50% would indicate that 50% of the total variation in the meta-analysis is due to heterogeneity, and a value

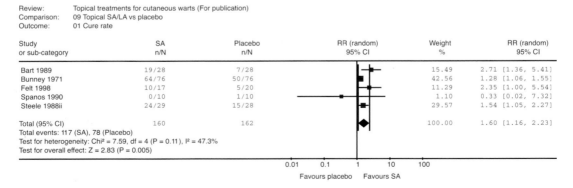

Figure 12.8 Visual assessment of heterogeneity (from Gibbs and Harvey, 2006). Copyright Cochrane Collaboration, reproduced with permission.

Review: Interventions for basal cell carcinoma of the skin
Comparison: 20 Imiquimod 5% cream vs vehicle
Outcome: 01 Early treatment failure within 6 months measured histologically

Study or sub-category	Imiquimod 5% n/N	Vehicle n/N	RR (random) 95% CI	Weight %	RR (random) 95% CI
Beutner 1999	4/24	10/11		7.08	0.18 [0.07, 0.46]
Geisse 2002	23/96	26/32		21.07	0.29 [0.20, 0.44]
Geisse 2004	70/364	349/360		30.98	0.20 [0.16, 0.25]
Schulze 2005	17/84	77/82		19.46	0.22 [0.14, 0.33]
Shumack 2002b	21/68	21/24		21.41	0.35 [0.24, 0.52]
Total (95% CI)	636	509		100.00	0.25 [0.19, 0.32]

Total events: 135 (Imiquimod 5%), 483 (Vehicle)
Test for heterogeneity: Chi² = 9.22, df = 4 (P = 0.06), I² = 56.6%
Test for overall effect: Z = 10.19 (P < 0.00001)

0.1   0.2   0.5   1   2   5   10
Favours Imiquimod   Favours vehicle

Figure 12.9   Visual assessment of heterogeneity (from Bath-Hextall *et al.*, 2007). Copyright Cochrane Collaboration, reproduced with permission.

of 100% would indicate that all the variation in the meta-analysis is due to heterogeneity. As a basic rule of thumb, one should not conduct a meta-analysis if the I^2 value is between 85% and 100%, as this means the studies are too different and not comparable. Using the warts example from above, the I^2 value was 47.3%, indicating that 47% of the total variation in the meta-analysis is due to heterogeneity.

Heterogeneity is not usually a problem if the confidence intervals from the studies overlap with each other and lie within the confidence intervals from the pooled result (diamond shape). Heterogeneity can be quantified using I^2.

Pooling the data in a meta-analysis

We are now at the point where we have identified all the studies, extracted all the data, plotted the results and assessed the degree of heterogeneity. Now we come to pooling the studies together to get the new single measure of effect called the 'summary statistic'. There are two main methods used to calculate the summary statistic and for the purpose of explanation, let's assume this is a relative risk. Using the warts example, the results from both methods are shown in Figure 12.10, so you can see the effect heterogeneity has on the pooled summary statistic.

Fixed effect method

The first method is called the 'fixed effect method'. This is the most commonly used method where a weighted average of the relative risk is calculated using data from all the different studies, where the weight is proportional to the size of the study. Therefore, the larger the study, the more influence it will have on the pooled relative risk. The fixed effect method assumes that all the available studies were trying to estimate a true value that is the same for all of them – that is, it does not vary according to where or when or in whom the study is done. The fixed effects model is probably appropriate when the estimates visually vary but their confidence intervals more or less overlap, so it is likely that they are all estimating the same thing. This validity of using the fixed effect method may be assessed also using the I^2 statistic, where a fixed effect model is appropriate when I^2 is between 0% and 30–40%. In the

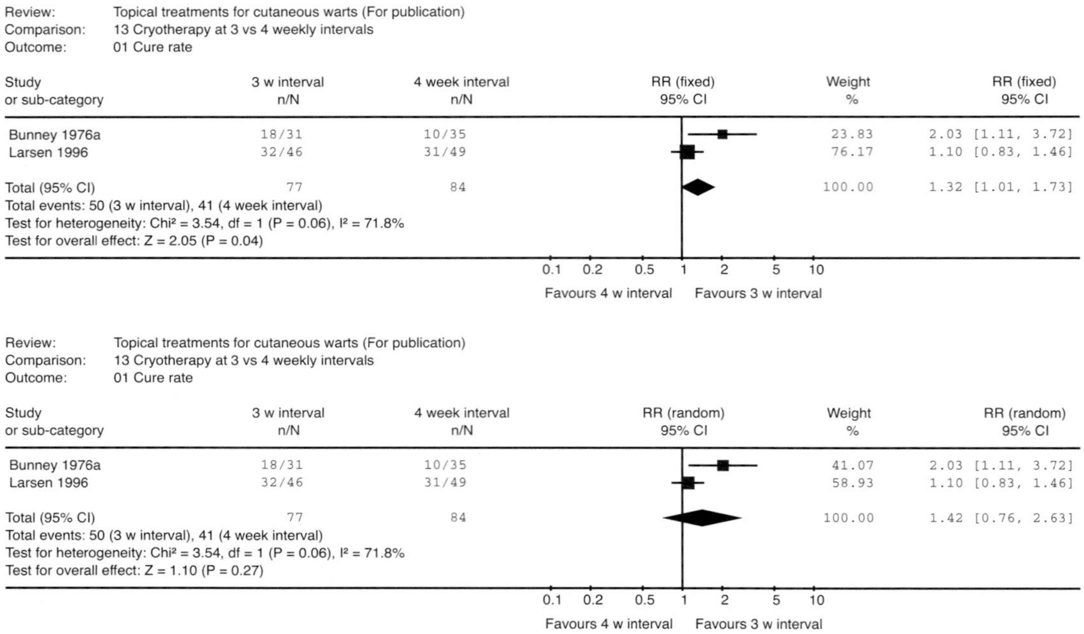

Figure 12.10 Fixed and random effect methods (from Gibbs and Harvey, 2006). Copyright Cochrane Collaboration, reproduced with permission.

figure above, the results from the fixed effect method are statistically significant ($p = 0.04$) since the p value is less than 0.05.

Random effect method

However, if moderate levels of heterogeneity are detected by I^2, that is, a value between 40 and 85%, then the 'random effect method' would be more appropriate method. This method accounts for some of the heterogeneity between studies. This is the more appropriate method when there are *a priori* grounds to suspect that the true pooled effect would differ between studies. Reasons would include different types of drug therapy or different levels of exposure being considered. Briefly, this is done by estimating the between-study variance and using this to modify the weighting of each study. In the figure above, the 95% confidence intervals are now a lot wider than was seen using the fixed effect method. As you can see from Figure 12.10, the p value for the pooled result is now 0.27, which is greater than 0.05, so the results are not statistically significant. Therefore the more appropriate method to use for this meta-analysis would be the random effect method. However, an I^2 value greater than 85–90% suggests extreme heterogeneity and implies that the studies are not comparable (Higgins and Green, 2008). Therefore the meta-analysis should be abandoned and instead the studies should be reported individually.

A fixed effect method is more appropriate when I^2 is between 0% and 30–40%. A random effect method should be used when I^2 is between 40% and 85%. If I^2 is greater than 85% then the meta-analysis should be abandoned.

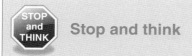

Stop and think

Last time you looked at a forest plot, did you consider if it was appropriate for the authors to conduct a meta-analysis?

Publication bias

A potential problem with meta-analysis is called publication bias, which can occur during the search strategy phase of the systematic review. Publication bias is where you are more likely to identify published studies which have found 'interesting' (usually positive) results, and which tend to be published earlier, than 'less interesting' (usually negative) ones. One way of looking for publication bias is to inspect the magnitude of published effects in relation to the order of their publication – if publication bias is present, then the earlier reports will tend to find larger effects than later studies.

A more formal approach to this question, which is not dependent on the time sequence of publication, is to use the 'funnel plot' of the magnitude of the odds ratio against the precision of the study (Egger and Smith, 1997). If no publication bias exists then the funnel plot will be approximately symmetrical. If we look at a hypothetical example of a funnel plot (Figure 12.11), we can see there is a definite asymmetry to the plot which suggests that there has

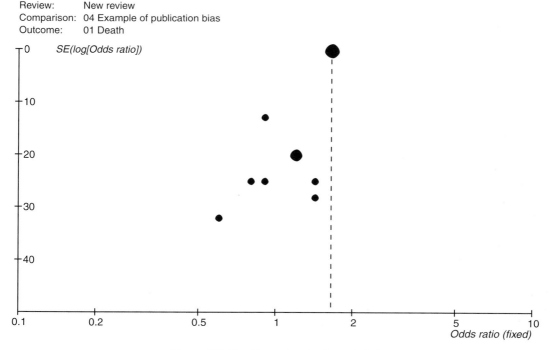

Review: New review
Comparison: 04 Example of publication bias
Outcome: 01 Death

Figure 12.11   Example of a funnel plot.

been considerable publication bias towards studies showing a protective effect. The effects of publication bias can be reduced by making sure that the review of published literature is as thorough as possible, and by additional hand searching through references quoted by each paper to make sure everything is found.

Funnel plots can be used to assess if there is the potential for publication bias. A comprehensive search strategy and retrieval of all sources of evidence reduce the potential for publication bias.

Summary

- Data are the observations collected on patients from scientific studies. There are two main types of data: numerical ('how much?') and categorical ('what type?').
- Effect measures are used to describe the relative harm or benefit a treatment can produce in a patient. The main measures of effect are odds ratio, relative risk and the mean difference.
- Researchers test hypotheses to see if one treatment is better than another, and decide whether the findings are likely to be real using statistical tests which generate p values. A p value less than 0.05 is taken as statistically significant, and thus unlikely to have occurred by chance.
- A meta-analysis pools data together from various scientific studies and yields a new pooled result; however, for a meta-analysis to be valid, an assessment of heterogeneity needs to be performed. There are two main methods that can be used to pool the data together: fixed effect and random effect. Publication bias can threaten the validity of the results from a meta-analysis.

Activity

1. Interpreting three odds ratios, relative risks and mean difference:
   Odds ratio = 1.20
   Relative risk = 0.90
   Mean difference = −20 cm
2. Deciding whether three p values are significant or not:
   p value = 0.04
   p value = 0.0001
   p value = 0.50
3. Interpreting 95% confidence intervals for two relative risks and two mean differences:
   Data presented as: RR (95% CI):
   RR 0.60 (95% CI 0.10–1.10)
   RR 3.00 (95% CI 2.10–3.90)
   Data presented as: MD (95% CI):
   MD 65.2 mol/l (95% CI 60.9–70.3)
   MD −0.99 g (95% CI −10.89 to 12.55)

Section 2

4. Interpreting the pooled result from three meta-analyses:
   Forest plot 1

Review: New review
Comparison: 01 Comparison between active drug X and placebo
Outcome: 01 Death

Study or sub-category	Active drug X n/N	Placebo n/N	OR (fixed) 95% CI	OR (fixed) 95% CI
Study 1	10/50	12/90		1.63 [0.65, 4.08]
Study 2	14/25	65/200		2.64 [1.14, 6.14]
Study 3	1/30	1/30		1.00 [0.06, 16.76]
Study 4	14/50	12/50		1.23 [0.50, 3.02]
Study 5	13/50	16/50		0.75 [0.31, 1.78]
Study 6	165/900	155/980		1.19 [0.94, 1.52]
Total (95% CI)	1105	1400		1.24 [1.00, 1.53]

Total events: 217 (Active drug X), 261 (Placebo)
Test for heterogeneity: Chi² = 4.85, df = 5 (P = 0.43), I² = 0%
Test for overall effect: Z = 2.00 (P = 0.05)

0.2 0.5 1 2 5
Favours active drugX   Favours placebo

Forest plot 2

Review: New review
Comparison: 01 Comparison between active drug X and placebo
Outcome: 02 Recurrence of disease

Study or sub-category	Active drug X n/N	Placebo n/N	OR (random) 95% CI	OR (random) 95% CI
Study 1	1/50	6/90		0.29 [0.03, 2.44]
Study 2	4/25	120/200		0.13 [0.04, 0.38]
Study 3	18/30	17/30		1.15 [0.41, 3.20]
Study 4	6/50	4/50		1.57 [0.41, 5.93]
Study 5	10/50	12/50		0.79 [0.31, 2.05]
Study 6	50/900	50/980		1.09 [0.73, 1.64]
Total (95% CI)	1105	1400		0.69 [0.34, 1.40]

Total events: 89 (Active drug X), 209 (Placebo)
Test for heterogeneity: Chi² = 15.21, df = 5 (P = 0.010), I² = 67.1%
Test for overall effect: Z = 1.03 (P = 0.30)

0.2 0.5 1 2 5
Favours active drugX   Favours placebo

Forest plot 3

Review: New review
Comparison: 01 Comparison between active drug X and placebo
Outcome: 03 Side effects

Study or sub-category	Active drug X n/N	Placebo n/N	RR (fixed) 95% CI	RR (fixed) 95% CI
Study 1	4/50	10/90		0.72 [0.24, 2.18]
Study 2	10/25	4/200		20.00 [6.78, 59.04]
Study 3	15/30	10/30		1.50 [0.81, 2.79]
Study 4	6/50	2/50		3.00 [0.64, 14.16]
Study 5	15/50	5/50		3.00 [1.18, 7.63]
Study 6	400/900	20/980		21.78 [14.03, 33.81]
Total (95% CI)	1105	1400		10.77 [8.07, 14.39]

Total events: 450 (Active drug X), 51 (Placebo)
Test for heterogeneity: Chi² = 82.73, df = 5 (P < 0.00001), I² = 94.0%
Test for overall effect: Z = 16.10 (P < 0.00001)

0.01 0.1 1 10 100
Favours active drugX   Favours placebo

Section 2

Reusable learning objects

Levels of measurement. www.nottingham.ac.uk/nursing/sonet/rlos/statistics/levels_measurement1/index.html

Descriptive statistics for interval and ratio scale data. www.nottingham.ac.uk/nursing/sonet/rlos/statistics/descriptive_stats/index.html:
- Levels of measurement – what you can and can't do arithmetically. www.nottingham.ac.uk/nursing/sonet/rlos/statistics/levels_measurement2/index.html
- Quantitative and qualitative research methods. www.nottingham.ac.uk/nursing/sonet/rlos/ebp/qvq/
- NNT and NNH. www.nottingham.ac.uk/nursing/sonet/rlos/ebp/nnt_nnh/
- Interpreting the results of clinical trials. www.nottingham.ac.uk/nursing/sonet/rlos/ebp/trial_results/
- Probability associated with inferential statistics. www.nottingham.ac.uk/nursing/sonet/rlos/statistics/probability/index.html
- Confidence intervals. www.nottingham.ac.uk/nursing/sonet/rlos/ebp/confidence_intervals/index.html
- Relative risk reduction (RRR) and absolute risk reduction (ARR). www.nottingham.ac.uk/nursing/sonet/rlos/ebp/risk_reduction/index.html
- Meta-analysis. www.nottingham.ac.uk/nursing/sonet/rlos/ebp/meta-analysis/index.html
- Presenting and interpreting meta-analyses. www.nottingham.ac.uk/nursing/sonet/rlos/ebp/meta-analysis2/

References

Bath-Hextall, F.J., Perkins, W., Bong, J. and Williams, H.C. (2007) Interventions for basal cell carcinoma of the skin. *Cochrane Database Syst Rev*, 1, CD003412).

Becker, B.J. (1994) Combining significance levels, in *The Handbook of Research Synthesis* (eds H. Cooper and L.V. Hedges), Russel Sage Foundation, New York.

Egger, M., and Smith, G.D. (1997) Meta-analysis: potential and promise. *BMJ*, **315**, 1371–1374.

Egger, M., Smith, G.D. and Phillips, A.N. (1997) Meta-analysis: principles and procedures. *BMJ*, **315**, 1533–1537.

Gibbs, S. and Harvey, I. (2006) Topical treatments for cutaneous warts. *Cochrane Database Syst Rev*, 3, CD001781).

Harris, M. and Taylor, G. (2005) *Medical Statistics Made Easy*, Martin Dunitz, London.

Higgins, J.P.T. and Green, S. (eds) (2008) *Cochrane Handbook for Systematic Reviews of Interventions* Version 5.0.0 [updated February 2008]. The Cochrane Collaboration. Available from www.cochrane-handbook.org.

Higgins, J.P.T., Thompson, S.G., Deeks, J.J. and Altman, D.G. (2003) Measuring inconsistency in meta-analyses. *BMJl*, **327**, 557–560.

Section 2

Huque, M.F. (1988) Experiences with meta-analysis in NDA submissions. Proceedings of the Biopharmaceutical Section of the American Statistical Association, vol. 2, pp. 28–33.

Laupacis, A., Sackett, D.L. and Roberts, R.S. (1988) An assessment of clinically useful measures of the consequences of treatment. *N Engl J Med*, **318** (26), 1728–1733.

Further Reading

Greenland, S. (1994) A critical look at some popular meta-analytic methods. *Am J Epidemiol*, **140**, 290–296.

Moher, D., Cook, D.J., Eastwood, S., *et al.*, for the QUOROM Group (1999) Improving the quality of reports of meta-analyses of randomised controlled trials: the QUOROM statement. *Lancet*, **354**, 1896–900.

Pogue, J. and Yusuf, S. (1998) Meta-analysis. *Lancet*, **351**, 47–45.

Stroup, D.F., Berlin, J., Morton, S., *et al.* (2000) Meta-analysis of observational studies in epidemiology. A proposal for reporting. *JAMA*, **283**, 2008–2012.

Section 2

13 How do we apply the evidence?

Learning outcomes

By the end of this chapter the reader should be able to:

- understand the relationship between evidence and practice
- have a better understanding about changing practice
- have an understanding of the PARIHS framework
- understand the range of approaches to promoting individual and organisational change
- understand what is meant by reflective practice.

Evidence in itself is of little benefit to those with healthcare needs if it does not influence what actually occurs in practice and therefore what patients experience. This brings us to the difficult process of implementing evidence in practice.

The relationship between evidence and practice

While increasing knowledge offers the promise of improved care and better healthcare outcomes, the wealth of evidence available to practitioners can often be overwhelming. For example, there are over 530,000 trials listed on the Cochrane Central Register of Controlled Trials with new reviews being added all the time. It is therefore not surprising that one of the most consistent findings in the research of health services is the gap between evidence and practice. As outlined in Chapter 8, studies suggest that 30–40% of patients do not receive the care that the present evidence suggests and about 20–25% of care provided is not needed or harmful (Schuster, McGlynn and Brook, 1998; Grol, 2001).

Seeing differences between theory and practice as a gap to be closed suggests that we can achieve a situation where there is no difference between the latest evidence and what goes on in practice. However, it is difficult to imagine a situation in which new research findings

The New Prescriber. Edited by J Lymn, D Bowskill, F Bath-Hextall, R Knaggs, © 2010 John Wiley & Sons.

will not suggest better ways of practising or that practitioners will not develop new ways of practising from their own observations and experience. It has been argued that, in fact, new innovations in care will always occur and that this leads to a dynamic tension between theory development and what is done in practice (Rafferty, Allcock and Lathlean, 1996). What is needed, therefore, is an understanding of the most effective ways of ensuring that the current best available evidence is used to inform our everyday practice.

Although some changes in practice can occur relatively quickly, changing practice is generally a complex process that can be a very challenging undertaking. Analyses of barriers to changing practice, such as a review of 76 studies in doctors, have shown that obstacles to change in practice can arise at different stages in the healthcare system – at the level of the patient, the individual professional, the healthcare team, the healthcare organisation, or the wider environment (Grol and Grimshaw, 2003). The idea that simply making research information available is enough for practitioners to change their practice is now accepted as unrealistic. Whilst the evidence contained in a guideline or a research-based publication may be important, it is unlikely to lead to changes in practice by itself. The best way of getting evidence into practice (evidence transfer) depends on the nature of the evidence and the context in which it is being applied.

 Stop and think

What are the limitations in seeing the differences between theory and practice as a 'gap' that can be closed?

Step 4: Getting the evidence into practice

Changing practice

It is widely accepted that change is a complex process that requires changes not only by individuals but also by the organisations in which they work. Change does not happen overnight; it is a long process that requires planning, lots of commitment and stacks of time and energy. It is important that anyone planning to implement a change in practice considers the wide range of factors that can affect the process of getting evidence into practice. There are several models/theories of change that can help us to think about the many factors that need to be considered when planning change. A review of all the models proposed would fill this entire book so we will concentrate on one particular framework that may be helpful.

The PARIHS framework

The Promoting Action on Research Implementation in Health Services (PARIHS) framework was first developed in 1998 and identified the multiple factors that can influence change (Kitson, Harvey and McCormack, 1998). The framework emerged from working with clinicians to help them improve practice. The main features and assumptions of the framework are described in Box 13.1.

Section 2

Box 13.1   The Main Features and Assumptions of the PARIHS Framework

- Evidence encompasses codified and non-codified sources of knowledge, including research evidence, clinical experience, including professional craft knowledge, patient preferences and experiences and local information.
- Melding and implementing such evidence in practice involves negotiation and developing shared understanding about the benefits, disbenefits, risks and advantages of the new over the old. This is a dialectical process that requires careful management and choreography and one that is not done in isolation; in other words, it is a team effort.
- Some contexts are more conducive to the successful implementation of evidence into practice than others. These include contexts that have transformational leaders, features of learning organisations, appropriate monitoring, evaluative and feedback mechanisms.
- There is an emphasis on the need for appropriate facilitation to improve the likelihood of success. The type of facilitation and the role and skill of the facilitator required are determined by the state of preparedness of an individual or team, in terms of their acceptance and understanding of evidence, the receptivity of their place of work or context in terms of the resources, culture and values, leadership style and evaluation activity. Facilitators work with individuals and teams to enhance the process of implementation.

From Kitson *et al*., 2008; licensee BioMed Central Ltd
under the Creative Commons Attributions License.

The framework suggests that successful implementation of evidence in practice can be explained by looking at three elements.

Evidence

Finding the evidence has already been covered in Chapter 10. Remember, in Chapter 9 we discussed how evidence-based practice (EBP) was made up of not only research evidence but also clinical expertise and patient preference. To maximise the uptake of evidence into practice, all three of the components of EBP should be subjected to scrutiny and found to be credible. This is one of the reasons why it is important to develop the ability to appraise the evidence that you are planning to implement – we covered appraisal in Chapter 12. In Chapter 11 we looked at different levels of evidence, placing systematic reviews and RCTs as the most valuable sources of research evidence when looking at issues of effectiveness of interventions. If, however, we wish to consider patients' experiences of a particular intervention to inform our implementation, other forms of research including qualitative approaches may provide more appropriate evidence, and different approaches to evaluating this type of research will be required. In Chapter 12 we suggested some useful websites where you can download checklists to appraise qualitative studies.

However, be aware that using different sources of evidence such as patients' preferences, research and clinical experience may not always lead to the same conclusions. As part of the process of appraising the evidence, unpinning any change, a process involving discussion of the strengths and limitations of the available evidence, needs to be conducted so that individuals and teams can come to a consensus about the evidence available and so that it can be valued as a valid source of evidence.

Context

The contexts in which healthcare takes place are hugely varied. In the PARIHS model context refers to the environment or setting in which healthcare services are provided and the proposed change is planned (Rycroft-Malone *et al.*, 2002). There are a number of factors that are identified as key characteristics of an environment that is conducive to implementing research:

- clearly defined boundaries
- clarity about decision-making processes
- clarity about patterns of power and authority
- adequate resources, information and feedback systems
- active management of factors that may promote or resist change
- systems in place that may enhance the dynamic processes of change and continuous development (Rycroft-Malone *et al.*, 2002).

Rycroft-Malone *et al.* (2002) suggest that it is important to have an understanding of the prevailing values and beliefs as a prerequisite to introducing and sustaining change. For change to be effectively managed and sustained, the organisation has to have the values and structures to support innovation. Organisations which value the contribution of individuals, are open and have decentralised decision making, for example, are more likely to be able to support change. A shared vision and organisational systems that promote innovation are also important.

Facilitation

Change can be challenging and may meet some resistance or opposition. Helping individuals and teams to see what changes are required to implement evidence in practice and how to go about it requires people who can lead and guide those changes, whether they are described as change agents, leaders or facilitators. Facilitation has been described as 'a technique by which one person makes things easier for others' (Kitson, Harvey and McCormack, 1998). The roles that facilitators can adopt can be quite varied and there is a lack of rigorous research into the facilitator's role.

Facilitators can take different approaches that can range from a specific focus on the particular change to a more general approach involving helping individuals and teams to reflect on their practice and to develop their knowledge and attitudes. However, there is a general opinion in the literature that inspirational and transformational leadership is an essential ingredient of developing practice.

Approaches to change

There is a range of approaches to promoting individual and organisational change which have been tried in various settings. Choosing an appropriate approach will depend on the nature of the change planned, the context and the role of facilitators. Therefore, considering the elements outlined in the PARIHS framework will help you to plan how you intend to apply the evidence to practice. A range of approaches has been used and described in the literature, including the following adapted from Haines (2001).

Section 2

Educational materials

Published or printed recommendations, including guidelines, audio-visual materials and electronic publications can all be used as part of education sessions, distributed locally or more widely. Passive dissemination of guidelines is, however, unlikely to bring about change in practice. Guidelines have been shown to be more likely to change practice if they take account of local circumstances, are disseminated by active educational interventions and are implemented with patient-specific reminders (NHS Centre for Reviews and Dissemination, 1999). A systematic review of guideline implementation strategies noted a median improvement of 8% across four cluster randomised trials (Grimshaw *et al.*, 2002).

Conferences

Participation of healthcare providers in conferences, lectures or workshops. It should be stated that learning doesn't necessarily lead to change in practice.

Local meetings/workshops

Involve your colleagues in the change process. This helps by generating a consensus about the nature and importance of the problem and the best way to approach it. You might want to do this to ensure that guidelines can be applied locally.

Educational outreach visits

Trained individuals can go out into practice to inform/provide evidence to practitioners. Evaluation of outreach visits in prescribing has consistently shown small changes in prescribing habits.

Local opinion leaders

Key local practitioners who are seen as likeable, trustworthy and influential can influence their colleagues.

Patient-mediated interventions

Patients and carers can influence change given appropriate information and by ensuring patients have a voice about their care. This might include patient information and educational interventions.

Audit

This is a process of gathering information about performance measured against a standard of care. This can be used to plan changes and then practice can be reassessed as part of an ongoing improvement process. Audit and feedback can be effective in improving professional practice. When it is effective, the effects are generally small to moderate. Grol and Grimshaw (2003) identified 16 reviews that looked at audit and feedback and noted mixed effects although the effects could be moderated by type of feedback offered, its source and format and the frequency or intensity of presentation. The relative effectiveness of audit and feedback is likely to be greater when baseline adherence to recommended practice is low and when feedback is delivered more intensively.

Reminders (Manual or computerised)

These are interventions that prompt the healthcare provider to perform in a particular way.

Multifaceted interventions

This involves multiple approaches. Some evidence suggests that multifaceted interventions are more likely to be successful although a review failed to identify any benefit (Grimshaw *et al.*, 2002).

While there are studies into the effectiveness of different approaches in bringing about change, it is important to look at the evidence for different approaches in relation to particular areas of practice. For example, a review of interventions to improve prescribing found that mailed educational materials alone were generally ineffective, educational outreach approaches and ongoing feedback were generally effective and there was insufficient evidence to determine the effectiveness of reminder systems and group education (Soumerai, McLaughlin and Avron, 1998).

The general messages from studies that have reviewed approaches to implementing evidence and changing practice suggest that any implementation programme requires:

● a systematic approach to change with good planning
● a period of information gathering and exploration of the situation. This might involve collecting routine data and surveys designed to obtain particular information
● the design of an appropriate strategy to disseminate and implement evidence
● use of a range of strategies that work together with adequate resources
● the identification of people with the appropriate skills
● plans to monitor and evaluate whether the proposed change is being achieved
● activity to maintain and reinforce the change.

 Stop and think

Think of a change in your own area of practice that you or a colleague implemented or that you were involved in.

● How successful was it?
● What was your reaction/the reaction of other staff to the change?
● What approach was taken to changing practice?
● What worked well and what didn't work?
● What do you think are the advantages and disadvantages of the approach used?
● What were the main problems encountered?

Section 2

The joanna briggs institute (JBI)

An integrated approach to getting evidence into practice is illustrated by the work of the Joanna Briggs Institute. The JBI was established in 1996 and is an international collaboration involving nursing, medical and allied health researchers, clinicians, academics and quality managers across 90 countries. It offers resources designed to meet the needs of service providers, health professionals and consumers by connecting the best available international evidence to the point of care. The Institute undertakes this work through processes designed to support the translation, transfer and utilisation of evidence.

The JBI collaborating centres carry out systematic reviews of the available information based on questions that are generated by practitioners. There are similarities between the approach that the JBI centres use to carry out systematic reviews and those developed by the Cochrane Collaboration. Indeed, if the reviews are purely about effectiveness of an intervention then JBI centres will often conduct reviews with the relevant Cochrane centres using Cochrane Collaboration methodology. However, JBI centres may also conduct reviews that look at a range of questions relating to the effectiveness, appropriateness, meaningfulness and feasibility of health practices and delivery methods.

The JBI is committed to ensuring that the best evidence is implemented in practice and that systems have been developed to help to transfer evidence into practice through COnNECT + (Clinical Online Network of Evidence for Care and Therapeutics) which has a number of elements.

The online manual builder allows organisations to enhance their own clinical decision support resources by creating evidence-based clinical practice manuals. Consumer sheets ensure patients/residents/clients are provided with the same information as health professionals to assist them in a more informed decision-making process while other systems support quality improvement by measuring compliance, implementing change and tracking and comparing outcomes.

Step 5: Evaluation and reflection

The assumption that providing new information or research will bring about changes in professional practice is based on the information deficit model of behaviour change. This model suggests that people will change their behaviour in the light of new information and understanding. Unfortunately, this is not always the case. Passive approaches to knowledge transfer have been shown to be ineffective and we know that knowledge is only one of the factors that influence changes in behaviour.

Adult learning theories emphasise the need for active learning strategies which engage the learner in reflection and problem solving. Indeed, this relates to discussions about the nature of evidence upon which we base our decisions about the best approach to practice. Many would argue that we need to base our practice on evidence drawn from clinical experience, patients, clients and carers and local context and environment as well as research.

Practical, know-how knowledge derived from experience is not necessarily clear cut and requires different approaches to enable this type of evidence to be incorporated into practice. Titchen (2000) describes a process for articulating, reviewing, generating and verifying professional craft knowledge through critical reflection. Reflection on practice can help practitioners to identify, discuss and reflect on their practice knowledge, helping to integrate it with other forms of knowledge. This is not always straightforward. Practice knowledge may reinforce and support evidence from research. However, if practitioners' beliefs and understandings, derived from their experiences, contradict evidence from research, it can be important to explore those beliefs to ensure they are not allowed to block necessary change. However, reflection on practice may also be an important source of understanding the context and particular circumstances that apply in a particular setting and can help to make appropriate decisions for specific individuals.

Summary

- Variations between practice and available evidence are often perceived as a 'gap' between theory and practice. As both are dynamic, it is perhaps unlikely that this gap will disappear completely and their relationship can perhaps be better characterised as a dynamic tension.
- Changing practice can be a complex activity requiring an understanding of the factors that influence change. Both individual and organisational factors are important.
- Implementing evidence in practice is unlikely to occur with just the passive provision of evidence; it needs to be an active planned activity.
- The PAHRIS framework suggests that successful implementation of evidence requires consideration of the nature of the evidence, the context and the facilitation.
- A range of approaches to promoting change and getting evidence into practice has been evaluated and strategies need to be carefully planned and based on available evidence.
- Reflective practice can help practitioners to identify, discuss and reflect on their practice knowledge, helping to integrate it with other forms of knowledge.

 Activity

1. Using the PARHIS framework, describe the three elements that need to be considered in order to bring about successful change.
2. List five factors that the evidence suggests are important in implementing change in clinical practice.

Useful websites

The Joanna Briggs Institute. www.joannabriggs.edu.au/about/home.php

NHS Institute for Innovation and Improvement. Improvement Leaders Guides. www.institute. nhs.uk/option,com_joomcart/Itemid,26/main_page,document_product_info/products_id,309. html

Foundation of Nursing Studies. www.fons.org/

Cochrane Effective Practice and Organisation of Care Group. www.epoc.cochrane. org/en/localrevs.html

Reusable learning objects

Why critique research? www.nottingham.ac.uk/nursing/sonet/rlos/ebp/research_critique/index.html

References

Grimshaw, J., Eccles, M., Walker, A. and Thomas, R. (2002) Changing physicians' behaviour: what works and thoughts on getting more things to work. *J Cont Educ Health Professions*, **22**, 237–243.

Grol, R. (2001) Successes and failures in the implementation of evidence-based guidelines for clinical practice. *Med Care*, **39**(suppl 2), 46–54.

Grol, R. and Grimshaw, J. (2003) From best evidence to best practice: effective implementation of change in patients' care. *Lancet*, **362**(9391), 1225–1230.

Haines, A. (2001) *Getting Research Findings into Practice*, BMJ Publishing Group, London.

Kitson, A.L., Harvey, G. and McCormack, B. (1998) Enabling the implementation of evidence based practice: a conceptual framework. *Qual Health Care*, **7**, 149–158.

Kitson, A., Rycroft-Malone, J., Harvey, G., *et al.* (2008) Evaluating the successful implementation of evidence into practice using the PARiHS framework: theoretical and practical challenges. *Implementat Sci*, **3**, 1. www.implementationscience.com/content/3/1/1

NHS Centre for Reviews and Dissemination (1999) Getting evidence into practice effective health care. www.york.ac.uk/inst/crd/.

Rafferty, A.M., Allcock, N. and Lathlean, J. (1996) The theory/practice 'gap': taking issue with the issue. *J Adv Nurs*, **23**, 685–691.

Rycroft-Malone, J., Kitson, A., Harvey, G., *et al.* (2002) Ingredients for change: revisiting a conceptual framework. *Qual Safe Healthcare*, **11**, 174–180.

Schuster, M., McGlynn, E. and Brook, R. (1998) How good is the quality of health care in the United States? *Milbank Q*, **76**, 517–563.

Soumerai, S.B., McLaughlin, T.J. and Avron, J. (1998) Improving drug prescribing in primary care: a critical analysis of the experimental literature. *Milbank Q*, **67**, 268–317.

Titchen, A. (2000) Professional craft knowledge in patient-centred nursing and the facilitation of its development. DPhil thesis, University of Oxford. Ashdale Press, Oxford.

Further reading

Ballantine, K. (2006) A realist synthesis of evidence relating to practice development: final report to NHS Education for Scotland and NHS Quality Improvement Scotland. www.nhshealthquality.org/nhsqis/files/Final%20report.pdf

Section 2: Evidence-based practice activity answers: Chapters 8–13

Chapter 8: What is evidence-based practice?

1.
    1. Asking the question.
    2. Finding the evidence that best answers the question.
    3. Appraising the evidence for its validity, impact and applicability.
    4. Acting on the evidence – that is, implementing the evidence in practice.
    5. Evaluation and reflection.

2. Best research evidence (BRE), clinical expertise (CE) and patient preference (PP).

3. 1992.

Chapter 9: How do we find the evidence?

1. AND, OR:

2.
    - National Library of Guidelines (including NICE guidance)
    - NICE guidance (only)
    - Protocols and Care Pathways Library
    - Clinical Knowledge Summaries
    - International Guidelines.

3. EMBASE, MEDLINE, PubMed, AMED, LILACS, CINAHL, PsycInfo, Cochrane Library and so on.

Chapter 10: What are the different types of study design?

1.
    Cohort study
    RCT
    Case–control study

2.
    Simple randomisation
    Block randomisation

Stratified randomisation
Minimisation

Chapter 11: Appraising the evidence

1.

Computer-generated random numbers
Table of random numbers
Tossing a coin

2.

The use of sealed opaque envelopes.
Central randomisation (i.e. away from the trial location).

Chapter 12: How do we interpret the evidence?

1. Interpreting the odds ratio, relative risk and mean difference.
Odds ratio = 1.20, 20% more likely to have event in the exposed group as compared to the unexposed group.
Relative risk = 0.90, 10% reduced risk of event in the exposed group as compared to the unexposed group.
Mean difference = –20 cm, 20 cm lower in the exposed group as compared to the unexposed group.

2. Deciding whether three p values are significant or not.

P value = 0.04	significant
P value = 0.0001	highly significant
P value = 0.50	not significant

3. Interpreting 95% confidence intervals for two relative risks and two mean differences.
Data presented as RR (95% CI).
RR 0.60 (95% CI 0.10–1.10).
We are 95% sure that the patients in the exposed group are between 90% less likely and 10% more likely to have the event than patients in the unexposed group.
RR 3.00 (95% CI 2.10–3.90).
We are 95% sure that the patients in the exposed group are between 2.1 times and 3.9 times more likely to have the event than patients in the unexposed group.
Data presented as MD (95% CI).
MD 65.2 mol/l (95% CI 60.9–70.3).
We are 95% sure that patients in the exposed group have between 60.9 mol/l and 70.3 mol/l more than patients in the unexposed group.
MD –0.99g (95% CI –10.89, 12.55).
We are 95% sure that patients in the exposed group are between 10.89 g less and 12.55 g more than patients in the unexposed group.

4. Interpreting the pooled result from three meta-analyses.

Forest plot 1

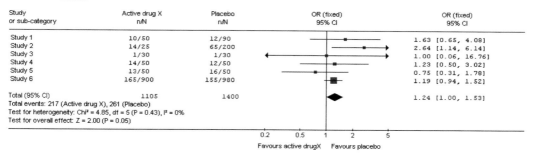

A fixed effect model is appropriate since there is no evidence of heterogeneity between the studies. Patients on active drug X are, on average, 24% more likely to die than patients on placebo. We are 95% sure that patients on active drug X are between 1 times and 1.53 times more likely to die (or between 0% and 53% more likely to die). The overall effect p value = 0.05, therefore the effect is not statistically significant since p is not less than 0.05.

Forest plot 2

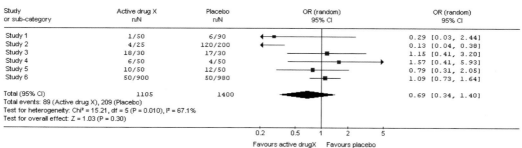

A random effect model is appropriate since there is evidence of heterogeneity between the studies. Patients on active drug X are, on average, 31% less likely to have a recurrence of disease than patients on placebo. We are 95% sure that patients on active drug X are between 66% less likely and 1.40 times more likely to have a recurrence of disease (or between 66% less likely and 40% more likely to have a recurrence of disease). The overall effect p value = 0.30, therefore the effect is not statistically significant since p is not less than 0.05.

Section 2

Forest plot 3

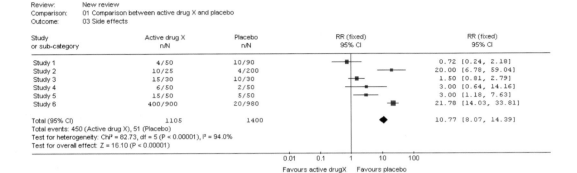

Review:	New review
Comparison:	01 Comparison between active drug X and placebo
Outcome:	03 Side effects

Study or sub-category	Active drug X n/N	Placebo n/N	RR (fixed) 95% CI	RR (fixed) 95% CI
Study 1	4/50	10/90		0.72 [0.24, 2.18]
Study 2	10/25	4/200		20.00 [6.78, 59.04]
Study 3	15/30	10/30		1.50 [0.81, 2.79]
Study 4	6/50	2/50		3.00 [0.64, 14.16]
Study 5	15/50	5/50		3.00 [1.18, 7.63]
Study 6	400/900	20/980		21.78 [14.03, 33.81]
Total (95% CI)	1105	1400		10.77 [8.07, 14.39]

Total events: 450 (Active drug X), 51 (Placebo)
Test for heterogeneity: Chi² = 82.73, df = 5 (P < 0.00001), I² = 94.0%
Test for overall effect: Z = 16.10 (P < 0.00001)

0.01 0.1 1 10 100
Favours active drugX   Favours placebo

This meta-analysis should be abandoned since there are extreme levels of heterogeneity between the studies. $I^2 = 94.0\%$, which is more than 85%.

Chapter 13: How do we apply the evidence?

1. Evidence, context, facilitation.

2. Any five of:
   a. a systematic approach to change with good planning
   b. a period of information gathering and exploration of the situation; this might involve collecting routine data and surveys designed to obtain particular information
   c. designing an appropriate strategy to disseminate and implement evidence
   d. use of a range of strategies that work together with adequate resources
   e. the identification of people with the appropriate skills
   f. plans to monitor and evaluate whether the proposed change has been achieved
   g. activity to maintain and reinforce the change.

Section 2

Section 2: Evidence-based practice glossary

AGREE: An international collaboration of researchers and policy makers who are looking to improve the quality and effectiveness of clinical practice guidelines.

Allocation concealment: This is when the person enrolling participants into a clinical trial is unaware to which group the next participant will be allocated.

Attrition bias: Differences in terms of losses of subjects between groups.

Bias: This is any process at any stage of inference tending to produce results that differ systematically from the true values.

Boolean operators: Boolean operators allow you to combine search terms using AND, OR and NOT.

Case–control study: A retrospective study which investigates the relationship between a risk factor and one or more outcomes.

Cases: Usually refers to patients but could also refer to hospitals, wards, countries, blood samples and so on.

CASP: Critical Appraisal Skills Programme.

Cochrane Collaboration: Prepares, maintains and disseminates reviews of the effects of healthcare based on randomised controlled trials.

Cohort study: The prospective cohort study starts with the identity and examination of a group of subjects (cohort) who are then followed up over a period of time looking for the development of a disease or other specified end-point.

Confidence interval: A range (interval) in which we can be fairly sure (confident) that the 'true value' lies.

Confounding: When the association between an outcome and an exposure variable is distorted by a third variable.

CONSORT statement (Consolidated Standards of Reporting Trials): A minimum set of recommendations for reporting RCTs. Developed to increase the quality of trials and their reporting.

Cross-sectional surveys: These studies look at one point in time and describe what is happening at that time.

The New Prescriber. Edited by J Lymn, D Bowskill, F Bath-Hextall, R Knaggs, © 2010 John Wiley & Sons.

Detection bias: Differences in how outcomes of the intervention are assessed for each of the participant groups.

Evidence-based practice: Provides a framework and process for the systematic incorporation of research evidence and patient preference into clinical decision making at the level of the individual practitioner and healthcare organisation.

Hypothesis: A statement which can be tested that predicts the relationship between variables.

Information bias: This type of bias arises when data on the outcome and/or exposure are collected, measured or classified differently in the groups being compared. May also be referred to as observation bias.

Interviewer bias: When interviewers do not interview individuals in the groups being compared in the same way.

Incidence: The rate or proportion of a group developing a condition within a given period of time.

Intention to treat (ITT): An intention to treat analysis is one in which patients are included in the analysis according to the group into which they were randomised, even if they withdrew from the study.

Joanna Briggs Institute: An International not-for-profit Research and Development Organisation specialising in Evidence-Based resources for healthcare professionals in nursing, midwifery, medicine, and allied health.

Mean: The sum of the observed values divided by the number of observations.

Mean difference: Calculated by subtracting means of the data in the two treatment groups.

Measure of effect: Used to describe how effective the treatments (or interventions) are when compared to each other.

Meta-analysis: A statistical technique that combines or integrates the results of several independent clinical trials considered to be combinable.

Misclassification bias: This is when participants are incorrectly classified according to exposure (cohort studies) or disease status (case–control studies).

National Library of Guidelines: The National Library of Guidelines is a collection of guidelines for the NHS. It is based on the guidelines produced by NICE and other national agencies.

Null hypothesis: A hypothesis that there is no difference between the groups being tested.

Number needed to harm (NNH): Used to assess how many patients need to be exposed to the treatment to cause harm to one patient who wouldn't have been harmed otherwise.

Number needed to treat (NNT): This tells you how many patients would need to receive the new treatment in order to prevent the event (bad outcome) occurring in one patient

Observational studies: Examples of these are case–control, cohort studies and cross-sectional surveys.

Odds ratio: These are calculated by dividing the odds of having been exposed to a risk factor by the odds in the control group.

p values: Used to test a *null hypothesis*, the *p* value gives the probability of any observed differences having happened by chance.

PARIHS: The Promoting Action on Research Implementation in Health Services framework – used to help clinicians improve practice.

Performance bias: Systematic differences in the care provided to the participants in the comparison groups other than the intervention under investigation.

Precision: Is reflected in the confidence intervals around the estimate of effect.

Primary research: Studies in which original data are collected to answer a specific question.

QUADAS tool: A tool for the quality assessment of studies of diagnostic accuracy included in systematic reviews.

Qualitative research: Used to gain insight into people's attitudes, behaviours, value systems, concerns, motivations, aspirations, culture or lifestyles.

Quantitative research: Quantitative research determines the relationship between one thing (an independent variable) and another (a dependent or outcome variable) in a population.

QUOROM (Quality of Reporting Of Meta-analysis): A checklist for improving the quality of reports of meta-analysis of randomised controlled trials.

Randomised controlled trial (RCT): Randomised controlled trials are experimental studies in which an intervention of some kind is evaluated. The most common design is one where participants are randomly allocated to one of two or more groups.

Recall bias: A problem found in case–control studies as participants are asked to recall events in the past.

Relative risk or risk ratio (RR): It is estimated by dividing the risk of the event in the new treatment group (exposed group) by the risk of the event in the conventional or control group (unexposed).

Retrospective cohort studies: These studies are based on cohorts that were formed in the past and rely on baseline and outcome data that were collected in the past.

Risk: The probability that an event will happen. It is calculated by dividing the number of events by the number of people at risk.

Risk reduction: Difference in the event rate between the two treatment groups.

Reusable Learning Object (RLO): An interactive WWW-based resource based on a single learning objective which can be used in multiple contexts.

Secondary research: Uses information from existing studies to answer a specific research question.

Selection bias: May lead to bias and distort treatment comparisons resulting from the way the comparisons groups are assembled in RCTs.

Section 2

Standard deviation (SD): A measure of the spread of scores away from the mean.

STARD: **STA**ndards for the **R**eporting of **D**iagnostic accuracy studies.

STROBE (STrengthening the Reporting of OBservational studies in Epidemiology): Guidelines on how to report observational studies.

Surveillance bias: When participants in the groups being compared are not managed in the same way.

Systematic review: A summary of the Health Care literature that uses explicit methods to perform a comprehensive literature search, critical appraisal of the individual studies and uses appropriate statistical techniques to combine the valid studies.

Validity: Validity of a study is the extent to which its design and conduct are likely to prevent systematic errors or bias.

Section 2

Section 3

Pharmacology

      Dave Skingsley

30   **Neurodegenerative disorders**   383
      Dave Skingsley

31   **Depression and anxiety**   394
      Dave Skingsley

32   **Schizophrenia**   406
      Dave Skingsley

33   **Epilepsy and anticonvulsant drugs**   416
      Michael Schachter

34   **Pain and analgesia**   427
      Roger Knaggs

35   **Antibacterial chemotherapy**   444
      Tim Hills

36   **Antibiotic resistance and *Clostridium difficile***   461
      Tim Hills

37   **Antifungal and antiviral drugs**   472
      Tim Hills

      Quiz answers   482

      Glossary   491

Section 3

Section introduction

Before starting to think seriously about pharmacological concepts, it is perhaps pertinent to give some consideration to what is meant by the term pharmacology.
Pharmacology is:

- the branch of medicine concerned with the uses, effects and action of drugs ('Compact Oxford English Dictionary')
- 1: the science of drugs including their origin, composition, pharmacokinetics, therapeutic use and toxicology
  2: the properties and reactions of drugs especially with relation to their therapeutic value ('Medline Plus Medical Dictionary').

As can be seen from the definitions above, pharmacology is essentially the study of how drugs act in the body to affect physiological function, so one of the main issues in terms of pharmacology and prescribing is around what constitutes a drug. A drug is:

- a chemical that affects physiological function in a specific way (Rang *et al.*, 2007)
- a medicine or other substance which has a marked effect when taken into the body ('Compact Oxford English Dictionary').

It is clear, then, that the term 'drug' actually covers any substance that is taken into the body in order to have a specific effect. Thus the term 'drug' encompasses a number of chemicals which may not be considered to be drugs in the conventional sense, particularly by patients, but which do impact on body function and thus have the potential to affect the action of other drugs (Section 3 Figure 1).

It is important therefore that the new prescriber gathers information on all substances that the patient may be taking before making prescribing decisions.

Terms printed in the main text in blue are defined in the glossary at the end of the section.

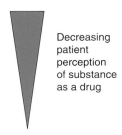

- Prescribed Medication
- Over the counter medications
- Substances of misuse (e.g. Cannabis, Cocaine, Heroin)
- Alcohol
- Nicotine
- Caffeine
- Vitamins & minerals
- Herbal preparations
- Cosmetic preparations (e.g. Botox)

Decreasing patient perception of substance as a drug

Section 3 Figure 1 'Drugs' which may be used by patients but may not be recognised or disclosed as such.

Section 3

14 General principles underlying drug action

Learning outcomes

By the end of this chapter the reader should be able to:

- identify the four main types of protein 'drug targets' and give examples of drugs which act on each target type
- define the terms agonist, antagonist, affinity, efficacy and potency and understand how they relate to clinical practice
- understand the difference between full and partial agonists and give examples of each type of agonist currently used in practice
- describe the effect of both competitive and irreversible antagonists and be able to differentiate between them
- understand the nature, and give examples, of non-competitive, chemical, physiological and pharmacokinetic antagonism
- understand the concept of the therapeutic index.

How do drugs exert their effects in the body?

One thing that drugs have in common is that in order to affect the physiological function of the body, they need to physically interact with specific components of cells in the body. There are some exceptions to this rule, for example antacids, which are simply chemicals which act to neutralise stomach acid (Chapter 26).

Drugs also need to exert some degree of specificity in terms of the cell types and/or cell constituents with which they interact in the body. This is obvious if we think about it – if it were not for the specificity between the drug and its 'target' then all drugs would interact with similar cellular components and would exhibit similar effects – this is clearly not true. This

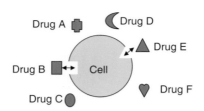

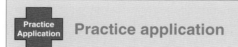

Figure 14.1 Schematic depicting the importance of shape in determining the specificity of interaction between drug and cell. Only drugs B and E would be able to interact with this particular cell type and each of these would only be able to interact with a specific site on the cell.

specificity is often determined by three-dimensional shape. All drugs have a specific shape and will bind to, or interact with, cell components which have a matching shape (Figure 14.1). This is termed the 'lock and key' hypothesis and is a useful analogy. While specificity between locks and keys is reciprocal (each key is specific for a particular lock and each lock recognises a specific key), it is not absolute; under certain circumstances a lock can be forced open with the wrong key and a badly cut key will not be able to open its particular lock. This is true also of drugs and their targets.

Essentially, when thinking about drug 'targets' we are looking at drug action at the molecular level. The immediate effects caused by the interaction between the drug and target would be considered the 'cellular' level of drug action while the impact of the drug on tissue and organ responses would be considered the 'tissue' and 'system' levels of drug action. While the action of drugs at the 'tissue' and 'system' levels is relatively clear, it is knowledge of drug action at the 'molecular' and 'cellular' levels which allows us to understand and explain some of the most important clinical aspects of drug activity.

Practice application

Drug side effects, contraindications and interactions can often be explained by knowledge of the action of a drug at the molecular and cellular levels.

Target molecules

The 'target' to which a drug binds in the body is almost always a protein. However, as with all good rules, there are exceptions, with the main exception being antitumour drugs which bind to DNA (deoxyribonucleic acid).

The proteins to which drugs bind fall into four categories:

● receptor molecules
● enzymes
● carrier molecules
● ion channels.

Examples of commonly used drugs which act on each of these four target types are shown in Box 14.1.

Box 14.1 Examples of Commonly Used Drugs (Grouped by BNF Chapter) which Act on Each of the Four Categories of Drug Target

Receptor Molecules

GI system – cimetidine, ranitidine

Cardiovascular system – atenolol, irbesartan, dobutamine

Respiratory system – salbutamol, ipratropium, montelukast, adrenaline

Central nervous system – diazepam, haloperidol, clozapine, cyclizine, domperidone, ondansetron, codeine, sumitriptan, bromocriptine

Endocrine system – insulin, rosiglitazone, prednisolone, ethinylestradiol, norethisterone

Eye – tropicamide, timolol

Enzymes

Cardiovascular system – enalapril, aspirin, heparin, simvastatin

Respiratory system – theophylline

Central nervous system – phenelzine, paracetamol, carbidopa, selegiline, donepezil

Infections – trimethoprim, rifampicin, ciprofloxacin, ritonavir, fluconazole

Obstetrics, gynaecology and urinary tract disorders – sildenafil

Carrier molecules

GI system – omeprazole

Cardiovascular system – digoxin, furosemide

Central nervous system – amitriptyline, citalopram

Ion channels

Cardiovascular system – amiloride, amlodipine

Central nervous system – ethosuximide, phenytoin

Non-target proteins

It is important to remember that not all proteins which drugs bind to or interact with actually represent drug targets. Plasma proteins such as albumin actually bind large numbers of different drugs but do not represent 'drug targets'. Plasma proteins are not drug targets for two reasons:

- they bind many different drug types and do not therefore exhibit any specificity
- binding of a drug to a plasma protein does not directly produce a physiological change in the body.

This is not to say that binding to plasma proteins is unimportant as this is not true – plasma protein binding can have profound effects on drug action within the body and we will discuss this further in Chapters 15 and 16.

Receptors

Before we can really start to think about how drugs interact with receptors, we need to understand what a receptor is. A receptor is a protein which occurs naturally in the body and acts as a recognition site for the body's normal, or endogenous, chemical mediators such as neurotransmitters, hormones and inflammatory mediators. The natural mediators interact with the receptor and stimulate a cellular response.

Many drugs used today are designed to look like, or mimic, these normal mediators so that they can act on these receptors and modulate physiological function.

Section 3

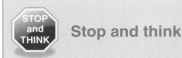

Stop and think

Do you think adrenaline, serotonin, histamine and dopamine interact with receptors in the body?

Drug–receptor interactions

Drugs which act on receptors can be divided into two classes called agonists and antagonists.

Agonists are drugs which bind to the receptor and induce the same cellular/physiological response as the normal chemical mediator. Thus agonists produce the same response as the endogenous mediator.

Antagonists are drugs which bind to the receptor but do not produce the normal cellular response; instead, they act to block the receptor, preventing the normal mediator from binding. Thus, antagonists act to reduce or inhibit the normal physiological response.

The interaction between drugs and receptors can be divided into two components: affinity and efficacy.

Affinity is the likelihood of the drug binding to the receptor. The higher the affinity of the drug for the receptor, the more likely it is to bind to that receptor.

Efficacy is the likelihood of the bound drug producing a cellular response or effect.

So an agonist has both affinity and efficacy while an antagonist has affinity but no efficacy (Figure 14.2).

Another term you may come across is potency, which is the combination of the affinity and efficacy of a drug.

$$\text{Potency} = \text{affinity} \times \text{efficacy}$$

Thus agonists are more potent than antagonists.

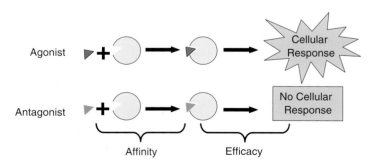

Figure 14.2   The agonist binds to the receptor and induces a cellular response. The antagonist binds to the receptor but does not induce a cellular response.

Section 3

Dose–response curves

Agonism

In terms of measuring drug action, we could measure drug binding directly but it is actually much more usual to measure the biological/physiological response to the drug. For example, if we were looking at bronchodilators we would measure peak flow and if we were looking at antihypertensives we would measure blood pressure. This allows us to determine the maximal response to a drug, known as E_{max}. The maximum biological response may be very different for different drugs and may or may not be the same as the maximum tissue response. If the maximum drug response is the same as the maximum tissue response then that drug is known as a full agonist. If we measure the biological response to different doses of drug, we can construct a dose–response curve. Dose response curves are sigmoidal or 'S' shaped (Figure 14.3).

Agonists can themselves be divided into two categories:

- full agonists which elicit a maximum tissue response (Figure 14.3)
- partial agonists which only ever exert a partial, or submaximal, tissue response even when all receptors are occupied.

A good analogy for a partial agonist is that of a badly cut key – it fits into the lock but will not always open it. In pharmacological terms, then, a partial agonist has similar affinity to, but has less efficacy than, a full agonist (Figure 14.4). While a partial agonist drug binds to the receptor, it does not always produce a cellular response; it is therefore acting as an antagonist as well as an agonist. These drugs could be described as 'partial antagonists'. Indeed, in terms of clinical application some of the 'beta-blockers' in clinical use act as partial agonists (e.g. pindolol).

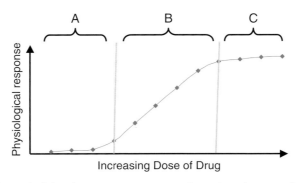

Figure 14.3   (a) At this end of the dose–response curve there is only a small physiological response because while the drug is binding to the receptor at the molecular level, this is not occurring at large enough concentrations to demonstrate a response at the tissue/organ level. (b) As the dose of drug increases, a physiological response becomes apparent and this part of the curve is actually linear. The physiological response increases proportionally to the dose of drug. (c) At this stage the maximum drug response has been reached and continuing to increase the drug dose does not result in increased physiological response. At this stage non-specific binding of the drug to other receptors may start to occur, resulting in the development of side effects.

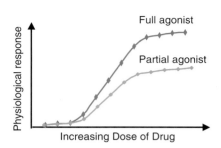

- Both dose response curves are sigmoidal in shape

- Partial agonist dose response curve is shifted to the right of the full agonist curve

- Maximal physiological response of a partial agonist is always lower than that of a full agonist and less than the maximal tissue response

Figure 14.4 Comparison of dose–response curves of a full agonist and a partial agonist.

Stop and think

Would a partial agonist be more or less potent than a full agonist?

Antagonism

An antagonist binds to the receptor in such a way as to block or prevent agonist binding – this is generally to prevent the binding of the body's natural, endogenous, mediator to the receptor and hence antagonists reduce the normal cellular/physiological response in the body.

Receptor antagonists can be divided into two categories.

Competitive antagonism

The binding which occurs between a drug and its target protein is generally weak and easily broken or 'reversible' and this type of binding is important in terms of competitive antagonism. The antagonist competes with the natural agonist for receptor binding so agonist occupancy is reduced in the presence of a competitive antagonist. This competitive antagonism is surmountable; in other words, it can be overcome. Increasing the concentration of the agonist enough will eventually overcome the action of the competitive antagonist and restore the tissue response (Figure 14.5). In terms of a full agonist dose–response curve then the presence of a fixed concentration of competitive antagonist acts to shift the curve to the right. The maximal tissue response, however, is not decreased – it just takes a larger dose of agonist to achieve this response (Figure 14.6)

Irreversible antagonism

While the binding between competitive antagonists and their target proteins is weak and reversible, a bit like using 'Blu-tack', the binding that occurs between an irreversible antagonist and its target protein is very strong and not easily overcome and could be thought of as a bit like using 'Super Glue'. Consequently, an irreversible antagonist only dissociates from its receptor very slowly or not at all. The receptor is effectively taken out of action. This means

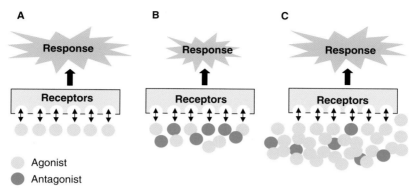

Agonist

Antagonist

Figure 14.5 Visual analogy for competitive antagonism. (a) Agonist binds to receptors and produces a cellular response. (b) Equal concentration of competitive antagonist added in, competes with the agonist for receptor binding, level of tissue response is reduced. (c) Increased concentration of agonist competes with competitive antagonist and restores level of tissue response.

that the addition of more agonist does not affect antagonist binding. This type of antagonism is non-surmountable (Figure 14.7). Thus these antagonists will have a long-acting effect on the physiological processes in the body. Indeed, in order to increase the likelihood of agonist binding, the body would have to make new receptors and this is a lengthy and time-consuming process. While most antagonists in clinical use are competitive and have a reversible action, there are a number of irreversible antagonists in clinical use (Table 14.1).

STOP and THINK Stop and think

Would irreversible antagonists have a longer or shorter duration of action than comepetitive antagonists?

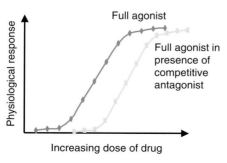

- Both dose response curves are sigmoidal in shape
- Agonist dose response curve is shifted to the right in the presence of a competitive antagonist
- Maximal physiological response of the agonist remains the same but it requires a higher concentration of agonist to produce it

Figure 14.6 Difference in dose–response curve of full agonist in the presence and absence of a competitive antagonist.

Section 3

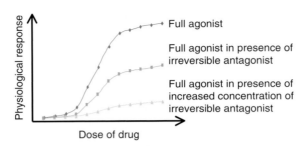

Figure 14.7 Maximum response of a full agonist is reduced in the presence of an irreversible antagonist.

Enzymes

An enzyme is a protein which speeds up a biological reaction without being chemically altered itself. Many reactions in the body occur only because of the action of an enzyme and enzymes are therefore critical for maintaining mammalian homeostasis. Enzymes are all highly specific for the type of reaction they catalyse and must interact with, or bind to, one of the substrates in order to catalyse the reaction. This interaction is another example of a 'lock and key' mechanism. Drugs which target enzymes inhibit their activity and they do this in a number of slightly different ways.

Competitive (Reversible) inhibition

The drug interacts with the active site of the enzyme in a similar way to the natural substrate binding to the enzyme. Thus the drug competes with the natural substrate for the binding site on the enzyme. This is essentially the same process as competitive antagonism, with the chemical bonds being weak and easily broken.

Table 14.1 Examples of drugs in clinical use which act as agonists, competitive antagonists and irreversible antagonists.

Drug action	Examples in clinical use
Agonist	Salbutamol (β_2-adrenoceptor agonist) Morphine (opioid receptor agonist) Norethisterone (progesterone receptor agonist)
Competitive antagonist	Atenolol (beta-adrenoreceptor antagonist) Cimetidine (histamine receptor antagonist) Ipratropium (muscarinic acetylcholine receptor antagonist) Ondansetron ($5HT_3$ receptor antagonist)
Irreversible antagonist	Phenoxybenzamine (α-adrenoceptor antagonist) Candesartan (angiotensin II receptor antagonist) Clopidogrel (ADP receptor antagonist)

Table 14.2   Examples of drugs in clinical use which act as reversible and irreversible enzyme inhibitors.

Drug action	Examples of drugs
Reversible enzyme inhibitors	Ibuprofen, enalapril, simvastatin, selegiline, aspirin
Irreversible enzyme inhibitors	Aspirin

Irreversible inhibition

In this situation the drug binds to the enzyme using strong covalent bonds which are not easily broken. Thus the enzyme is irreversibly inhibited in much the same way that an irreversible antagonist acts on a receptor. The action of an irreversible enzyme inhibitor is very long-lived and in order to overcome this inhibition, the body will need to make new enzyme.

Most drugs in clinical use act by competitive or reversible inhibition but there are a small number of drugs which use irreversible inhibition (Table 14.2).

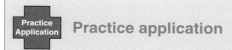

Practice application

Aspirin and ibuprofen both act by inhibiting the enzyme cyclooxygenase (COX) but only aspirin has an irreversible effect. It is this difference that makes aspirin, but not ibuprofen, an effective antiplatelet drug.

Carrier proteins

Ions and a number of other small molecules such as neurotransmitters are too polar to readily cross cell membranes and so use carrier proteins to move them across membranes (Chapter 15). The carrier proteins contain a recognition site which makes them specific for particular ions or molecules and these recognition sites can be targeted by drugs which bind to the recognition site and prevent the interaction between carrier protein and its specific ion/molecule. Once again, the action of drugs on these carriers can be either reversible, using weak binding forces, or irreversible, using covalent binding. Most drugs act reversibly or competitively on the carrier molecule; however, proton pump inhibitors act to irreversibly inhibit the proton pump.

Ion channels

Ion channels are proteins which act as 'gated tunnels' to allow the passage of ions across membranes. These proteins can be targeted by drugs to block the ion channel, preventing the passage of ions across the membrane as is the case with local anaesthetics. Alternatively, drugs can bind to a different area on the ion channel and modulate its activity, either by promoting channel opening, 'keeping the gate open' (e.g. benzodiazepines), or by reducing channel opening, 'shutting the gate' (e.g. dihydropyridines).

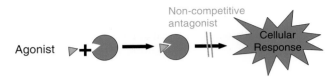

Figure 14.8   Site of action of a non-competitive antagonist.

Drug antagonism

There are a number of forms of drug antagonism, other than antagonism by receptor blockade, which also impact on clinical practice.

Non-competitive antagonism

This type of antagonism refers to the situation where the 'antagonist' interferes with the cellular response to an agonist. The 'antagonist' does not interact at receptor level so agonist binding occurs normally. Instead, the 'antagonist' acts to inhibit part of the cellular response to the agonist (Figure 14.8). Examples of drugs which act as non-competitive antagonists include calcium channel blockers such as nifedipine. Normally the binding of noradrenaline or angiotensin II to their specific receptors results in increased calcium concentration and leads to smooth muscle contraction. Calcium channel blockers do not interfere with the agonist (such as noradrenaline or angiotensin II) binding to its receptor but instead they prevent calcium entering the cell and therefore inhibit cell contraction.

Chemical antagonism

A chemical antagonist binds to a drug in solution, either in gastric fluid or in plasma, to produce a complex which has no activity. An example of a drug which acts as a 'chemical antagonist' is protamine which binds to heparin in the plasma and forms an inactive complex. The activity of heparin in the plasma is then lost. Protamine is used as an antidote to overanticoagulation with heparin.

Pharmacokinetic antagonism

This refers to the situation where the 'antagonist' reduces the acitivity of the drug by modulating the pharmacokinetic processes. This can occur in a number of ways.

● The 'antagonist' reduces the absorption of the active drug from the GI tract.
● The 'antagonist' increases the metabolism of the active drug in the liver.
● The antagonist' increases the rate of excretion of the active drug from the body.

An example of a drug which acts as a pharmacokinetic antagonist is rifampicin which speeds up the metabolism of a number of other drugs, thus reducing their activity. These types of interactions are very important in the clinical context (further information in Chapter 19).

Physiological antagonism

This refers to the situation where the physiological antagonist has the opposite effect to another drug in the body. Thus the activities of both the 'physiological antagonist' and the 'drug' are effectively cancelled out.

Physiological antagonism occurs more frequently in patients who are taking large numbers of drugs (polypharmacy), such as the elderly.

Therapeutic index

Rather than measuring a drug's value purely in terms of the desired response, a more appropriate measure of drug activity would take into account both the 'wanted' and 'unwanted' effects. The therapeutic index or TI is such a measure, taking into account both beneficial and toxic effects. The TI can be defined as the median toxic dose of a drug (the dose which produces unwanted effects in 50% of the population) divided by the median effective dose (the dose which produces a therapeutic effect in 50% of people).

$$TI = \frac{\text{Median toxic dose}}{\text{Median effective dose}} \qquad TI = \frac{TD_{50}}{ED_{50}}$$

If the median toxic dose is much larger than the median effective dose then the drug will have a large TI and hence a large safety margin. Drugs which have a small TI need to be monitored regularly to ensure that toxicity does not develop.

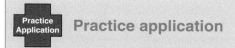

Practice application

Most drugs in clinical practice have a large TI. However, some drugs, including warfarin, phenytoin and theophylline, have a small TI and their levels in the body need monitoring.

Summary

- Drugs generally need to interact with target molecules to exert an effect.
- Drug targets are generally one of the following types of proteins: receptors, enzymes, ion channels, carrier molecules.
- Receptors are recognition sites for the body's natural chemical mediators.
- Agonists bind to receptors and induce a physiological response while antagonists bind to receptors but do not produce a response.
- Affinity is the likelihood of a drug binding to a receptor while efficacy is the likelihood of this binding resulting in a physiological response.
- Potency describes the product of a drug's affinity and efficacy.
- Partial agonists always give a submaximal response even when all receptor sites are bound.

Section 3

- Competitive antagonism is surmountable and involves weak binding such as ionic and hydrogen bonds; irreversible antagonism involves strong covalent bonds and is not surmountable.
- Non-competitive antagonism does not inhibit receptor binding but instead acts on the signalling response induced by the agonist.
- Chemical antagonism is the combination of an 'antagonist' and drug in solution resulting in the production of an inactive complex.
- Pharmacokinetic antagonists act to reduce drug absorption or increase drug metabolism or excretion.
- Physiological antagonism can be the result of polypharmacy.
- The therapeutic index is a measure of the safety of a drug.

Activity

1. Which of the following is not a drug target?
   A. Receptor
   B. Carrier protein
   C. Lipid
   D. Enzyme
2. Which of the following statements about partial agonists is untrue?
   A. They only ever give a submaximal response.
   B. They have similar potency to a full agonist.
   C. The dose–response curve of a partial agonist is shifted to the right of the dose–response curve of a full agonist.
   D. They have a high receptor affinity.
3. Which of the following drugs acts as an irreversible receptor antagonist?
   A. Salbutamol
   B. Atenolol
   C. Simvastatin
   D. Candesartan
4. Which of the following forms of drug antagonism describes the action of protamine on heparin?
   A. Receptor blockade
   B. Non-competitive antagonism
   C. Chemical antagonism
   D. Pharmacokinetic antagonism
5. Which of the following drugs acts to irreversibly inhibit enzyme activity?
   A. Aspirin
   B. Ibuprofen
   C. Simvastatin
   D. Enalapril
6. Which of the following statements is incorrect?
   A. Agonists mimic the body's normal physiological response.
   B. Agonists have affinity and efficacy.
   C. Irreversible antagonists use covalent binding.
   D. Antagonists have similar efficacy to agonists.

Reusable learning objects

- Lock and key hypothesis.
  www.nottingham.ac.uk/nursing/sonet/rlos/bioproc/lock_and_key/index.html
- Atomic bonding.
  www.nottingham.ac.uk/nursing/sonet/rlos/bioproc/atomic_bonding/index.html
- Drug–receptor interaction.
  www.nottingham.ac.uk/nursing/sonet/rlos/bioproc/drug-receptor/index.html

Reference

Rang, H.P., Dale, M.M., Ritter, J.M. and Flower, R. (2007) *Rang and Dale's Pharmacology*, 6th edn, Churchill Livingstone, Edindurgh.

Further reading

Birkett, D.J. (2002) *Pharmacokinetics Made Easy*, 2nd edn, McGraw-Hill, Australia.

British Medical Association and Royal Pharmaceutical Society of Great Britain (2010) *British National Formulary*, 59th edn, BMJ Publishing, London

Cattaneo, M. (2006) P2Y12 receptor antagonists: a rapidly expanding group of antiplatelet agents. *Eur Heart J*, **27**, 1010–1012.

Foster, R.W. (2003) *Basic Pharmacology*, 4th edn, Arnold, London.

Kenakri, T. (1997) *Molecular Pharmacology. A Short Course*, Blackwell, Oxford.

McGavock, H. (2005) *How Drugs Work. Basic Pharmacology for Healthcare Professionals*, 2nd edn, Radcliffe Publishing, Oxford.

Page, C.P., Curtis, M.J., Sutter, M.C., *et al.* (2006) *Integrated Pharmacology*, 3rd edn, Mosby, London.

Sica, D.A. (2001) Clinical pharmacology of the angiotensin receptor antagonists. *J Clin Pharmacol*, **3**, 45–49.

Smith, H.J. (2006) *Smith and Williams' Introduction to the Principles of Drug Design and Action*, 4th edn, Taylor and Francis, Boca Raton.

Section 3

15 Pharmacokinetics 1 – absorption and distribution

Learning outcomes

By the end of this chapter the reader should be able to:

- describe the mechanisms used by drug molecules to cross cell membranes
- understand the influence of environmental pH on lipid solubility and drug absorption
- define the terms absorption and distribution and differentiate between them
- list the five major drug compartments in the body
- understand the nature of plasma protein binding and its effect on drug distribution
- describe the concept of 'volume of distribution' and how lipid solubility might affect this.

Pharmacokinetics is essentially about what the body does to the drug or, perhaps more specifically, how the body handles the drug. Pharmacokinetics can be divided into four separate processes:

Absorption

Distribution

Metabolism

Excretion.

The first letter of each of these processes has been highlighted in bold because you may see the acronym ADME referred to in drug literature or other textbooks. ADME refers to the processes of absorption, distribution, metabolism and excretion.

The New Prescriber. Edited by J Lymn, D Bowskill, F Bath-Hextall, R Knaggs, © 2010 John Wiley & Sons.

Section 3

This chapter is going to concentrate on the first two of these processes – absorption and distribution.

In Chapter 14 we described how drugs need to be present at an adequate concentration at the target in order to exert a pharmacological effect. It is the processes of absorption and distribution which are key to ensuring that this occurs.

How do drugs get into the body?

Almost all drugs need to cross cell membranes in order to get into the body. For example, drugs which are given orally will need to cross the membranes of the cells in the GI tract, while drugs administered by transdermal patch will need to cross the membranes of skin cells in order to reach the bloodstream.

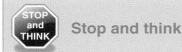

Stop and think

Not all routes of administration require drug absorption to occur. Why do you think the intravenous and inhaled routes do not strictly require drug absorption to occur?

Cell membranes

If you remember some basic biology, you will recall that cell membranes consist of a lipid bilayer or two layers of lipid molecules. Each lipid molecule consists of a polar, or water-loving, head and a non-polar, or water-hating, tail (Figure 15.1). The majority of the lipids contained in mammalian cell membranes are cholesterol, phospholipids and glycolipids. Perhaps the most interesting thing about lipid bilayers is that they will form spontaneously in aqueous solutions as the lipid molecules will automatically arrange themselves so that the hydrocarbon tails are facing away from the aqueous environment.

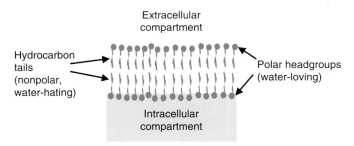

Figure 15.1 The lipid bilayer which makes up the cell plasma membrane.

Section 3

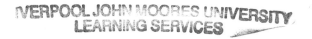

Mechanisms of crossing cell membranes

Now that we know why drugs need to cross cell membranes, we need to turn our attention to how they do it. There are two main mechanisms by which drugs can cross cell membranes:

- diffusion directly through lipid
- combination with a carrier protein.

Diffusion through lipid

This is exactly what it says it is – the drug literally diffuses through the membrane from an area of high concentration to an area of lower concentration. The ability of drugs to use this mechanism is very dependent on their chemical nature. So what do we mean when we say that a drug's ability to diffuse through lipid depends on its chemical nature? Essentially, it means that 'like dissolves in like' – non-polar substances dissolve in freely in non-polar solvents. Lipids are non-polar so non-polar substances will dissolve freely in lipids. In Figure 15.1 we show that cell membranes consist of a lipid bilayer so non-polar substances will diffuse freely across cell membranes while polar or charged molecules will not (Figure 15.2).

Examples of 'like dissolves in like' are common in general life – particularly in relation to cooking. If you added a few drops of red food dye to a pan of water, they dissolve,completely, making the water pink. On the other hand, when cooking pasta you might add a few drops of oil to the pan of water; this does not dissolve in the water no matter how hard you try – it remains in small discrete globules which are easily visible in the water. If you added a few drops of olive oil to a pan of vegetable oil, however, it would dissolve completely. So in terms of pharmacokinetics, the most important chemical factor which determines a drug's ability to diffuse across cell membranes is its lipid solubility.

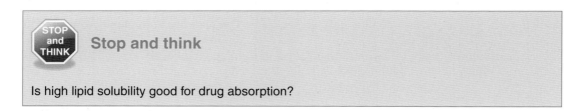

Stop and think

Is high lipid solubility good for drug absorption?

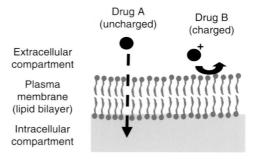

Figure 15.2   Diffusion through lipid (adapted from Rang *et al.,* 2007).

Box 15.1   Explanation of the multitude of terms which can be used to describe lipid solubility.

Lipid soluble	Non-polar
	Unionised
	Lipophilic
	Hydrophobic
	Uncharged
Water soluble	Polar
	Ionised
	Lipophobic
	Hydrophilic
	Charged

There are a number of terms which are often used interchangeably to describe a drug's lipid solubility (Box 15.1) and it is important to be aware of all these terms and what they mean.

Acid–base relationships and lipid solubility

In reality, however, many drugs are weak acids or weak bases which means they exist as a mixture of non-polar and polar forms. The ratio of non-polar to polar forms is defined by something called the pKa of the drug – this is the pH at which the drug exists at a 50:50 equilibrium between the non-polar (unionised) and polar (ionised) forms. Remember, only the non-polar form is lipid soluble and hence only this form will readily diffuse across cell membranes.

A basic knowledge of acids and bases is important for pharmacology because the pH of the environment the drug is in will affect the amount of drug in the non-polar, lipid-soluble form, thus affecting the extent and rate at which it is able to cross membranes. This has an impact on both absorption and excretion (Chapter 16). Weak acids in solution are able to give up a hydrogen ion (H^+) and become ionised (negatively charged) while weak bases are able to accept a hydrogen ion and become ionised (positively charged). On the other hand, strong acids, like the hydrochloric acid in the stomach, are permanently ionised and exist as H^+ and Cl^-.

pH refers to the acidity or alkalinity of a solution, or the number of free hydrogen ions (H^+); the higher the concentration of H^+, the lower the pH, or the more acidic the solution. A change in the pH of the environment from the pKa of the weak acid or base (as might occur with the movement of drug from the stomach to the intestine) will substantially affect the proportion of the non-polar (unionised) form. A change of 1 pH unit below the pKa of a weak acid will result in 90% of the drug being unionised while a change of 2 pH units below the pKa will result in 99% of the drug being unionised. Similarly, a change of 1 pH unit above the pKa of a weak base will result in 90% of the drug being ionised and a change of 2 pH units will result in 99% being ionised.

In an acid environment like the stomach, there are plenty of free H^+ ions and hence there is no need for a weak acid to give up its own H^+. Thus drugs which are weak acids tend to exist in the unionised (non-polar) form in the stomach and can start to be absorbed across the stomach membranes.

Section 3

Table 15.1   Key facts concerning degree of ionisation of drugs which are weak acids and weak bases.

	Weak acids	Weak bases
Acid environment (e.g. stomach)	Unionised	Ionised
Basic environment (e.g. gut)	Ionised	Unionised

Drugs which are weak bases, however, will be more inclined to accept H^+ from the plentiful supply in the stomach acid and will as a result exist mainly in the ionised (polar) form and will not start to be absorbed until further down the GI tract when the pH of the environment is more favourable.

It might be simpler just to think of this as acidic drugs are unionised in acidic conditions while basic drugs are unionised in basic conditions and ionised in acidic conditions (Table 15.1).

 Practice application

If you know the pKa of a drug and the pH of the environment, you can work out its exact degree of ionisation using simple calculators available on the internet such as: www.manuelsweb.com/pka.htm.

Examples of common drugs which are acidic and basic in chemical nature are identified in Table 15.2.

Use of a carrier molecule

In this case the drug will bind to (interact with) the carrier protein on the outer surface of the plasma membrane. This interaction between drug and carrier protein leads to a conformational change, or change in the shape, of the carrier protein, resulting in the protein essentially

Table 15.2   Examples of commonly used drugs which are either acidic or basic in nature.

Acidic drugs	Basic drugs
Aspirin	Caffeine
Phenytoin	Theophylline
Warfarin	Morphine
Methotrexate	Pethidine
Ascorbic acid (vitamin C)	Erythromycin
Zidovudine	Amphetamine
Penicillin V	Propranolol
Tetracycline	Trimethoprim

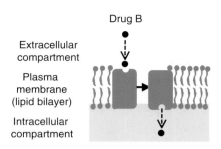

Figure 15.3   A drug crossing a cell membrane by using a carrier molecule (adapted from Rang *et al.*, 2007).

flipping over so that the drug binding site is located on the inner surface of the plasma membrane. The drug is then released from the carrier protein into the intracellular compartment. This release of drug again causes a conformational change in the protein so that it flips back to its original position and is thus ready to bind to and carry another drug molecule across the membrane (Figure 15.3).

Since this method of crossing cell membranes requires the drug to interact with the carrier protein at a specific binding site, it can show saturation kinetics at high drug concentrations. Essentially, then, the rate of absorption across the cell membrane is determined by the number of available carrier molecules.

It may be easier to understand what is meant by saturation using visualisation. If, for example, the cell membrane contains 10 carrier molecules and there are five drug molecules then these will all be carried across the cell membrane within a specific time period. Similarly, if there are 10 drug molecules then these could all be carried across the cell membrane within the same time period – this would appear to increase the rate of absorption of the drug. However, if the number of drug molecules increases to 30, the rate of absorption remains constant, or saturated, because there are only a fixed number of carrier molecules which can only carry a fixed number of drug molecules within a fixed time period (Figure 15.4).

 Practice application

Carrier molecules can act as drug targets (Chapter 14). Drugs can bind to carrier molecules thus preventing other drugs from using these carrier molecules.

For example, probenicid used to be given with penicillin to prolong its action – probenicid binds to the carrier molecules in the kidney tubule, thus preventing penicillin from binding. In this way the excretion of penicillin from the body was delayed and hence it remained active in the body for longer.

Carrier molecules are important:

● in the GI tract – levodopa (a drug used to treat Parkinson's disease) and fluorouracil (an anticancer drug) both use carrier molecules to cross the intestinal mucosa

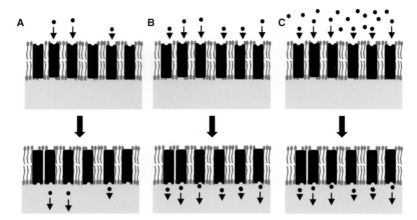

Figure 15.4 Saturation of carrier protein and its impact on drug absorption. (a) Complete drug absorption occurs. (b) Complete drug absorption occurs (rate appears to increase). (c) Carriers are saturated, rate of absorption remains fixed.

- in the biliary tract – a considerable number of drugs and metabolites of drugs are transported from the liver into the bile using carrier proteins
- at the blood–brain barrier – levodopa is carried across the blood–brain barrier
- in the renal tubule – acidic and basic carrier proteins exist in the kidney and act to carry drugs into the renal tubule.

Drug absorption

Absorption is defined as the passage of the drug from its site of administration into the plasma. Drug absorption is essential for almost all drugs, except those given intravenously and inhaled anti-asthma drugs. This is because drugs given IV enter the plasma directly and therefore bypass the need to cross cell membranes while anti-asthma drugs given by the inhaled route are delivered directly to the cells in the lungs on which they will act.

While drug absorption can start in the stomach (specifically weak acids), the majority of absorption occurs in the intestine. This is because the intestine has a much larger surface area, due to the villi and microvilli of the ileum (approximately 200 m^2 compared to 1 m^2 in the stomach), and also because drugs tend to be in the intestine for a much longer period of time compared to the stomach.

Most drugs are administered orally and are influenced by factors which affect GI function. The absorption of drugs from other routes can also be affected by a number of factors (Chapter 18).

Drug distribution

Drug distribution refers to the specific localisation of drugs within the body. Once drugs have been absorbed into the plasma, they are carried around the body in the bloodstream prior to

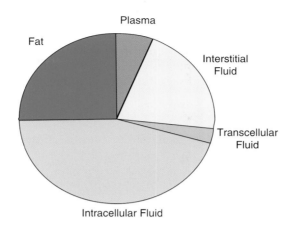

Figure 15.5   The relative proportions of drug compartments in the body.

reaching their specific site of action. Drugs can be distributed within a number of different compartments of the body including:

- plasma
- interstitial fluid (fluid which surrounds the cells)
- transcellular fluid (e.g. digestive secretions, cerebrospinal fluid)
- intracellular fluid (fluid contained in the cells)
- fat.

The relative proportions of these drug compartments is shown in Figure 15.5.

Drug distribution exhibits a number of patterns depending on which of these compartments the drug localises in, and may be classified as follows:

- remains within the vascular system
- distributes in body water
- concentrates in specific tissues
- distributes throughout body water and tissues.

These distribution patterns in turn are dependent on:

- plasma protein binding
- accumulation in tissues.

Plasma protein binding

As discussed previously in this chapter, many drugs exist as weak acids or bases consisting of a mixture of ionised and unionised forms. While the unionised form is good for absorption, passing readily through the plasma membranes, it is relatively insoluble in the aqueous environment of the plasma and needs to bind to plasma proteins in order to move around the body in the plasma.

Section 3

It is important to remember that plasma proteins do not represent drug targets as they do not show specificity in terms of their binding nor does drug binding to them induce a physiological response; they are essentially a transport system.

The major plasma proteins are albumin, acid-glycoprotein and beta-globulin with albumin being arguably the most important of these. Examples of drugs bound to plasma proteins are shown in Box 15.2.

Box 15.2 Examples of drugs that bind to the plasma proteins albumin and acid-glycoprotein.

Albumin	Acid-glycoprotein
Aspirin	Propranolol
Warfarin	Lidocaine
Indometacin	Imipramine
Phenytoin	Chlorpromazine
Diazepam	

Drugs bind readily and reversibly to plasma proteins according to the following equation:

$$\text{Unbound drug} + \text{free plasma protein} \leftrightarrow \text{plasma protein-drug complex}$$

It is important to be aware that only the unbound, or free, drug is available to act on its specific drug target and exert a pharmacological effect. As the unbound drug passes into the tissues, there is a corresponding release of plasma protein-bound drug. The extent of plasma protein binding is different for individual drugs (Table 15.3) but may be as high as 99%, in which case the fraction of free, unbound drug available to have a pharmacological effect will only be 1%.

It is possible, therefore, that a reduction in the concentration of plasma proteins in the body (hypoalbuminaemia) can affect the activity of highly plasma protein-bound drugs such as warfarin and phenytoin (Figure 15.6). Hypoalbuminaemia can occur in patients suffering from cirrhosis, nephritic syndrome, severe burns, chronic inflammation and malnutrition.

Table 15.3 Examples of drugs across the range of plasma protein concentrations.

Drug	Plasma protein binding (%)
Warfarin	99
Diazepam	96
Propranolol	90
Phenytoin	87
Fentanyl	80
Theophylline	40
Digoxin	30
Gentamicin	<10

Section 3

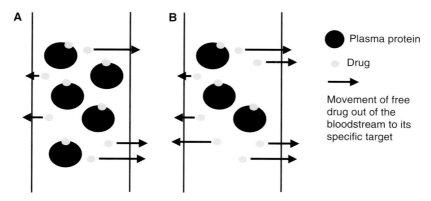

Figure 15.6 (a) A normal plasma protein concentration with 50% of drug free and able to leave the bloodstream to reach its specific target. (b) A reduced plasma protein concentration but the same drug dose; in this situation 70% of the drug is free and available to act on its target.

Plasma protein binding may also be affected by competition between drugs. Albumin has two major drug-binding sites (site I and site II) which bind acidic drugs. Drugs which bind to the same site will compete with each other for the binding site, resulting in drug displacement.

Warfarin and non-steroidal anti-inflammatory drug (NSAIDs) both bind to site I and the NSAID will displace warfarin from the albumin binding site, resulting in an increase in the free warfarin concentration. This is the reason why NSAIDs should not be used in patients taking warfarin.

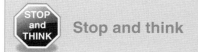 **Stop and think**

What is the likely pattern of distribution for drugs which are very tightly bound to plasma proteins or are very large in size?

Accumulation in tissues

Most drugs have their effects in body tissues and the degree of accumulation of drugs in the tissues depends on the lipid solubility of the drug. As discussed previously, the more lipid soluble a drug, the more readily it will cross plasma membranes. Drugs which can cross cell membranes often tend to be distributed throughout body fluids and tissues. Some highly lipid-soluble drugs such as the benzodiazepines can accumulate in body fat. Remember, body fat is a highly non-polar body compartment.

Blood flow to the tissue

In just the same way that blood flow impacts on drug absorption, it also affects drug distribution. Drugs will distribute to the most highly vascularised tissue such as the heart, lungs and brain first. This is followed by tissues which have a moderate blood flow such as muscle

Section 3

and then lastly tissues such as fat which have a low blood supply. Benzodiazepines take some time to accumulate in body fat because of the low blood flow to this area, hence accumulation only occurs following chronic use of these drugs. However, this low blood supply also means that these drugs are only slowly released from fat stores once drug administration has ceased.

Specific drug accumulation

Some drugs have a high affinity for particular areas of the body and will accumulate in these areas. For example, tetracycline has a high affinity for calcium and consequently accumulates in areas of the body which have high levels of calcium such as bones and teeth.

Practice application

Accumulation of tetracycline in developing teeth results in discolouration which is permanent and may affect bone growth. This is why we do not give tetracycline to children or pregnant women.

Similarly, the drug chloroquine is used to prevent malaria and for the treatment of rheumatoid arthritis and systemic lupus erythematosus. It has, however, been shown to have a high affinity for melanin-containing tissues and can accumulate in the retina of the eye, causing retinopathy. This can occur in up to 16% of rheumatoid patients and the Royal College of Ophthalmologists has issued guidelines for screening to prevent ocular toxicity for patients on long-term treatment.

Volume of distribution

The volume of distribution (Vd) is defined as the total volume of plasma that would be required to contain the total body content of the drug at the same concentration at which it is present in the plasma. This is not a real volume but rather represents a theoretical volume and describes the ability of the drug to distribute throughout body tissues. Consequently it is referred to as the apparent volume of distribution. It is measured in litres and can be calculated from the equation below:

$$\text{Vd (apparent)} = \frac{\text{amount of drug in the body}}{\text{plasma drug concentration}}$$

Drugs which are retained within the plasma, because of either their size or their protein binding, will have a Vd similar to that of plasma volume and drugs which distribute throughout body tissues will have a Vd similar to that of total body water. However, drugs which have high affinity for specific peripheral tissues may show very low plasma concentrations and hence will have a Vd which is much larger than that of total body water (Figure 15.7). In general, then, lipid-soluble drugs will tend to have a larger Vd than more water-soluble polar drugs.

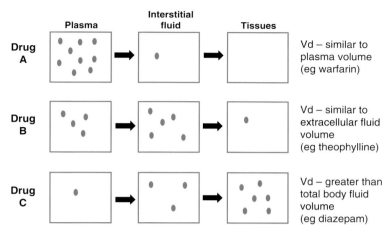

Figure 15.7   Different patterns of drug distribution in the body and examples of each.

The Vd is important clinically:

- in calculating the loading dose of drugs
- in overdose – drugs with a small Vd could be treated by dialysis as they are relatively contained within the plasma while drugs with a larger Vd cannot as these have left the plasma compartment and are distributed throughout body tisues.

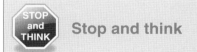 **Stop and think**

Why is it that overdoses of digoxin (Vd 500 l) and nortriptyline (Vd 1500 l) cannot be managed by dialysis?

Summary

- Lipid-soluble drugs are readily absorbed.
- Most drugs are weak acids or weak bases and exist in a mixture of charged and uncharged forms.
- Environmental pH will affect the proportion of charged forms of weak acids and bases.
- The rate of absorption of polar drugs which use carrier molecules is saturable.
- Absorption of oral drugs occurs in the intestine.
- Drug absorption is not required for drugs given IV or for inhaled respiratory drugs.
- Many drugs are carried around the body bound to plasma proteins.
- Plasma proteins are not drug targets.
- Only drug which is not bound to plasma protein (free drug) can exert a pharmacological effect.
- Drug distribution is affected by plasma protein binding, lipid solubility and blood flow.

Section 3

- Drugs are distributed to the brain, heart and lungs first and fat last.
- Drugs which are very large or with a high affinity for plasma proteins will remain within the plasma.
- Lipid-soluble drugs will distribute more readily to tissues and will show a larger Vd than polar drugs.
- Vd is important for calculating loading dose.

✎ Activity

1. The passage of a drug molecule across a lipid membrane is influenced by the:
   - lipid solubility of the drug — True / False
   - route of administration — True / False
   - degree of ionisation of the molecule — True / False
   - pH of the surrounding medium — True / False
   - presence of carrier molecules — True / False
2. With regard to drug absorption, which of the following statements are correct?
   - Is required for drugs given by all routes — True / False
   - The rate and extent of absorption following oral administration are dependent on the pH of the gut — True / False
   - Always starts in the stomach — True / False
   - Is unaffected by the lipid solubility of a drug — True / False
   - The rate of absorption of very polar drugs may depend on carrier molecules — True / False
3. With regard to plasma protein binding, which of the following statements are correct?
   - Drugs bound to plasma proteins readily cross cell membranes — True / False
   - Albumin, acid-glycoprotein and beta-globulin are all plasma proteins — True / False
   - Plasma protein concentrations can be reduced in malnutrition — True / False
   - Plasma proteins are important drug targets — True / False
   - Plasma protein binding can restrict the pattern of drug distribution — True / False
4. With regard to volume of distribution, which of the following statements are correct?
   - It represents the total volume of the body. — True / False
   - Is generally larger for lipid-soluble compared to polar drugs — True / False
   - Is important for calculating a loading dose — True / False
   - Is not affected by the size of the drug or its plasma protein binding — True / False
   - Describes the ability of a drug to distribute throughout body tissues — True / False

Useful websites

Ocular toxicity and hydroxychloroquine: guidelines for screening 2004. www.rcophth.ac.uk/docs/publications/published-guidelines/Oculartoxicity2004.pdf

Reusable learning objects

- Acids, alkalis and bases: an introduction.
  www.nottingham.ac.uk/nursing/sonet/rlos/science/acid_base_intro/index.html

- Acids, alkalis and bases: further application.
  www.nottingham.ac.uk/nursing/sonet/rlos/science/acid_base_further_app/
- Concentration gradients.
  www.nottingham.ac.uk/nursing/sonet/rlos/bioproc/gradients/index.html
- Plasma proteins and drug distribution.
  www.nottingham.ac.uk/nursing/sonet/rlos/bioproc/plasma_proteins/index.html
- Volume of distribution. www.nottingham.ac.uk/nursing/sonet/rlos/bioproc/vd/

Further reading

Abelow, B. (1998) *Understanding Acid-Base*, Lippincott, Williams and Wilkins, Philadelphia.

Bertagnolio, S., Tacconelli, E., Camilli, G. and Tumbarello, M. (2001) Case report: retinopathy after malaria prophylaxis with chloroquine. *Am J Trop Med Hyg*, **65**, 637-638.

Birkett, D.J. (2002) *Pharmacokinetics Made Easy*, 2nd edn, McGraw-Hill, Australia.

British Medical Association and Royal Pharmaceutical Society of Great Britain (2010) *British National Formulary*, 59th edn, BMJ Publishing, London.

Browning, D.J. (2002) Hydroxychloroquine and chloroquine retinopathy: screening for drug toxicity. *Am J Ophthalmol*, **133**, 649-656.

Foster, R.W. (2003) *Basic Pharmacology*, 4th edn, Arnold, London.

Lindup, W.E. and Orme, M.C.L.E. (1981) Plasma protein drug binding. *BMJ*, **282**, 212-214.

McGavock, H. (2005) *How Drugs Work. Basic Pharmacology for Healthcare Professionals*, 2nd edn, Radcliffe Publishing, Oxford.

Page, C.P., Curtis, M.J., Sutter, M.C., *et al.* (2006) *Integrated Pharmacology*, 3rd edn, Mosby, London.

Rang, H.P., Dale, M.M., Ritter, J.M. and Flower, R. (2007) *Rang and Dale's Pharmacology*, 6th edn, Churchill Livingstone, Edinburgh.

Smith, H.J. (2006) *Smith and Williams' Introduction to the Principles of Drug Design and Action*, 4th edn, Taylor and Francis, Boca Raton.

Warren, S.E. and Fanestil, D.D. (1979) Digoxin overdose. Limitations of haemoperfusion-haemodialysis treatment. *JAMA*, **242**, 2100-2101.

Section 3

16 Pharmacokinetics 2 – metabolism and excretion

Learning outcomes

By the end of this chapter the reader should be able to:

- understand the terms metabolism and excretion and differentiate between them
- understand the nature and relevance of drug metabolism with particular reference to:
    inducers and inhibitors
    pharmacogenetics
    active metabolites
    toxic metabolites
    pro-drugs.
- understand the concepts of first-pass metabolism and bioavailability and how they are related
- describe how drug metabolism may be affected by age and disease
- understand the fundamental processes involved in drug excretion via the kidneys
- understand how renal drug excretion can be affected by pH, age and disease
- understand the nature of biliary excretion and the importance of enterohepatic recycling
- understand the concept of drug clearance
- understand the concept of half-life.

Drug elimination

This is the irreversible loss of drug from the body and is made up of the two processes of metabolism and excretion. Metabolism is defined as the enzymatic conversion of one drug entity to another while excretion is the removal of the drug from the body. It is important to recognise that the definition of metabolism is not concerned with inactivating drugs. Drug

The New Prescriber. Edited by J Lymn, D Bowskill, F Bath-Hextall, R Knaggs, © 2010 John Wiley & Sons.

metabolism is often referred to in physiology textbooks as being 'detoxification'; this is not entirely accurate as drug metabolism does not always result in pharmacological inactivation, as we shall see later.

Drug metabolism

In Chapter 15 we defined lipid solubility as the key determinant of a drug's ability to cross cell membranes and stated that lipid solubility was good for absorption. However, drugs cannot distinguish between the cell membranes of the GI tract and the renal tubules so lipid-soluble drugs are readily reabsorbed from the renal tubules back into the circulation. Consequently, lipid-soluble drugs are not excreted efficiently by the kidneys. Lipid solubility is therefore good for drug absorption but bad for drug excretion. Hence the purpose of metabolism is to make drugs more polar, less lipophilic, thereby enhancing the body's ability to excrete them.

Drug metabolism occurs primarily in the liver, although some can occur in the gut, lungs and plasma. Drug metabolism in the gut wall is important for oral drugs and we will discuss this in more detail later in the chapter. Above we defined metabolism as the enzymatic conversion of one chemical entity to another; the most important enzyme system involved is called the cytochrome P450 system. Drug metabolism can be divided into two different phases, simply called phase I metabolism and phase II metabolism. These two phases can occur singly or sequentially (phase I followed by phase II). Both of these types of reaction reduce lipid solubility, thereby increasing excretion efficiency.

Phase I drug metabolism reactions can be divided into three types of chemical reactions:

- oxidation
- reduction
- hydrolysis.

The cytochrome P450 enzymes are involved in phase I oxidation and reduction enzymes. The key point to remember about phase I metabolism is that while it reduces lipid solubility, it does not necessarily result in inactivation of the drug.

Phase II drug metabolism involves the process of conjugation – this means the attachment of a polar chemical group (glucuronyl, methyl, acetyl, sulphate or glutathione) to the drug or phase I metabolite. Unlike phase I metabolism, while phase II metabolism reduces lipid solubility it almost always results in drug inactivation (Figure 16.1).

Cytochrome P450 enzyme system

Location

The cytochrome P450 enzymes are located in the smooth endoplasmic reticulum of liver cells (hepatocytes) and the gut wall. This represents the ideal location since in order for drugs to reach these enzymes, they must cross the cell membrane and find their way to the endoplasmic reticulum. Only lipid-soluble drugs will be able to do this easily. Drug metabolism is more important for lipid-soluble drugs because without metabolism, they will not be excreted efficiently, so where better to house the metabolising enzymes than this highly membranous structure within the cells?

Section 3

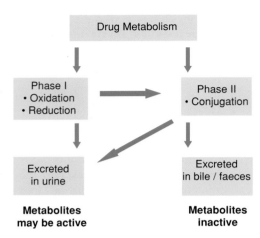

Figure 16.1 Depicts the phases of, and enzymatic processes involved in, drug metabolism.

Activity

The cytochrome P450 family of enzymes is actually a large superfamily of related enzymes which are involved in the metabolism of drugs, steroids and carcinogens. While there are around 74 families of cytochrome P450, there are only three main families involved in human drug metabolism. These are referred to as CYP1, CYP2 and CYP3. Each family contains a number of individual enzymes which are represented by the addition of a further letter and number, for example CYP1A2, CYP2C9, CYP2D6, CYP3A4. Each of these individual enzymes has distinct drug substrate specificities, although there may be some overlap in these specificities with more than one enzyme acting on the same substrate but at different rates (Table 16.1).

Inducers

The activity of specific cytochrome P450 enzymes can be induced, or 'speeded up', by a variety of drugs, foodstuffs and herbal supplements. This is hugely important because induction

Table 16.1 Examples of drugs which are substrates for individual cytochrome P450 enzymes.

CYP1A2	CYP2C19	CYP2C9	CYP2D6	CYP3A4
Amitriptyline	Amitriptyline	Amitriptyline	Amitriptyline	Amlodipine
Clozapine	Citalopram	Diclofenac	Carvedilol	Clarithromycin
Olanzapine	Diazepam	Fluoxetine	Fluoxetine	Diazepam
Paracetamol	Lansoprazole	Glibenclamide	Lidocaine	Domperidone
Propranolol	Omeprazole	Ibuprofen	Metoclopramide	Fentanyl
Theophylline	Phenytoin	Losartan	Paroxetine	Lidocaine
Verapamil	Propranolol	Ondansetron	Propranolol	Nifedipine
Warfarin	Warfarin	Phenytoin	Timolol	Ondansetron
		Tramadol		Propranolol
		Warfarin		Simvastatin

Drugs in blue are metabolised by more than one isoform of cytochrome P450. A more complete list of cytochrome P450 enzymes and their drug substrates can be found at www.medicine.iupui.edu/flockhart/table.htm.

Section 3

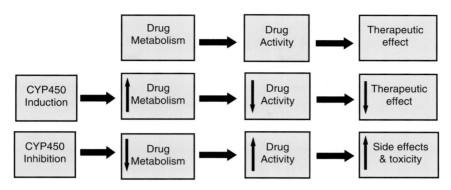

Figure 16.2 Possible effects of cytochrome P450 induction and inhibition on the metabolism and activity of substrate drugs.

of a cytochrome P450 enzyme will result in the metabolism of drugs which are substrates of that enzyme being speeded up, resulting in their reduced activity (Figure 16.2). This is the mechanism which underlies a number of important drug–drug interactions. Examples of cytochrome P450 inducers are shown in Table 16.2.

> **Practice application**
>
> Rifampicin speeds up (induces) the activity of CYP3A4. Oestradiol, an oestrogen in combined oral contraceptive pills, is a substrate of CYP3A4. Rifampicin speeds up the metabolism and hence reduces the activity of oestradiol, leading to possible contraceptive failure. This is the reason why the dose of oral contraceptive may be increased along with the use of additional contraceptive precautions in women taking a short course of rifampicin.

Table 16.2 Examples of drugs, foodstuffs and herbal supplements which either induce or inhibit cytochrome P450 activity.

	Cytochrome P450 inducers	Cytochrome P450 inhibitors
Drugs	Rifampicin (CYP2B6, CYP2C8, CYP2C19, CYP2C9, CYP3A4) Carbamazepine (CYP2C19, CYP3A4) Phenytoin (CYP3A4) Glucocorticoids (CYP3A4)	Fluconazole (CYP2C9, CYP3A4) Fluoxetine (CYP2C19, CYP2D6) Erythromycin (CYP3A4) Cimetidine (CYP1A2, CYP2C19, CYP2D6)
Foods	Leafy green vegetables (CYP1A2) Cigarette smoke (CYP1A2) Ethanol (CYP2E1)	Grapefruit juice (CYP3A4) Cranberry juice (CYP3A4) Watercress (CYP2C9, CYP2C19, CYP2D6, CYP3A4)
Herbals	St John's wort (CYP3A4) Valerian (CYP3A4) Gingko (CYP1A2)	St John's wort (CYP2D6, CYP2C9, CYP2C19) Gingko (CYP2C9) Ginseng (CYP2D6, CYP2C19) Echinacea (CYP3A4)

Section 3

Inhibitors

The activity of specific cytochrome P450 enzymes can be inhibited or reduced by a variety of drugs, foodstuffs and herbal supplements. This is hugely important because inhibition of a cytochrome P450 enzyme will result in the metabolism of drugs which are substrates of that isoform being reduced, resulting in increased drug activity and possible side effects or toxicity (Figure 16.2). This mechanism underlies a number of important drug–drug interactions. Examples of cytochrome P450 inhibitors are shown in Table 16.2.

Practice application

Grapefruit juice inhibits CYP3A4 activity, reducing the metabolism of simvastatin which is a substrate of this enzyme. This results in an increase in the activity of simvastatin and the side effect profile, particularly muscle effects. This is why concomitant use of simvastatin and grapefruit juice should be avoided.

Pharmacogenetics

Pharmacogenetics can be defined as clinically important hereditary variation in the response to drugs. The large number of cytochrome P450 enzymes makes genetic variation in these enzymes almost inevitable and this genetic variation can be important therapeutically. Genetic variations in, or polymorphisms of, specific cytochrome P450 enzymes can result in patients being either slow (poor) metabolisers (their CYP450 enzyme is less effective than the norm) or fast metabolisers (their CYP450 enzyme is more efficient than the norm). For slow metabolisers this may result in increased drug activity within the body and possible side effects/toxicity while for fast (extensive) metabolisers there may be a lack of therapeutic effect. The most important cytochrome P450 enzymes in terms of clinical impact of polymorphisms are CYP2C9, CYP2C19 and CYP2D6 and these polymorphisms are more common in specific ethnic groups (Table 16.3), making ethnicity an important issue for safe and effective prescribing.

Perhaps one of the best examples of the effect of genetic polymorphisms on clinical therapeutics is that of debrisoquine which was used in the treatment of essential hypertension. The use of debrisoquine resulted in excessive hypotension in a number of patients and this was related to their lack of ability to metabolise the drug. The enzyme involved in debrisoquine metabolism is CYP2D6 and studies suggested that up to 8% of Caucasians had this 'poor metaboliser' polymorphism and this impacted greatly on the clinical use of this drug, resulting in it falling out of favour (Caldwell, 2004).

Stop and think

Would you use the same dose of proton pump inhibitor for Caucasian, Asian and Ethiopian patients?

Table 16.3 Examples of polymorphisms in cytochrome P450 isoforms, prevalence in different ethnic groups and clinical impact.

CYP isoform	Polymorphism	Drugs affected by polymorphism
CYP2C9	PM 11% Caucasians 0% Asians	Increased activity of warfarin, candesartan, losartan, diclofenac, ibuprofen, fluvastatin and phenytoin
CYP2C19	PM 20% Asians	Increased activity of proton pump inhibitors
	EM 18% Ethiopians	Decreased activity of proton pump inhibitors
CYP2D6	PM 8% Caucasians	Increased activity of tramadol, venlafaxine and metoprolol
	UM 28% North Africans	Lack of therapeutic effect of tramadol, venlafaxine and metoprolol

PM, poor metaboliser; EM, extensive metaboliser; UM = ultra-rapid metaboliser.

Active and toxic metabolites

As mentioned earlier in the chapter, phase I metabolism does not always inactivate drugs. There are a number of drugs including diazepam, morphine, imipramine, verapamil and propranolol which, following phase I metabolism, exhibit active metabolites. This means that the pharmacological activity is retained even after the parent drug has disappeared from the plasma.

 Stop and think

Why should drugs with active metabolites be used with caution in the elderly and/or patients with renal failure?

Phase I drug metabolites can also be toxic. The most important example of a drug with a toxic metabolite is paracetamol. The majority (95%) of paracetamol undergoes phase II metabolism to an inactive metabolite. The remainder (5%) undergoes phase I metabolism and results in the production of the toxic metabolite N-acetyl-p-benzo-quinoneimine (NAPQI). Under normal circumstances this is not a problem as the NAPQI rapidly undergoes phase II metabolism, being conjugated to glutathione which inactivates it. In overdose situations problems arise because the liver's store of glutathione becomes depleted and can no longer inactivate the NAPQI (Figure 16.3).

Pro-drugs

A pro-drug is one which is administered in an inactive form and only becomes active following metabolism. This is an ideal drug design as it allows the inactive parent drug to be administered

Section 3

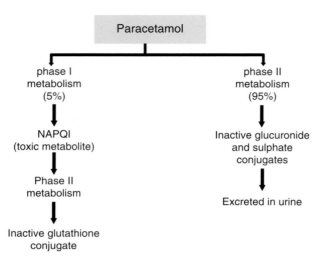

Figure 16.3   The metabolism of paracetamol and production of toxic metabolite.

in a lipid-soluble form which would be readily absorbed. The active metabolite is then released following metabolism, at which point the drug is also more polar in nature and therefore more readily excretable (Box 16.1).

First-pass metabolism and bioavailability

First-pass metabolism (sometimes called presystemic metabolism) is defined as the metabolism of the drug which occurs in the gut wall and the liver prior to that drug reaching the systemic circulation and only affects drugs which are given orally. Orally administered drugs are absorbed through the GI tract and enter the hepatic portal system, passing through the liver prior to entering the systemic circulation (Figure 16.4).

Bioavailability is defined as the proportion of administered drug which is available in the systemic circulation. Bioavailability is therefore affected by the degree of both drug absorption and first-pass metabolism. Drugs which undergo high first-pass metabolism have low bioavailability and drugs which undergo little or no first-pass metabolism exhibit high bioavailability.

Box 16.1	**Examples of common pro-drugs and their active metabolites.**

Pro-drug	Active metabolite
Enalapril	Enalaprilat
Abacavir	Carbovir monophosphate
Famciclovir	Penciclovir
Simvastatin	6-hydroxy simvastatin acid
Codeine	Morphine

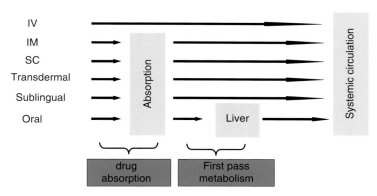

Figure 16.4 Whether changes in absorption and first-pass metabolism affect different routes of drug administration.

The percentage bioavailability of a drug is important in determining the dose required in relation to the route of administration. Drugs which are given intravenously are defined as having 100% bioavailability because the entire drug dose is delivered directly into the systemic circulation, thus avoiding problems with absorption and first-pass metabolism. If the oral bioavailability of a drug is only 20% then you would need to administer five times the dose of the same drug given IV to ensure similar drug levels within the systemic circulation. An example of a drug which requires a much higher dose when given orally compared to IV is morphine.

The degree of first-pass metabolism which occurs between individuals for the dose of drug can be very variable and this can result in wide variations in the oral bioavailability of the drug. The use of other drugs or dietary supplements which induce cytochrome P450 enzymes will result in decreased bioavailability while cytochrome P450 inhibitors will result in increased bioavailability.

First-pass metabolism can also be affected by age and disease which again will result in changes in oral bioavailability and unpredictability in terms of therapeutic effects.

Factors affecting drug metabolism

Age

Both liver size and hepatic blood flow decrease with increasing age. There is an additional decline in the activity of cytochrome P450 enzymes in the liver with age. The effect of these changes is to reduce drug metabolism which will result in increased drug activity within the body. Furthermore, changes in liver function will also act to reduce first-pass metabolism which could lead to increased bioavailability of certain oral drugs.

The activity of cytochrome P450 enzymes is reduced in neonates, resulting in decreased drug metabolism. Conversely, the activity of cytochrome P450 enzymes in children is often greater than that of adults, resulting in increased drug metabolism and possible loss of therapeutic effect.

Disease

A number of diseases can affect drug metabolism. Most obviously, diseases affecting the liver, such as cirrhosis, alcoholic liver disease and carcinoma, affect drug metabolism through a

Section 3

reduction in functional hepatocytes. This seems to result in a decrease in the activity of the cytochrome P450 enzymes involved in phase I metabolism but not on the activity of the conjugating enzymes involved in phase II metabolism. Infectious diseases can also result in the reduction of cytochrome P450 enzyme activity and decrease drug metabolism. Similarly, diseases which result in decreased blood flow to the liver, such as heart failure and shock, will necessarily result in reduced drug metabolism.

Drug excretion

The two main routes of drug excretion are via the kidneys (in the urine) and via the biliary system (in the faeces).

Renal excretion

The rate at which individual drugs are excreted by the kidneys is highly variable but is essentially determined by the rates of glomerular filtration, tubular secretion and passive diffusion as depicted in the following equation:

$$\text{Renal excretion} = \text{glomerular filtration} + \text{tubular secretion} - \text{passive diffusion}$$

Glomerular filtration

About 20% of renal blood flow passes through the glomerulus of the kidney and the leaky nature of the glomerular capillaries results in plasma diffusing through the capillary walls into the renal tubule. This is known as the glomerular filtrate and contains not just plasma but free, unbound drugs, which are contained within that plasma. Drugs which are bound to plasma proteins cannot diffuse through the glomerular capillaries because of their size. Very large drugs such as heparin will similarly be retained within the bloodstream as they will also be too big to pass through the glomerular capillaries.

Tubular secretion

The remaining 80% of the renal blood flow passes through to the peritubular capillaries of the proximal tubule. Here there are two major carrier systems which carry drugs from the bloodstream into the renal tubule: the acidic carrier system which carries weak acids (e.g. furosemide, indometacin, thiazide diuretics, penicillin) into the renal tubule, and the basic carrier system which carries weak bases (e.g. amiloride, dopamine, pethidine) into the renal tubule.

These carrier systems can operate against a gradient and consequently represent the most efficient mechanism of renal excretion. They can reduce drug concentrations in the plasma to almost zero. However, they are subject to competitive inhibition and this may lead to drug interactions and unwanted effects. As mentioned previously (Chapter 15), penicillin and probenecid both compete for the acidic carrier. The presence of probenecid reduces the renal excretion of penicillin, prolonging its activity in the body, and probenecid was given with penicillin for this very reason. On the other hand, both uric acid and thiazide diuretics compete for this acidic carrier system. This can result in reduced renal excretion of uric acid and is the mechanism underlying the possible side effect of gout in patients taking diuretics.

Passive diffusion

The nature of the kidney is such that most of the plasma filtered through the glomerular capillaries is reabsorbed as it passes through the renal tubule. As plasma is reabsorbed, the concentration gradient between drug in the renal tubule and unbound drug in the plasma changes and drugs which are lipid soluble will be reabsorbed across the membranes of the renal tubule into the plasma. As a result, very lipid-soluble drugs are only slowly excreted by the kidneys while polar, water-soluble drugs cannot readily cross membranes and are retained in the tubule.

Factors affecting renal drug excretion

pH of the environment

Just as drug absorption can be affected by environmental pH, so can renal drug excretion. Essentially the concept remains the same – alteration of the pH changes the proportion of drug in the unionised, lipid-soluble form. While in Chapter 15 we were interested in increasing the concentration of the lipid-soluble form to enhance drug absorption, in terms of renal excretion it is important to reduce the concentration of the lipid-soluble form, thus reducing passive diffusion and enhancing excretion.

Modulation of urinary pH has been used to promote drug excretion in overdose situations (Table 16.4).

 Stop and think

Why do you think aspirin overdose is sometimes treated by alkalinisation of the urine?

Age

Both renal mass and renal perfusion are reduced with increasing age. This decreased blood flow through the kidneys and reduction in the number of functional nephrons results in decreased renal excretion of drugs. Similarly, both glomerular filtration and tubular secretion are reduced with increasing age which also reduces renal excretion of drug.

Table 16.4   Effect of modulation of urinary pH on the renal excretion of weak acids and bases.

	Weak acids	Weak bases
Acidic urine	Reabsorbed into bloodstream	Excreted
Alkaline urine	Excreted	Reabsorbed into bloodstream

Section 3

Disease

Reduced renal blood flow, as can be seen in shock, will reduce the delivery of drug to the kidney and hence result in reduced renal excretion. Similarly, renal disease will result in reduced renal mass, thus reducing drug excretion, and may require a reduction in drug dosage in patients, particularly for drugs which are excreted unchanged or have active metabolites.

Biliary excretion

Biliary excretion is the major route of excretion for large, ionised molecules, particularly glucuronide and sulphate conjugates. These phase II metabolites are transferred from hepatocytes to the bile by non-specific carrier systems which can be competitively inhibited in a manner similar to that seen in the renal tubule. Negatively charged drugs/metabolites compete with other negatively charged drugs/metabolites while positively charged drugs/metabolites compete with other positively charged drugs/metabolites.

Drugs are then delivered by the biliary system to the small intestine where they may be excreted in the faeces or may undergo enterohepatic recycling.

Enterohepatic recycling

Drugs which have been conjugated in phase II metabolism are often transferred into the bile and delivered to the small intestine as described above. Bacteria within the small intestine can then hydrolyse some of the conjugate, releasing the original free drug. A portion of this free (unconjugated) dug can then be reabsorbed through the membranes of the GI tract and returned to the liver and systemic circulation prior to being remetabolised and re-excreted as a conjugate (Figure 16.5). This 'recirculation' of drug can occur many times before the drug is finally eliminated from the body and creates a 'reservoir' of drug.

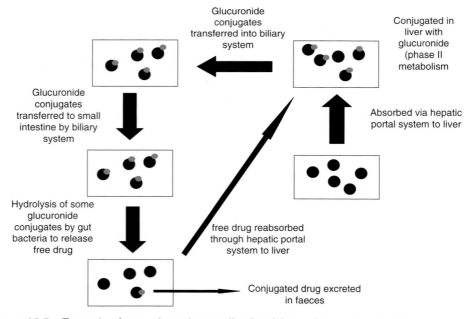

Figure 16.5 Example of enterohepatic recycling involving a drug conjugated to a glucuronide.

This recycling is very important for a number of prescribed drugs including rifampicin, morphine, benzodiazepines and the oestrogen of oral contraceptives.

In terms of oral contraceptives, disruption of enteroheptic recycling, because of either diarrhoea or disruption of the normal bacterial flora of the small intestine following broad-spectrum antibiotic use, can result in a reduction in oestrogen levels and possible contraceptive failure.

Drug clearance

Drug clearance is defined as the rate of drug elimination divided by the plasma concentration. Drug clearance is concerned with the rate at which the active parent drug is removed from the body and consists of both metabolism and excretion. Metabolic or hepatic clearance is the conversion of the active parent drug to a metabolite while renal clearance is the removal of the drug by the kidneys.

The relative importance of hepatic and renal clearance depends on the nature of the individual drug. Drugs which are highly lipid soluble will probably undergo extensive hepatic clearance while for drugs which are polar in nature, renal clearance will be more important. The main determinants of renal clearance are the rate of active tubular secretion and the rate of passive diffusion. Drugs which undergo mainly renal clearance should be used with care in patients whose renal function may be impaired. Examples of drugs which undergo mainly renal clearance are shown in Box 16.2.

Half-life

Half-life ($t_{1/2}$) is defined as the time taken for the plasma concentration of the drug to fall by half (Figure 16.6) and for most drugs this remains constant regardless of the dose of drug administered. Half-life is dependent on the clearance of the drug and its volume of distribution. If a drug is rapidly cleared by either hepatic or renal clearance then the half-life of the drug will be short. However, if the drug is only slowly cleared from the body then the half-life will be longer. Similarly, drugs which have a very large volume of distribution are likely to have a longer half-life than drugs with a small volume of distribution. Anything which reduces clearance, such as increasing age or disease, will increase the half-life of a drug and anything which increases clearance, such as cytochrome P450 induction, will decrease drug half-life. Similarly, changes in the volume of distribution of a drug, as might be seen in the elderly, will affect half-life. Half-life is important in determining the time interval between drug doses

Box 16.2   **Examples of drugs which undergo mainly renal clearance**

Furosemide
Atenolol
Benzylpenicillin
Cimetidine
Digoxin
Gentamicin

Section 3

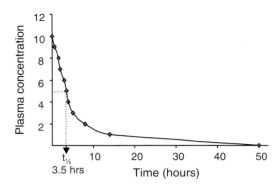

Figure 16.6 The change in concentration of drug in plasma with time and a determination of half-life.

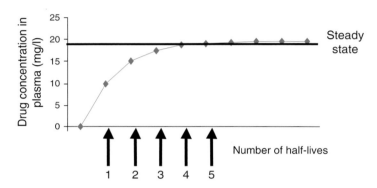

Figure 16.7 Concentration of drug in plasma. Half-life of drug is 2 hours – steady state is reached after 5 half-lives (10 hours).

and the time taken for drug concentrations to reach steady state in the plasma. Drugs such as ibuprofen ($t_{1/2} = 2$ hours) which have short half-lives need to be given frequently whereas drugs such as ethosuximide ($t_{1/2} = 50$ hours) which have long half-lives need only be given once daily. Steady state is reached when the plasma drug concentration does not drop below therapeutic levels between doses; this usually takes 3–5 half-lives to be achieved (Figure 16.7).

Summary

- The purpose of drug metabolism is to make drugs more polar and therefore easier to excrete.
- The cytochrome P450 superfamily of enzymes are important in phase I metabolism while phase II metabolism involves conjugation.
- Phase I metabolism can result in the production of active and/or toxic metabolites.
- Ethnicity can impact on drug metabolism and hence on drug activity.
- Cytochrome P450 enzyme activity can be both induced (speeded up) and inhibited (slowed down) by other drugs, dietary components and herbal preparations.

- Pro-drugs are inactive until they are metabolised.
- First-pass metabolism is metabolism of oral drugs in the gut wall and liver prior to reaching the systemic circulation.
- Bioavailability is the percentage of administered drug which is available in the systemic circulation.
- Renal excretion consists of glomerular filtration, tubular secretion and passive diffusion.
- Renal excretion is affected by environmental pH, age and disease.
- Biliary excretion is common for drugs which are conjugated either to glucuronide and sulphate.
- Enterohepatic recycling of glucuronide conjugates creates a reservoir of drug.
- Drug clearance involves both hepatic and renal clearance.
- Half-life is the time taken for the plasma concentration of the drug to drop by half.

Activity

1. Which of the following statements regarding drug metabolism are correct?
   - Is increased in children compared to adults   True / False
   - Is decreased by rifampicin   True / False
   - Is decreased by grapefruit juice   True / False
   - Is decreased in elderly patients   True / False
   - Is more important for lipid-soluble drugs   True / False
2. Which of the following statements regarding first-pass metabolism are correct?
   - Affects bioavailability   True / False
   - Affects drugs given orally, SC and IM   True / False
   - Never affects drugs administered IV   True / False
   - Occurs prior to the drug entering the systemic circulation   True / False
   - Can be reduced in elderly patients   True / False
3. Which of the following statements regarding passive diffusion of drug in the renal tubule are correct?
   - Depends on the pH of the urine   True / False
   - Depends on the rate of glomerular filtration   True / False
   - Depends on the degree of plasma protein binding   True / False
   - Depends on the age of the patient   True / False
   - Depends on the lipid solubility of the drug   True / False
4. Which of the following statements regarding biliary excretion and enterohaptic recycling are correct?
   - Affects drugs which undergo only phase I metabolism   True / False
   - Can be disrupted by broad-spectrum antibiotics   True / False
   - Results in drug excretion in the faeces   True / False
   - Is more important for unionised molecules   True / False
   - Is important for oral contraceptives   True / False
5. Which of the following statements regarding half-life are correct?
   - Determines the time to reach steady state   True / False
   - Increases with increasing drug clearance   True / False
   - Is longer in drugs with a large volume of distribution   True / False
   - Determines the dosing schedule of drugs   True / False
   - Can be affected by increasing age   True / False

Useful websites

Flockhart DA. Drug Interactions: Cytochrome P450 Drug Interaction Table. Indiana University School of Medicine. www.medicine.iupui.edu/flockhart/table.htm

Reusable learning objects

- Bioavailability.
  www.nottingham.ac.uk/nursing/sonet/rlos/bioproc/bioavailability/home.htm
- Half-life of drugs. www.nottingham.ac.uk/nursing/sonet/rlos/bioproc/halflife/index.html
- Kidney anatomy.
  www.nottingham.ac.uk/nursing/sonet/rlos/bioproc/kidneyanatomy/index.html
- Physiology of the kidneys.
  www.nottingham.ac.uk/nursing/sonet/rlos/bioproc/kidneyphysiology/index.html
- Liver anatomy.
  www.nottingham.ac.uk/nursing/sonet/rlos/bioproc/liveranatomy/index.html
- Physiology of the liver.
  www.nottingham.ac.uk/nursing/sonet/rlos/bioproc/liverphysiology/index.html
- The kidneys and drug excretion.
  www.nottingham.ac.uk/nursing/sonet/rlos/bioproc/kidneydrug/index.html
- The liver and drug metabolism.
  www.nottingham.ac.uk/nursing/sonet/rlos/bioproc/liverdrug/index.html
- Understanding first-pass metabolism.
  www.nottingham.ac.uk/nursing/sonet/rlos/bioproc/metabolism/default.html
- Introduction to drug clearance.
  www.nottingham.ac.uk/nursing/sonet/rlos/bioproc/clearance1/index.html

Reference

Caldwell, J. (2004) Pharmacogenetics and individual variation in the range of amino acid adequacy: the biological aspects. *J Nutr*, **134**, 1600S–1604S.

Further reading

Birkett, D.J. (2002) *Pharmacokinetics Made Easy*, 2nd edn, McGraw-Hill, Australia.

British Medical Association and Royal Pharmaceutical Society of Great Britain (2010) *British National Formulary*, 59th edn, BMJ Publishing, London.

Foster, R.W. (2003) *Basic Pharmacology*, 4th edn, Arnold, London.

Frye, R.F., Zgheib, N.K., Matzke, G.R., *et al.* (2006) Liver disease selectively modulates cytochrome P450-mediated metabolism. *Clin Pharmacol Ther*, **80** (2), 235–245.

Herrlinger, C. and Klotz, U. (2001) Drug metabolism and drug interactions in the elderly. *Best Pract Res Clin Gastroenterol*, **15**, 897–918.

Ingelman-Sundberg, M. (2004) Human drug metabolising cytochrome P450 enzymes: properties and polymorphisms. *Naunyn Schmiedebergs Arch Pharmacol*, **369**, 89–104.

Ingelman-Sundberg, M., Sim, S.C., Gomez, A. and Rodriguez-Antona, C. (2007) Influence of cytochrome P450 polymorphisms on drug therapies: pharmacogenetic, pharmacoepigenetic and clinical aspects. *Pharmacol Ther*, **116**:496–526.

McGavock, H. (2005) *How Drugs Work. Basic Pharmacology for Healthcare Professionals*, 2nd edn, Radcliffe Publishing, Oxford.

Nakajima, M., Yoshida, R., Shimada, N., *et al.* (2001) Inhibition and inactivation of human cytochrome P450 isoforms by phenethyl isothiocyanate. *Drug Metab Dispos*, **29**, 1110–1113.

Nowack, R. (2008) Cytochrome P450 enzyme, and transport protein mediated herb–drug interactions in renal transplant patients: grapefruit juice, St John's wort – and beyond! *Nephrology*, **13**, 337–347.

Page, C.P., Curtis, M.J., Sutter, M.C., *et al.* (2006) *Integrated Pharmacology*, 3rd edn, Mosby, London.

Rang, H.P., Dale, M.M., Ritter, J.M. and Flower, R. (2007) *Rang and Dale's Pharmacology*, 6th edn, Churchill Livingstone, Edinburgh.

Sim, S.C., Risinger, C., Dahl, M.-L., *et al.* (2006) A common novel CYP2C19 gene variant causes ultrarapid drug metabolism relevant for the drug response to proton pump inhibitors and antidepressants. *Clin Pharmacol Ther*, **79**, 103–113

Smith, H.J. (2006) *Smith and Williams' Introduction to the Principles of Drug Design and Action*, 4th edn, Taylor and Francis, Boca Raton.

Strolin Benedetti, M., Whomsley, R. and Canning, M. (2007) Drug metabolism in the paediatric population and in the elderly. *Drug Discov Today*, **12**, 599–610.

Section 3

17 Routes of administration

Learning outcomes

By the end of this chapter the reader should be able to:

- describe the potential barriers to drug absorption from the oral route
- understand why first-pass metabolism and gastric instability may lead to drugs being given via the sublingual administration route
- describe how the rectal, transdermal, ocular and inhalation routes can result in both local and systemic drug action
- discuss the differences in rate of absorption, bioavailability and advantages of the three different parenteral routes of drug administration.

The extent to which an individual drug undergoes the processes of absorption, distribution, metabolism and excretion largely depends on its physical characteristics and chemical properties. This chapter will discuss why the different routes of administration are available for drugs and why the route chosen may be determined by the pharmacokinetics of the drug. Drugs can act to give both a local and a systemic effect on the body and the route of administration chosen is in part determined by the effect required (Box 17.1).

Oral administration

Oral administration is probably the easiest and most convenient route of administration for most people. Drugs can be administered as solids or solutions, making this a suitable route for most patients, including children and the elderly.

Excipients and binding agents are added to the active ingredient in tablets and can contribute to the taste of some oral drug formulations, although sometimes this can be overcome by using a sugar or film coating. Flavourings can be added to liquid preparations to make them more palatable to children; however, the use of sugar in these preparations is being discouraged to

The New Prescriber. Edited by J Lymn, D Bowskill, F Bath-Hextall, R Knaggs, © 2010 John Wiley & Sons.

Box 17.1 Routes of administration available and whether they are routinely used for local or systemic drug effect.

Local drug effect	Systemic drug effect
Oral (vancomycin)	Oral
Rectal	Sublingual
Transdermal	Rectal (not always reliable)
Ocular	Transdermal
Inhalation	Subcutaneous injection
	Intramuscular injection
	Intravenous injection

reduce the possibility of dental caries. Similarly, it is not wise to make drugs too palatable for children as this may encourage overuse. Some drugs (e.g. phenoxymethylpenicillin, penicillin V) are relatively unstable in solution and have to be stored in powder form prior to use; some also have to be kept refrigerated until the course is finished.

Practice application

You should be aware that patients may be allergic to the excipients, such as colourings, added to the drug and not necessarily to the drug itself.

Oral administration is the most complex route of administration in terms of presenting the greatest number of barriers to the drug prior to it reaching the systemic circulation. Ideally, drugs should be relatively stable in the acidic environment of the stomach and should be lipid soluble to be effectively absorbed from the gastrointestinal tract. Highly polar acids and bases are only absorbed slowly and incompletely with much of the drug being eliminated in the faeces. After absorption from the gut, the drug travels to the liver via the portal circulation and may undergo substantial first-pass metabolism, thus reducing the amount of active drug reaching the circulation.

Stop and think

Why is penicillin V but not penicillin G given by the oral route?

Drugs administered by the oral route generally have a systemic effect but can be utilised for local effects. Vancomycin is poorly absorbed orally but can be used to eradicate *Clostridium difficile* from the gut of patients with pseudomembranous colitis.

Section 3

Factors affecting absorption of orally administered drugs

Rate of gastric emptying

The majority of drug absorption occurs in the intestine rather than the stomach and hence the rate at which drug is delivered to the intestine will affect the rate of absorption.

Drugs taken after meals are usually more slowly absorbed because progress to the small intestine is delayed. Intake of fluid with orally administered drugs will affect rate of gastric emptying and hence alter the rate of absorption. The absorption of drugs which cause gastric stasis (e.g. morphine) will be delayed and these drugs are often given by other routes.

 Practice application

Metoclopramide (an antiemetic) is often prescribed in combination with analgesic medication for the treatment of migraine. In addition to treating the nausea often associated with migraine, metoclopramide has an action on the stomach muscle, speeding up the emptying of the stomach and thus the passage of the analgesic into the intestine, thereby increasing its rate of absorption.

Disease

Drug absorption can be affected by diseases which affect the available surface area of the gastrointestinal tract. Inflammatory bowel disease, bowel cancers and coeliac disease can all affect absorption of drugs due to damage to the intestinal wall. This may reduce drug absorption through reduced surface area. Sometimes it may paradoxically result in increased drug absorption because it is thought that the damaged mucosa becomes quite leaky and allows drug molecules to pass through more quickly.

Transit time in gastrointestinal tract

In Chapter 15 we established that the majority of drug absorption occurs in the intestine, even for weak acids which start to be absorbed from the stomach. Consequently the length of time the drug is in the intestine is important for absorption. Normal transit time in the intestine can be anything between 4 and 10 hours but most drugs are absorbed relatively rapidly, within an hour.

 Practice application

Patients with severe diarrhoea may have significantly reduced drug absorption after oral administration simply because drugs taken orally pass through the gastrointestinal tract so quickly.

Presence of other substances in the GI tract

The absorption of drugs from the gastrointestinal tract can be affected by the presence of other drugs or ions. Tetracycline antibiotics such as tetracycline, oxytetracycline and demeclocycline should not be given with milk because these drugs bind to the calcium ions in the milk to form large insoluble complexes which cannot be readily absorbed across the GI tract, reducing the absorption of the antibiotic.

Similarly, tetracycline should not be given with antacids as it binds to the magnesium, aluminium or calcium ions contained in the antacid. This results in the production of large insoluble complexes, again leading to reduced absorption. Antacids will also act to alter the pH of the local environment, thus affecting the amount of drug in the unionised form and impacting on drug absorption.

 Stop and think

The interaction between antacids and tetracycline is an example of which form of drug antagonism?

Sublingual administration

Drugs are administered by the sublingual route when a rapid response is required, particularly when the drug is either unstable at gastric pH or rapidly metabolised by the liver. Drugs absorbed from the mouth pass straight into the systemic circulation without entering the hepatic portal system and so escape the effects of first-pass metabolism. The degree of first-pass metabolism which occurs with a drug may be a determining factor in the route of administration. For example, glyceryl trinitrate (GTN) undergoes very high first-pass metabolism with around 99% of the orally administered drug being metabolised on its first pass through the liver and only 1% of the administered dose reaching the systemic circulation. It is for this reason that GTN is often administered sublingually or transdermally; drug absorption from both of these routes enters the systemic circulation directly, thus avoiding the first-pass effect.

Rectal administration

Administration of drugs via the rectum can be used for local or systemic effects. Rectal administration may be an alternative for patients who are vomiting or unable to swallow. Diazepam can be administered rectally to children in status epilepticus where intravenous access is difficult. While the surface area for absorption is small, the rectal mucosa is well supplied with blood vessels, making drug absorption into the systemic circulation from this route theoretically possible. Unfortunately, however, blood flow is variable, making drug absorption erratic and consequently rectal absorption gives more variable plasma concentrations than oral administration.

Transdermal adminstration

Drugs administered by the transdermal route may have a local effect on the skin or a systemic effect (Box 17.2). Drug absorption from the skin is primarily dependent on the lipid solubility

---

Box 17.2   Transdermal preparations separated into those used for local drug effect and those used for systemic drug action.

Transdermal formulations for local drug action	Transdermal formulations for systemic drug action
Creams Ointments Gels Lotions Plasters	Patches

---

of the drug with only very lipid-soluble drugs being able to penetrate this tough outer body layer for a systemic effect. These drugs can be delivered by transdermal patch whereas drugs applied to the skin as creams, lotions, ointments or gels generally have a local effect on the skin itself. Transdermal patches are being increasingly used (e.g. oestrogen in hormone replacement therapy and nicotine in cigarette addiction withdrawal). This produces a steady rate of delivery and avoids first-pass metabolism. Development costs are large and hence patch formulations tend to be expensive and are only suitable for very lipid-soluble drugs which are active in small quantities. The integrity of the skin is probably the most important factor in the absorption of these drugs as the dermis is well supplied with blood vessels and a break in the skin will allow topical drugs to be taken into the systemic circulation.

Ocular administration

Administration of drugs to the eye relies on absorption through the epithelium of the conjunctival sac. Often it is possible to have desirable local effects without causing systemic side effects (e.g. dorzolamide lowers ocular pressure in glaucoma but avoids the acidosis caused by oral administration), but systemic effects can occur (e.g. timolol used for glaucoma can result in bronchospasm in asthmatic patients).

Inhalation

Drugs used for their effects on the lung are given by inhalation. This allows high local concentrations in the lungs to be obtained with minimal systemic effects. Importantly, drug delivery by inhalation can avoid the first-pass metabolism effects seen when these drugs are given orally. However, beta2-adrenoceptor agonists (e.g. salbutamol) used in high concentrations can be absorbed into the systemic circulation and induce side effects. Muscarinic antagonists such as ipratropium have a quaternary ammonium ion which makes them both highly charged and large in size; thus they are poorly absorbed across membranes and do not generally enter the systemic circulation.

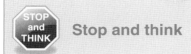

Stop and think

Why is the dose of salbutamol given by inhalation in the microgram range while the dose of oral salbutamol is in the milligram range?

Particles of solid or liquid droplets inhaled are deposited in the lungs by impaction. Only a proportion of inhaled drug actually reaches the lower respiratory tract, with the majority being deposited in the mouth and pharynx. This drug will then be swallowed, potentially being absorbed into the systemic circulation and resulting in side effects. It is possible to increase the proportion of a dose that reaches the required site. Patient education on correct use of an inhaler includes synchronising the operation of the spray during inhalation and teaching the patient to hold the breath after administration. Use of a spacer device also increases the amount of drug deposited in the lower airways.

Parenteral drug administration

Drugs given by subcutaneous, intramuscular and intravenous injection reach the systemic circulation by diffusion through body tissues and penetration of blood capillaries. Collectively, these processes are referred to as parenteral absorption. Drug absorption following parenteral administration is usually quite rapid and often comparable with absorption from an oral preparation. Parenteral drug administration avoids the problems and variability associated with oral administration, including first-pass metabolism and gastric instability.

Intramuscular injection

Intramuscular administration generally results in reliable plasma concentrations being attained. The rate of absorption following intramuscular administration depends on local blood flow and the site of injection. If a drug is distributed throughout a large volume of muscle, the rate of absorption is increased. Dispersion of drug within tissue can be enhanced by massage of the injection site. Transport away from the muscle depends on local blood flow. Blood flow is greater in muscles of the upper arm than in the gluteal mass or thigh. Muscle blood flow is not constant and increases with exercise and can decrease in shock and heart failure.

The pH of the injected solution can also greatly affect drug absorption. The pH changes gradually from its initial value to that of interstitial (tissue) fluid (pH 7.4). According to the pH partition hypothesis (Chapter 16), drugs are more rapidly absorbed when a significant proportion of the drug exists as the free unionised molecule.

Subcutaneous injection

Absorption following subcutaneous injection is influenced by the same factors that determine intramuscular injections. Absorption of drugs via these routes is dependent on the blood flow

Section 3

to these areas. However, as cutaneous blood flow is lower than in muscle so subcutaneous absorption will tend to be slower and consequently drugs given by intramuscular injection generally have a faster onset of action than drugs given SC simply because muscle is more highly perfused than subcutaneous tissues.

The major advantage of this route of administration is that it is possible to teach patients how to undertake subcutaneous injections safely and hence this route is suitable if self-administration is required (e.g. regular insulin injections for diabetes mellitus). The main disadvantage of subcutaneous injection is that the volume that can be injected is smaller than for intramuscular injection. As with intramuscular injection, drugs given by the subcutaneous route will show a slower rate of absorption in patients suffering from hypovolaemic shock as the blood flow to these areas is reduced to protect essential organs.

Intravenous injection

Injection directly into a vein is the fastest and most reliable route of administration to give a highly predictable plasma concentration. Intravenous administration does not exhibit the same variability of absorption as other routes of administration. As with other parenteral routes of administration, intravenous injection avoids first-pass metabolism effects and also avoids problems associated with drug instability at gastric pH.

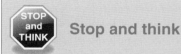

Stop and think

What is the bioavailability of drugs administered intravenously?

Intravenous administration is useful for drugs which are not absorbed from the gastrointestinal tract because of size or being very polar in nature or too irritant to be given by other routes. However, if given too quickly, plasma concentrations may rise at such a rate that normal mechanisms of distribution and excretion are saturated, resulting in toxicity and side effects. Given that intravenous administration requires cannulation of a vein, it is not suitable for routine self-administration.

Summary

- Oral administration is the most convenient route for drugs which have a systemic effect.
- The rate of drug absorption from the oral route can be decreased by gastric stasis, bowel disease and diarrhoea.
- Interaction with other drugs or foodstuffs in the GI tract can reduce the absorption from the oral route.
- Sublingual drug administration avoids first-pass metabolism and problems associated with gastric instability.
- Systemic absorption from the rectal route is erratic and as such results in variable plasma drug concentrations.

- Only drugs which are very lipid soluble and have a high potency can be given transdermally for a systemic effect.
- Ocular administration and inhalation can be used for local drug action in the eye and the lungs respectively.
- While the use of the ocular and inhalational routes reduces the likelihood of systemic side effects, it does not prevent them.
- Drug absorption from the intramuscular and subcutaneous route is dependent on local blood flow.
- Intravenous drug administration avoids the variability in absorption associated with other routes but can result in side effects and toxicity.

✏ Activity

1. Which of the following routes are routinely used to give systemic effects?
   - Oral   True / False
   - Intravenous   True / False
   - Inhalation   True / False
   - Ocular   True / False
   - Transdermal   True / False
2. Drug absorption from the oral route can be decreased by which of the following?
   - Diarrhoea   True / False
   - The use of metoclopramide   True / False
   - Gastric stasis   True / False
   - Antacids   True / False
   - Taking with food   True / False
3. Which of the following routes of drug administration avoid first-pass metabolism?
   - Inhaled   True / False
   - Oral   True / False
   - Sublingual   True / False
   - Transdermal   True / False
   - Intramuscular   True / False
4. Which of the following statements concerning intramuscular drug administration are correct?
   - Results in 100% bioavailability   True / False
   - Is affected by blood flow   True / False
   - Is unaffected by shock   True / False
   - Is used to produce systemic effects   True / False
   - Is dependent on the pH of the injected solution   True / False
   - Ocular   True / False

Further reading

British Medical Association and Royal Pharmaceutical Society of Great Britain (2010) *British National Formulary*, 59th edn, BMJ Publishing, London.

Cates, C.J., Crilly, J.A. and Rowe, B.H. (2006) Holding chambers (spacers) versus nebulisers for beta-agonist treatment of acute asthma. *Cochrane Database Syst Rev*, 2, CD000052.

Section 3

Eadala, P., Waud, J.P. and Matthews, S.B., *et al.* (2009) Quantifying the 'hidden' lactose in drugs used for the treatment of gastro-intestinal conditions. *Aliment Pharmacol Ther*, **29**, 677–687.

Irving, P.M., Shanahan, F. and Rampton, D.S. (2008) Drug interactions in inflammatory bowel disease. *Am J Gastroenterol*, **103**, 207–219.

Lavorini, F., Magnan, A., Dubus, J.C., *et al.* (2007) Effect of incorrect use of dry powder inhalers on management of patients with asthma and COPD. *Respir Med*, **102**, 593–604.

Orme, M. (1984) Drug absorption in the gut. *Br J Anaesth*, **56**, 59–67.

Page, C.P., Curtis, M.J., Sutter, M.C., *et al.* (2006) *Integrated Pharmacology*, 3rd edn, Mosby, London.

Rang, H.P., Dale, M.M., Ritter, J.M. and Flower, R. (2007) *Rang and Dale's Pharmacology*, 6th edn, Churchill Livingstone, Edinburgh.

Roberts-Thomson, P.J., Chan, A., Kupa, A., *et al.* (1984) Urticaria and angio-oedema. *Med J Aust*, **1**, S34–S37.

Wilson, C.G. and Washington, N. (1989) *Physiological Pharmaceutics. Biological Barriers to Drug Absorption*, Ellis Horwood, Chichester

Section 3

18 Variations in drug handling

Learning outcomes

By the end of this chapter the reader should be able to:

- understand and explain the pharmacokinetic differences in response to drugs from birth to old age
- understand the pharmacodynamic differences in response to drugs in the elderly
- understand the implications for drug dose and choice in neonates, paediatric and elderly patients
- understand the reasons for the differences in response to drugs in those patients with renal or hepatic impairment
- understand the implications for drug dose and choice in patients with renal or hepatic impairment.

Why is there variability?

There is a saying 'no two people are alike'; this is true in many ways, including the way different people respond to drugs. This is because of differences in their biological and chemical make-up.

Although individuals vary widely in their response to drugs, there are broad themes which apply to different groups of people, mainly different age groups. There are also differences in the way people with kidney and liver failure respond to drugs.

Pharmacokinetic variability with age

Neonates

It is important to remember that neonates exhibit variability in their ability to handle drugs which are specific to them. Neonates are not 'young children' and it is important to remember

The New Prescriber. Edited by J Lymn, D Bowskill, F Bath-Hextall, R Knaggs, © 2010 John Wiley & Sons.

Section 3

this when calculating drug dosages for neonates. Preterm neonates are particularly unique, as they may be born with immature body systems and therefore have reduced ability to handle drugs. There are specific reference texts giving dosage advice for neonatal patients and the British National Formulary for Children (BNF-C) often gives separate doses for neonates.

Absorption

Enteral drug absorption is erratic in the neonate because the stomach does not always empty effectively. In an ill neonate there may be no enteral absorption. In a preterm neonate of 28 weeks or less, the skin is very thin and acts as a poor barrier to water loss and there is increased absorption of topical agents and anything else which comes into contact with the skin, for example skin cleansers which contain alcohol. Neonates have small muscle bulk, so the intramuscular route is generally avoided.

 Practice application

The most reliable routes of absorption in the neonate are intravenous, inhaled (if direct action in the lung is required), rectal and buccal.

Distribution

Distribution into fat or water-based tissue is affected by the amount of fat or water tissue available. Neonates have variable amounts of fat tissue. Preterm neonates of 29 weeks or less and those who have not been able to grow fully in the uterus may have little body fat. Term neonates still have proportionally higher amounts of body water than adults. This affects the distribution of lipid-soluble drugs, for example diazepam, where the volume of distribution is decreased in neonates with a smaller proportion of body fat. Practically, this means the drug is less likely to accumulate in the body fat, and the elimination half-life of the drug may be decreased, requiring lower doses or longer dose intervals. Conversely, neonates born to diabetic mothers may have a larger than average amount of body fat. Practically, this means the drug accumulates in the body fat, creating a 'reservoir' and the elimination half-life of the drug may be increased.

 Stop and think

Why might benzodiazepine withdrawal be a problem in a neonate born to a diabetic benzodiazepine addict mother?

Protein binding of the drug to albumin in the plasma is also affected in the neonate, as preterm neonates born at 27 weeks or less have albumin concentrations which are only two-thirds of those seen in adults. This reduces the proportion of each dose which is bound to plasma albumin and hence increases the proportion of 'free, unbound, drug' which can then act on the target sites. An example of a drug affected by this is furosemide and practically it means lower doses are required.

Metabolism

At birth many enzyme systems involved in drug metabolism are not completely mature. Therefore the metabolism of most drugs is reduced.

Phase I metabolising enzymes (cytochrome P450 enzymes) generally reach adult capacity around the age of 6 months although the enzymes involved in phase II conjugation reactions take longer to reach adult levels, with glucuronidation pathways not reaching adult levels until around 3 years of age. It is this lack of conjugating activity that can result in 'grey baby syndrome' following the use of chloramphenicol in neonates. Some neonates are born with hyperbilirubinaemia, where there are high levels of unconjugated bilirubin in the blood. As bilirubin competes for binding sites involved in the metabolism of drugs in the liver, the metabolism of some drugs may be reduced, resulting in longer half-lives.

Excretion

Neonates have reduced kidney function, which will cause slow elimination of most drugs. Therefore half-lives are longer, and dose intervals should be extended or doses reduced. For drugs which have a narrow therapeutic index, close monitoring of plasma drug levels should be carried out.

 Practice application

Gentamicin, an antibiotic commonly used in neonates, is usually dosed at 24- or 36-hour intervals.

Paediatrics

As with neonates, it is important to remember when calculating drug dosages that children are not 'small adults'! Their body systems may still be immature, which affects their ability to handle drugs. The standard reference source for drug doses in children is the BNF-C.

Absorption

Very young children have a reduced concentration of gastric acid in their stomachs, and reduced gut motility when compared to older children. This results in longer dissolution times of some solid dosage forms that need gastric acid to be absorbed and increased time in the stomach for absorption. On balance, a longer absorption time has a greater clinical effect, increasing the peak plasma levels of some drugs. Older children have similar oral absorption rates to adults. As in neonates, topical absorption of drugs is dependent upon skin thickness, and younger children have relatively thin skin, leading to increased absorption of drugs and other agents by the topical route. Absorption from inhaled drugs is similar to that in adults, provided the child has an adequate inhaler technique.

Distribution

Children under the age of 1 year still have proportionally higher amounts of body water than adults. This affects distribution in a similar way to neonates. Protein binding of drugs in young children is reduced, again due to low albumin levels.

Metabolism

The immaturity of enzyme systems involved in metabolism is corrected as the child gets older and, due to the relative increase in hepatic blood flow and liver size in children compared to adults, these systems actually function more efficiently. When looked at in terms of doses in mg/kg, children require a higher dose of theophylline than adults, as the metabolism is more efficient in children until their enzyme systems are fully mature.

Excretion

In young children the kidneys are still immature, resulting in lower rates of glomerular filtration and tubular secretion (glomerular filtration rates do not reach adult levels until 6 months of age while tubular secretion does not reach adult levels until around 8 months of age). Practically this increases the half-life of renally cleared drugs, for example gentamicin. However, once children reach about 8 months old, kidney function is mature and the excretion of renally cleared drugs is comparable to that of adults.

 Practice application

Doses for children are usually in mg/kg, divided into age categories. This takes into account the pharmacokinetic differences in different age groups.

Elderly

As adults grow older changes occur in their body composition and ability to handle drugs. There are no specific reference texts for dosing of drugs in the elderly, but the BNF sometimes lists dosing schedules for the elderly alongside those for adults.

Absorption

Older people have a reduced concentration of gastric acid, so their gastric fluid is less acidic than in younger adults, which may increase the dissolution time of drugs in the stomach. Gastric emptying is delayed as peristalsis slows, and can result in drugs being present in the stomach for longer. These factors have a counteracting effect on each other when it comes to drug absorption. There is also reduced blood flow to the GI tract, which in theory reduces the amount of drug carried away from the GI area to the rest of the body. In practice, there is no real change in drug absorption as a person gets older.

Distribution

The balance of body water to body fat changes as a person gets older, with an increase in the body fat. This affects distribution of water- and lipid-soluble drugs. There is also a reduction in muscle mass. Benzodiazepines (e.g. diazepam) are lipid soluble, and so they deposit into the increased body fat to create reservoirs. This increases the length of time the drug is in the body to exert an effect, and so longer dosing intervals are needed. Cimetidine is water soluble, and there are higher plasma concentrations in older people after a standard dose. Digoxin is highly bound to muscle and therefore it has a reduced volume of distribution due to reduced lean body mass. This leads to increased plasma concentrations after a standard dose. There is also a lower concentration of plasma proteins, including albumin, in the elderly. This means there are fewer plasma proteins for drugs to bind to, for example warfarin, resulting in a higher proportion of the drug dose being 'free' and able to exert an effect. These distribution effects are usually only important when starting a drug or increasing the dose, as once steady state is achieved the body will balance the effect of distribution with metabolism and elimination.

Metabolism

Metabolism of drugs is generally reduced, because of reduced hepatic blood flow and a reduced liver mass and functioning liver cells. There may also be altered first-pass metabolism as liver function is reduced. Drugs which are pro-drugs and need converting by the liver to their active forms are less effective. Drugs which are not pro-drugs but undergo first-pass metabolism, for example nifedipine, will undergo less metabolism, so higher plasma concentrations are available to exert a therapeutic effect.

As the elderly usually have concomitant medical conditions and exact liver function is hard to measure, it is hard to predict the exact effect on the metabolism of specific drugs.

Excretion

The glomerular filtration rate declines by about 1% per year from the age of 40, so the effects of excretion can be seen in adults from a relatively early age. Some reporting labs now report estimated glomerular filtration rate (eGFR) (Chapter 25) as standard and this, once recalculated to take into account body surface area, is used to measure renal function when deciding upon the degree of renal failure a patient has. This is a recent method of calculating renal failure,and there is not much experience in drug dosing against the eGFR value. Most reference texts use creatinine clearance (CrCl), calculated using the Cockroft–Gault equation (Box 18.1), to calculate and quantify renal function for drug dosing. The Cockroft–Gault equation is not completely accurate for the older patient, although age and weight are factors in it. Older people have less muscle mass, as discussed earlier, and so produce less creatinine from muscle breakdown. So they may have artificially low creatinine levels, and therefore a lower CrCl than their actual renal function. However, it is the best practical tool we have to measure renal function for drug dosing in a patient, even the elderly.

Section 3

Box 18.1   Cockroft–Gault Equation

$$CrCl = \frac{(140 - age)\,(weight)\,(sex\ factor)}{Serum\ creatinine}$$

Sex factor – males = 1.23
Females = 1.04

Renal function is often adversely affected in the short term by dehydration and urinary tract infections, so in general drug doses for newly started drugs are not altered until the patient is fully hydrated and CrCl is remeasured. Drugs the patient has been on for some time with no problem may need their doses decreasing in the short term if the patient develops an infection, to avoid toxicity, for example digoxin. Drugs may also affect renal function, for example NSAIDs, so caution is needed when using these drugs at all in the elderly.

 Stop and think

Why is the BNF dose of imidapril in the elderly listed as initially 2.5 mg, maximum 10 mg daily?

Pharmacodynamic variability

Pharmacodynamic changes can be described as changes in the responsiveness of the organs of the body which cause the changes in effect of the drugs.

Elderly

The elderly can show either an increased or decreased effect of the drug, when compared to younger adults (Table 18.1).

Liver failure

A patient with impaired hepatic function will have limited ability to metabolise drugs. The drug plasma level then builds up and becomes toxic. In order to avoid this, the dosing interval is usually extended and sometimes the dose will need to be decreased. Some drugs undergo first-pass metabolism in the liver in order to become active. Their bioavailability will be decreased and doses may have to be increased. Other drugs undergo extensive first-pass metabolism and their bioavailability will be increased, with more drug available to have an effect. Doses may have to be decreased.

Drugs interact with the liver in three basic ways. They can either induce or inhibit liver enzymes, and therefore affect the metabolism of themselves and other drugs, and they can

Table 18.1 Pharmacodynamic changes in the elderly.

Drug class	Pharmacodynamic change	Effect	Action taken
Benzodiazepines	Increased affinity or increased numbers of benzodiazepine binding sites	Increased sensitivity to the therapeutic and side effects	Use lower doses and short-acting drugs, for example lorazepam
Beta-blockers	Fall in the responsiveness of beta-receptors	Reduced sensitivity to the therapeutic effects	Avoid monotherapy and use other drug classes where possible
	Reduced cardiac reserves	Heart failure	Avoid non-selective beta-blockers, use cardioselective ones with caution
Anticholinergics	Reduced number of cholinergic neurons	Increased sensitivity to side effects, for example confusion	Avoid where possible
Tricyclics, phenothiazines and levodopa	Reduced responsiveness of baroreceptors to blood pressure changes	Greater risk of falls due to postural hypotension	Avoid where possible – monitor postural hypotension if drug is used

cause drug-induced liver disease in which case their metabolism can be affected as described above and careful drug choice in liver disease is necessary.

Inducing or inhibiting liver enzymes

Some drugs are metabolised by enzyme systems in the liver. The main system involved is the cytochrome P450 system (Chapter 16), although others are involved too. Drugs can have an effect on a patient's liver enzymes. They can either induce their activity (make them work more) or inhibit their activity (make them work less), to have an effect on the metabolism of the drug, other hepatically metabolised drugs and anything else metabolised by the enzyme. A drug which inhibits enzymes will also inhibit its own metabolism along with other things. If one of these enzyme-inducing or -inhibiting drugs is prescribed, you will need to consider their effect on the other drugs prescribed and may need to alter the drugs used or change doses. It is important to slowly increase the doses of enzyme-inducing drugs until the target dose is reached.

 Stop and think

Phenytoin is an enzyme inducer. What effect might be seen if phenytoin is added to the prescription of a patient who used the oral contraceptive pill?

Section 3

Drug-induced liver disease

Drugs can cause actual liver disease or they can change a patient's liver function test results without causing frank illness. An example of this is rifampicin, commonly used to treat tuberculosis, which can cause a benign rise in liver function tests, but sometimes liver impairment.

Drug choice in liver disease

It is hard to quantify a patient's degree of liver failure and therefore predict their response to drug doses. When prescribing from a class of drugs, those with shorter half-lives are preferable to those with longer half-lives. Patients with liver failure may develop hepatic encephalopathy, which is a complication typified by a reduced level of consciousness and confusion. Drugs which have side effects of drowsiness or confusion should be avoided in these patients, to allow prompt diagnosis of encephalopathy and to prevent worsening of the drowsiness. The symptoms of liver failure include fluid retention and an increased risk of GI bleeds. Drugs which can cause fluid retention or GI bleeds should be avoided in liver failure, for example NSAIDs.

 Stop and think

Sulphonylureas, used to treat diabetes, have varying half-lives. The symptoms of hypoglycaemia include drowsiness. Which is the better drug to treat diabetes in liver disease: gliclazide (short half-life) or glibenclamide (long half-life)?

Some patients with liver failure also develop kidney failure, as a result of portal hypertension. Extra care is needed in these patients to avoid worsening both their kidney and liver failure.

Kidney failure

It is possible to quantify kidney failure using the patient's serum creatinine to estimate GFR, as discussed earlier. There are many reference sources that give information on drug doses in the varying degrees of kidney failure, of which the drug specific details in each monograph of the BNF is the most simple. Most reference sources need kidney function to be estimated using the Cockroft–Gault equation.

A patient with impaired renal function will have limited ability to excrete renally cleared drugs. The drug plasma level then builds up and becomes toxic. In order to avoid this, the dosing interval is usually extended and sometimes the dose needs to be decreased. As with liver failure, drugs with shorter half-lives are preferable to those with longer half-lives in the same class. Drugs which act on the kidney will have reduced efficacy, for example thiazide diuretics and nitrofurantoin. Alternatives should be used. As a general rule, drugs which can cause or worsen kidney failure should be avoided. If the patient is on dialysis, either haemodialysis or peritoneal dialysis, the drug dose and choice may be affected. There are specialist reference sources which give advice in these situations.

Summary

- Neonates, particularly very preterm neonates, have different pharmacokinetics and require different dosing schedules from children.
- Drug distribution in the tissues of the neonate is variable and can affect the half-lives of both water- and lipid-soluble drugs.
- Neonates have a reduced concentration of plasma albumin, which affects the distribution of protein-bound drugs.
- Due to immaturity of kidney and liver cells, neonates have impaired metabolism and elimination. This tends to increase the half-life of drugs.
- Older children have more mature body systems than younger children.
- Doses for children are usually in mg/kg, divided into age categories. This takes into account the pharmacokinetic differences in different age groups.
- The proportion of body water to body fat changes in the elderly, resulting in changes in the distribution of both water- and lipid-soluble drugs.
- The elderly have a reduced concentration of plasma albumin, which affects the distribution of protein-bound drugs.
- The function of liver and kidney cells deteriorates with age, which affects ability to metabolise and eliminate drugs.
- The elderly also undergo pharmacodynamic changes in the way they handle drugs. This is due to changes in responsiveness of the organs of the body which cause the changes in effect of the drugs.
- Drugs whose side effects mimic the symptoms of liver failure should be avoided in patients with liver failure.
- Patients with liver failure will have reduced liver enzyme induction or inhibition, which may affect the interaction of drugs with each other.
- Kidney failure can be quantified using the estimated glomerular filtration rate, eGFR, but calculated CrCl using Cockroft Gault may also be used when working out drug doses.
- Drugs which act directly on the kidney may have a reduced effect in kidney failure and should be avoided.
- Drugs which can worsen kidney failure should be avoided in patients with pre-existing kidney failure.

✎ Activity

1. Which of the following statements regarding drug dosing in neonatal patients are correct?

The skin is more permeable to agents.	True / False
Body systems are mature.	True / False
Plasma albumin concentration is reduced.	True / False
Gentamicin dose intervals are increased.	True / False
Therapeutic drug monitoring is not performed.	True / False

2. Which of the following statements regarding drug dosing in children are correct?

The skin is more permeable to agents.	True / False
Young children have a high amount of body water.	True / False
Doses of albumin-bound drugs need altering.	True / False

Section 3

The adult BNF can be used for children's doses.	True / False
Children's doses are usually quoted in mg/kg.	True / False
3. Which of the following statements regarding drug dosing in the elderly are correct?	
Generally lower doses are used.	True / False
Generally shorter dosage intervals are used.	True / False
Renal function improves with age.	True / False
Lower loading doses of warfarin are used.	True / False
Short-acting benzodiazepines are preferred.	True / False
4. Which of the following statements regarding drug dosing in renal impairment are correct?	
No dose amendments are required.	True / False
Renal function cannot be easily categorised.	True / False
NSAIDs are drugs of choice.	True / False
Drug dose is not affected by dialysis.	True / False
Generally longer dosage intervals are used.	True / False
5. Which of the following statements regarding drug dosing in liver impairment are correct?	
NSAIDs are drugs of choice.	True / False
Degree of liver impairment can be calculated.	True / False
Long-acting drugs are preferred.	True / False
Drugs which cause drowsiness are preferred.	True / False
Enzyme activity can be affected by drugs.	True / False

Further reading

Armour, D. and Cairns, C. (2002) *Medicines in the Elderly*, Pharmaceutical Press, London.

British Medical Association and Royal Pharmaceutical Society of Great Britain (2010) *British National Formulary*, 59th edn, BMJ Publishing, London.

British Medical Association and Royal Pharmaceutical Society of Great Britain (2009) *British National Formulary for Children*, BMJ Publishing, London.

Corsonello, A., Pedone, C., Corica, F., *et al.*, Gruppo Italiano di Farmacovigilanza nell'Anziano (GIFA) Investigators. (2005) Concealed renal insufficiency and adverse drug reactions in elderly hospitalized patients. *Arch Intern Med*, **165**, 790-795.

Kanneh, A. (2002) Paediatric pharmacological principles: an update. Part 2. Pharmacokinetics: absorption and distribution. *Paediatr Nurs*, **14**(9), 39-43.

Kanneh, A. (2002) Paediatric pharmacological principles: an update. Part 3. Pharmacokinetics: metabolism and excretion. *Paediatr Nurs*, **14**(10), 39-43.

Lichtman, S.M. (2007) Pharmacokinetics and pharmacodynamics in the elderly. *Clin Adv Hematol Oncol*, **5**, 181-182.

Rang, H.P., Dale, M.M., Ritter, J.M. and Flower, R. (2007) *Rang and Dale's Pharmacology*, 6th edn, Churchill Livingstone, Edinburgh.

Ritter, J.M., Lewis, L.D. and Mant, T.G.K. (1999) *A Textbook of Clinical Pharmacology*, 4th edn, Arnold, London.

Turnheim, K. (2003) When drug therapy gets old: pharmacokinetics and pharmacodynamics in the elderly. *Exp Gerontol*, **38**, 843–853.

Walker, R. and Whittlesea, C. (2007) *Clinical Pharmacy and Therapeutics*, 4th edn, Churchill Livingstone, Edinburgh.

Waller, D.G., Renwick, A.G. and Hillier, K. (2002) *Medical Pharmacology and Therapeutics*, W.B. Saunders, Edinburgh.

Winter, M. (2004) *Basic Clinical Pharmacokinetics*, 4th edn, Lippincott, Williams and Wilkins, Philadelphia.

19 Adverse drug reactions and interactions

Learning outcomes

By the end of this chapter the reader should be able to:

- describe the differences between a type A and a type B adverse drug reaction
- understand which patient groups are more susceptible to adverse drug reactions
- understand the different mechanisms of common adverse drug reactions
- identify and manage possible adverse drug reactions
- understand which adverse drug reactions must be reported to the MHRA using the Yellow Card system
- understand the different mechanisms of common drug and food interactions
- identify and manage drug–drug and drug–food interactions.

Adverse drug reactions – some definitions

An (adverse drug reaction) (ADR) is any undesirable effect of a drug which is not an anticipated therapeutic effect, occurring during clinical use. The World Health Organization (WHO) definition of an adverse drug reaction is 'a response to a drug which is noxious, unintended and occurs at doses used in man for prophylaxis, diagnosis or therapy'. The UK Commission on Human Medicines defines an ADR as 'an unwanted or harmful reaction experienced after the administration of the drug or combination of drugs under normal conditions of use and suspected to be related to the drug'. Patients often call ADRs 'side effects'.

Classification of ADRs

Adverse drug reactions are usually classified into two types: A and B. Type A reactions are exaggerated (Augmented) responses to the normal pharmacological action of the drug given

Table 19.1 Characteristics of type A and type B ADRs (adapted from Walker and Whittlesea, 2007).

	Type A (augmented response)	Type B (bizarre response)
Pharmacologically predictable	Yes	No
Dose dependent	Yes	No
Incidence	High	Low
Time of occurrence	Soon after first dose or dose increase	Variable, can be months or even years into (or after) treatment
Morbidity	High	Low
Mortality	Low	High
Management	Dose reduction	Stop drug
Rechallenge	Yes with caution	No

at a therapeutic dose. These reactions are usually dose dependent: the higher the dose, the more likely a type A reaction is to occur. An example of this occurs with glicazide, where too high a dose can cause hypoglycaemia. This can be managed by reducing the dose.

Type B reactions are *Bizarre* effects that are not predictable according to the drug's pharmacological action, and occur at any dose. An example of this is malignant hyperthermia after anaesthesia. These reactions can result in severe illness and death. Table 19.1 highlights other differences between these types of reactions.

Susceptible patient groups

There are certain patient groups that are particularly susceptible to ADRs (Table 19.2).

Table 19.2 Susceptible patient groups.

Patient group	Reason why
Polypharmacy	Multiple disease states and multiple drugs combine to cause interactions and ADRs
Elderly	Usually have polypharmacy, also altered pharmacokinetics and pharmacodynamics
Young children	Altered pharmacokinetics and pharmacodynamics, also unlicensed and off-label use of drugs
Gender	Women are at greater risk of ADRs than men due to altered pharmacokinetics and pharmacoynamics
Concomitant disease	Multiple disease states and multiple drugs combine to cause interactions and ADRs. Also altered pharmacokinetics
Race and genetics	Altered pharmacokinetics and pharmacodynamics

Section 3

Practice application

Patients with liver failure who take a loop diuretic, for example furosemide, are prone to the ADR of hypokalaemia (low serum potassium). Such patients may be given a combination of a loop diuretic and a potassium-sparing diuretic, for example amiloride, in the form of co-amilofruse. The amiloride does not have a large diuretic effect but it does prevent loss of potassium ions, as an ADR.

Mechanisms of ADRs and examples

Pharmaceutical causes

Adverse drug reactions can occur due to drug formulation, release characteristics from the dosage form and alterations in amount of drug in the dosage form. A common example of this is symptoms of opioid overdose in heroin users when a particularly pure preparation of heroin is circulating on the streets. Another example is pain following too rapid administration of clarithromycin injection; this is due to the excipients in the injection form.

Poor formulations of drugs (e.g. the use of diethylene glycol as a solvent which caused many deaths in the USA in the 1930s) can cause ADRs. Nowadays it is less likely for excipients to cause ADRs, as they are strictly tested. The warnings associated with enoxaparin injection used in pregnant women, due to a toxic excipient, show that mistakes can still be made, even when strict quality control processes are in place. The increasing availability of fake or counterfeit drugs in the UK may see an increase in ADRs due to poor quality control and the use of banned excipients.

Pharmacokinetic causes

Changes in pharmacokinetic parameters will cause changes in the concentration of drug at its site of action. Any increase in concentration of the drug may cause a type A ADR as there will effectively be an increased dose of the drug available to act on the target receptors. Elimination and metabolism are the main pharmacokinetic stages where changes can lead to ADRs.

Examples of metabolism ADRs include those associated with the cytochrome P450 enzyme system. This enzyme system metabolises many drugs and changes in the activity of the cytochrome P450 enzyme system, usually due to genetic differences, can result in impaired metabolism of certain drugs, leading to an increase in plasma levels and type A ADRs. There are also many drug interactions via this system which will be discussed later in the chapter. A drug commonly affected by this is warfarin. Other enzyme systems are affected by genetics and some drugs which produce ADRs via this method include isoniazid, hydralazine, paracetamol and oestrogens.

Examples of elimination ADRs include when a patient has renal impairment which leads to reduced elimination of the drug, and therefore a type A ADR, for example with digoxin and gentamicin. Doses of renally cleared drugs must be reduced in patients with renal impairment (Chapter 25).

Pharmacodynamic causes

Glucose 6 phosphate dehydrogenase (G6PD) deficiency is a common cause of ADRs in a small group of patients. G6PD is an enzyme required to maintain the stability of red blood cells and there are some patients who have an inherited deficiency of this enzyme. These patients are at risk of haemolysis when exposed to certain drugs, for example sulphonamides and nitrofurantoin, and these drugs should be avoided in patients with G6PD deficiency. There is a specific section in the BNF listing which drugs should be avoided. There are other genetic enzyme deficiencies and changes which can cause apparently idiosyncratic or bizarre (type B) ADRs.

Malignant hyperthermia is a type B ADR following administration of anaesthetics and muscle relaxants. It is thought to be due to an abnormal release of calcium following administration of these drugs and occurs, unpredictably, in a few patients only. Another type B ADR due to pharmacodynamic causes is cholestatic jaundice which can be caused by many drugs, including oral contraceptives and some antibiotics, including flucloxacillin. This is an unpredictable reaction, which is not always reversible on withdrawal of the drug, and can occur some weeks after the causative drug has been stopped.

 Stop and think

Patients who undergo GI surgery may be given a dose of co-amoxiclav as a prophylactic antibiotic. Both co-amoxiclav and anaesthetic agents can cause cholestatic jaundice. How would you establish which drug had caused the ADR?

There are also immunological reactions, sometimes known as hypersensitivity reactions. These are classed as type B reactions and include symptoms of a typical allergic reaction, blood dyscrasias, serum sickness, vasculitis, Stevens Johnson syndrome and contact dermatitis. These reactions usually have no relation to the pharmacological effects of the drug, can be seen at very small doses if rechallenge is undertaken, usually disappear on withdrawal of the drug and sometimes occur as a delayed response after the first dose of the drug. Some drugs can cause an ADR upon withdrawal of the drug; examples of these are rapid withdrawal of beta-blockers, corticosteroids and benzodiazepines.

Identification and management of ADRs

Patients who present with an ADR will often be coming to you for treatment of a new symptom. They will not realise that their symptom is an ADR. It is up to you as a prescriber to identify a suspected ADR to a specific drug and then manage it accordingly.

The first step in identifying an ADR is to take a thorough history from the patient. Include questions about the length of treatment of the drugs they are on, whether they have been treated with drugs in the same class before, how long they have had the symptoms, whether they are worse or better in relation to doses of drugs and questions to exclude a non-ADR reason for the symptoms.

For type A reactions, you will usually be able to discover a clear time association between starting a new drug or increasing a dose and the onset of the symptoms. The drug's summary of product characteristics (SPC) will list all the adverse reactions seen during the clinical trials for the suspected drug and maybe reactions seen during postmarketing surveillance. However, if you strongly suspect a symptom is associated with a particular drug, and this is not listed in the SPC, you could be observing a new ADR to that drug.

 Practice application

A patient on many antihypertensives who presents with dizziness should have their blood pressure monitored as part of the patient assessment. If it is low, the patient is experiencing a type A reaction to their antihypertensives and the doses should be reduced.

For Type B reactions, it is usually harder to make an association between drugs and symptoms, and these are usually diagnosed at the end of a process of eliminating other possible diagnoses.

The management of ADRs involves making a risk/benefit decision, in conjunction with the patient if possible, about what the risks are in stopping the drug or continuing with it and suffering the ADR. Some patients will prefer to continue with a drug if they are seeing a benefit, and put up with the inconvenience of a minor ADR.

 Stop and think

If you are taking a loop diuretic for heart failure, and experiencing the ADR of increased frequency of urination, would you want to continue with the diuretic?

If the ADR is serious, then the drug would usually be stopped. This is one of those rare situations where drugs can be abruptly stopped without tapering the dose down, for example beta blockers. Sometimes a drug from the same class will not have the same side-effect profile and can be substituted. However, other ADRs are class effects and so a drug from a different class must be used.

Some ADRs resolve on their own once the causative drug is stopped, although other ADRs may take longer to resolve and the patient may prefer to take another drug to treat the ADR whilst they wait for the symptoms to subside. This is particularly the case with skin reactions, which can take some time to settle, and may be treated with steroid creams or oral steroids.

Occasionally an ADR can be predicted, and if the drug is necessary then prophylactic drugs to treat the ADR symptoms can be given. An example of this is antiemetics given alongside emetogenic chemotherapy or a proton pump inhibitor given to prevent the GI side effects of NSAIDs.

Table 19.3   Types of ADRs to be reported to the MHRA via the Yellow Card system.

	Report
Drug type	
New (black triangle in BNF)	All suspected ADRs
Herbal medicines	All suspected ADRs
Older drugs	If fits patient group or ADR type
Patient group	
Elderly	All suspected ADRs
Children	All suspected ADRs
Other patient groups	If fits drug or ADR type
ADR type	
Fatal	All suspected ADRs
Life threatening	All suspected ADRs
Disabling or incapacitating	All suspected ADRs
Hospitalisation	All suspected ADRs
Prolonging hospital stay	All suspected ADRs
Congenital abnormality	All suspected ADRs
Other ADR	If fits drug type or patient group

It is important to remember to record any suspected ADRs and action taken in the patient's shared medical notes, to prevent other prescribers using the same drug in the future.

Yellow Card scheme

If an ADR to a particular drug is noticed, it is important for the wider health community that the ADR is recorded nationally. The Medicines and Healthcare products Regulatory Agency (MHRA) is a government agency that ensures that all UK medicines, amongst other things, are of an acceptable standard in terms of safety, quality, performance and effectiveness. The MHRA and the Commission on Human Medicines, another government committee, run the Yellow Card scheme in the UK for reporting suspected ADRs to drugs, blood products, vaccines, herbal products and radiation contrast media. Anyone suspecting an ADR, including a patient, can complete a Yellow Card and send it to the MHRA. Yellow Cards can be found in the back of BNFs, and also online at the MHRA website. The MHRA collates the information sent on the Yellow Card reports and uses this information to produce monthly drug safety updates and maintain a database of all Yellow Card reports for all drugs. Table 19.3 gives details of the types of ADRs that the MHRA is interested in receiving Yellow Cards for. The general motto is – if in doubt, report it.

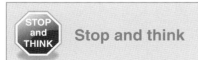 **Stop and think**

Would you report an ADR of a rash caused by furosemide in an elderly person? Should you?

Section 3

Drug interactions

A drug interaction occurs when the effects of one drug are changed by the presence of another drug, food or drink. The changes can be pharmacokinetic or pharmacodynamic.

Pharmacokinetic interactions

Absorption

Drugs which change the pH of gastrointestinal fluid can change the rate and amount of absorption of other drugs. If a drug relies on the acidic environment of the stomach to undergo dissolution and absorption, then the action of another drug which raises the pH of the gastrointestinal fluid will reduce the rate and amount of absorption of the first drug. Examples of drugs which are affected by this type of interaction are proton pump inhibitors reducing the oral absorption of ketoconazole.

Some drugs have a tendency to react directly with the contents of the stomach, either food or other drugs, to form a chelate or a complex which is not absorbed. Tetracyclines will form a chelate with calcium ions found in milk, and also with iron. This results in greatly reduced absorption of the tetracycline, and a reduced action in the body.

 Practice application

Patients who are being fed with an enteral feed, for example a nasogastric feed, must have their feeds turned off 2 hours before a dose of ciprofloxacin, and the feed restarted 2 hours after the dose. The nasogastric line must be flushed well with water before and after the ciprofloxacin dose.

Drugs which have an effect on gastrointestinal motility, for example metoclopramide, may change the rate and amount of oral absorption of some drugs. The absorption rate may be either increased or decreased, depending upon where the drug is absorbed in the GI tract.

Distribution

If two drugs are given which are highly bound to plasma protein, they will compete for the binding sites on the plasma proteins. The drug which is less successful at binding to plasma proteins will have a higher proportion of free drug available to have a therapeutic action. Phenytoin is a drug which is particularly affected by this mechanism of interaction.

Metabolism

Most drug metabolism takes place in the liver, by liver enzymes. The action of these liver enzymes can be inhibited or enhanced (induced) by the presence of other drugs. In the presence of a strong enzyme inducer, other drugs normally metabolised by the same enzyme system will be metabolised to a much greater extent, therefore reducing the plasma concentration of those drugs. Conversely, in the presence of a strong enzyme inhibitor, the plasma concentration of other drugs can be increased.

The cytochrome P450 enzyme system is particularly susceptible to enzyme inhibition or induction by drugs. There are many subtypes of the cytochrome P450 enzyme and drugs which are metabolised by a particular subtype are usually affected by the presence of other drugs metabolised by the same subtype (Chapter 16). An example of this type of interaction is where rifampicin induces liver enzymes, resulting in possible contraception failure where patients are taking oral contraceptives. Warfarin metabolism is also affected by both enzyme inducers and inhibitors; it is usual to monitor the international normalised ratio (INR) more closely when a known interacting drug is added to the regime of a patient taking warfarin. There are also drug-food interactions because of the cytochrome P450 enzyme system. Grapefruit juice is an inhibitor of one of the enzyme cytochrome P450 subtypes, and so patients who are taking drugs which are also metabolised via this subtype should be advised not to drink grapefruit juice. This includes some statins and cyclosporin.

Elimination

Drugs can affect various stages of elimination. Particular interactions to note are listed in Table 19.4.

Pharmacodynamic interactions

As you know from Chapter 14, drugs can be either agonists or antagonists at receptors. So logically, we can see that if a patient is given a drug that is an agonist and another drug that is an antagonist at the same receptor, these two drugs will antagonise each other. An example of this is giving an asthmatic patient who uses a beta agonist inhaler, for example salbutamol, a beta-blocker. There are many other examples of such interactions, some of which are used therapeutically.

Table 19.4 Drug interactions caused by alteration to elimination.

Drug 1	Drug 2	Mechanism of interaction	Outcome
Salicylates	Methotrexate	Competition for the same renal tubular secretion pathway	Methotrexate toxicity
NSAIDs	Lithium	Changes in renal blood flow due to reduced prostaglandins	Increased lithium levels
Sodium bicarbonate	Salicylates	Alkalinisation of urine	Increased elimination
Digoxin	Verapamil	Inhibition of drug transporter proteins	Increased digoxin levels

Section 3

Practice application

Naloxone is an opioid antagonist and is used in opioid overdose to compete for the opioid receptors, displace the opioid and prevent it having a further effect.

If two drugs which act in a similar way are given to a patient, their action could be additive or synergistic and result in an excessive therapeutic effect. Examples of these are NSAIDs, warfarin and clopidogrel, which can have an additive effect on increasing bleeding risk if given together. Another example is drugs which can prolong the QT interval on an ECG, for example terfenadine and fluconazole, which when given together can cause a serious cardiac arrhythmia called torsade de pointes. Terfenadine has fallen out of common use because of this serious drug interaction.

Antidepressants are particularly problematic when it comes to drug interactions. Drugs which affect serotonin, for example SSRIs, can cause serotonin syndrome if they are given concurrently or abruptly stopped. MAOI antidepressants also affect serotonin, so for this reason they are rarely given in combination with an SSRI. MAOIs are also the subject of interactions with foods containing tyramine, an amino acid. The body requires MAO to metabolise tyramine into inactive metabolites and in patients who are taking MAOIs, this metabolism cannot take place. Ecstasy and some drugs which can be bought over the counter in a pharmacy, for example pseudoephedrine, can also cause an interaction with the MAOI, resulting in hypertensive crisis.

Management of interactions

The appendix in the back of the BNF gives a good summary of drug interactions. When prescribing a new drug for a patient, consider the other drugs the patient is on and ensure there will be no serious interaction in the combination you are proposing. If there is an interaction, it is important to consider the possible effect on your specific patient and if there is an alternative drug which can be used, this should be chosen.

If a patient has been maintained on two drugs which are known to interact, it is likely that the doses of both drugs have been adjusted for the interaction. It is not usually necessary to change the therapy of such patients, unless they start to exhibit signs or symptoms of an interaction.

Summary

- Adverse drug reactions can be split into two classes: type A and type B.
- Type A ADRs are predictable, dose dependent and usually reversible when the causative drug is stopped.
- Type B ADRs are unpredictable, can occur at any dose, sometimes occurring after the causative drug has been stopped and may be irreversible.
- Pharmaceutical causes of ADRs are usually related to dangerous excipients or a poor manufacturing process.
- Pharmacokinetic causes of ADRs usually occur in the metabolism and elimination stages.

- The cytochrome P450 enzyme system is affected by genetic changes, and drugs metabolised by this system can cause ADRs in certain patient groups.
- Pharmacodynamic causes of ADRs usually result in type B ADRs.
- Patients presenting with suspected ADR should have a thorough history of drug use taken in order to identify the causative drug.
- Management of an ADR involves careful risk/benefit analysis to decide whether the causative drug should be continued or not.
- The MHRA collects data about ADRs through the Yellow Card scheme.
- A drug interaction occurs when the effects of one drug are changed by the presence of another drug, food or drink.
- Pharmacokinetic mechanisms of drug interactions can occur at any stage of the pharmacokinetic process.
- Pharmacodynamic mechanisms of drug interactions include synergistic or additive effects, agonist and antagonist effects and specific effects upon the neurotransmitter systems.
- When adding a new drug into a patient's therapy, it is important to consider potential drug interactions.
- Patients who have been maintained on two interacting drugs will probably be stabilised and do not necessarily need their therapy changing.

Activity

1. Which of the following statements regarding type A adverse drug reactions are correct?
   - Predictable — True / False
   - Low incidence — True / False
   - Low mortality — True / False
   - Managed by dose reduction — True / False
   - Low morbidity — True / False
2. Which of the following statements regarding the pharmacokinetic mechanisms of adverse drug reactions are correct?
   - Dose reduction is necessary in renal impairment. — True / False
   - Increases in plasma concentration result in type A ADRs. — True / False
   - The cytochrome P450 enzyme system is important in ADRs. — True / False
   - Pharmacokinetic ADRs result mainly in type B ADRs. — True / False
   - There is genetic variation in the way isoniazid is metabolised. — True / False
3. Which of the following statements about how ADRs should be managed are correct?
   - The patient will know exactly which drug is causing their ADR. — True / False
   - The causative drug must always be stopped. — True / False
   - The causative drug must always be slowly withdrawn. — True / False
   - You must only report definite ADRs to the MHRA. — True / False
   - Anyone can report an ADR to the MHRA. — True / False
4. Which of the following statements about drug interaction mechanisms are correct?
   - Synergy is where the effects of two drugs cancel each other out. — True / False
   - The formation of chelates in the GI tract aids drug absorption. — True / False
   - Methotrexate and aspirin have an important interaction. — True / False
   - Cytochrome P450 interactions affect the metabolism of various drugs. — True / False
   - Patients taking oral contraceptives must use extra contraceptive methods when they are taking rifampicin. — True / False

Section 3

5. Which of the following statements about the management of drug interactions are correct?
   - Patients taking MAOIs must not eat foods containing tyramine.   True / False
   - When starting new drugs, prescribers must disregard any other drugs the patient is
     taking.   True / False
   - The BNF is a useful reference source for identifying drug interactions.   True / False
   - Patients taking simvastatin must drink lots of grapefruit juice.   True / False
   - There are no drug interactions with warfarin.   True / False

Useful website

Medicines and Healthcare products Regulatory Agency website. www.mhra.gov.uk

Reference

Walker, R. and Whittlesea, C. (2007) *Clinical Pharmacy and Therapeutics*, 4th edn, Churchill Livingstone, Edinburgh.

Further reading

Baxter, K. (2007) *Stockley's Drug Interactions*, 8th edn, Pharmaceutical Press, London.

British Medical Association and Royal Pharmaceutical Society of Great Britain (2010) *British National Formulary*, 59th edn, BMJ Publishing, London.

Dunn, N. (2003) 10 Minute consultation: adverse drug event. *BMJ*, **326**, 1018.

Hersh, E.V., Pinto, A. and Moore, P.A. (2007) Adverse drug interactions involving common prescription and over-the-counter analgesic agents. *Clin Ther*, **29**, 2477–2497.

Pirmohamed, M., Breckenridge, A.M., Kitteringham, N.R. and Park, B.K. (1998) Fortnightly review: adverse drug reactions. *BMJ*, **316**, 1295–1298.

Rawlins, M.D. and Thompson, J.W. (1977) Pathogenesis of adverse drug reactions, in *Textbook of Adverse Drug Reactions* (ed. D.M. Davies), Oxford University Press, Oxford.

Routledge, P.A., O'Mahony, M.S. and Woodhouse, K.W. (2004) Adverse drug reactions in elderly patients. *Br J Clin Pharmacol*, **57**, 121–126.

White, R. (2008) Nutrition – drug–nutrient interactions. *Hosp Pharm*, **15**, 243–244.

Wijnen, P.A., Op den Buijsch, R.A., Drent, M., *et al.* (2007) The prevalence and clinical relevance of cytochrome P450 polymorphisms. *Aliment Pharmacol Ther*, **26**(Suppl 2), 211–219.

20 Introduction to the autonomic nervous system

Learning outcomes

By the end of this chapter the reader should be able to:

- describe the role of the autonomic nervous system within the body
- name the two branches of the autonomic nervous system, the neurotransmitters they release and the receptors they bind to
- describe the effects of the autonomic nervous system on the major organs of the body
- understand the mechanism of neurotransmission within the autonomic nervous system and how this may be terminated.

The nervous system

The nervous system of the body can be divided into two branches (Figure 20.1):

- the central nervous system (CNS) which consists of the brain and spinal cord
- the peripheral nervous system which comprises all the other nerves in the body and connects the central nervous system and body tissues.

The peripheral nervous system can itself be divided into two components: the somatic nervous system and the autonomic nervous system.

The main difference between these two systems is that the somatic system can be described as regulating voluntary movements – those movements which we choose to make. The autonomic nervous system, on the other hand, is involved in regulating involuntary body systems.

In other words, the somatic nervous system acts to relay messages between the central nervous system and the skin and skeletal muscles and is involved with regulating responses

The New Prescriber. Edited by J Lymn, D Bowskill, F Bath-Hextall, R Knaggs, © 2010 John Wiley & Sons.

Section 3

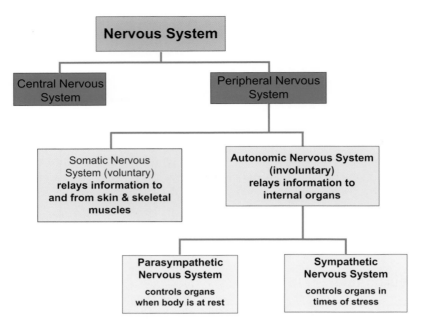

Figure 20.1   Divisions of the nervous system.

over which we have conscious control. The autonomic nervous system is responsible for relaying messages between the central nervous system and the internal organs of the body and as such regulates responses which occur without any conscious control on our part.

The autonomic nervous system

The main functions of the autonomic nervous system are regulation of:

- the heartbeat
- the contraction and relaxation of smooth muscle
- energy metabolism
- the production of exocrine (and some endocrine) secretions.

The autonomic nervous system also plays a role in regulating both renin release from the juxtaglomerular cells of the kidney and histamine release from mast cells.

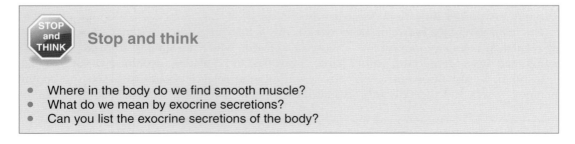

Stop and think

- Where in the body do we find smooth muscle?
- What do we mean by exocrine secretions?
- Can you list the exocrine secretions of the body?

The autonomic nervous system itself can be further divided into two components.

The parasympathetic nervous system

This is most active when the body is relaxed and is often referred to as the 'rest and digest' system – imagine lying on the settee watching the television after lunch on a Sunday.

The sympathetic nervous system

This is referred to as the 'fight/flight/fright' system and is at its most active when the body is under stress – imagine sitting in a pharmacology lecture!

It should be remembered, however, that both of these systems are operating continuously and together, to effectively regulate body function.

Action of the autonomic nervous system on body organs

The parasympathetic and sympathetic nervous systems produce opposing responses on a number of organs of the body (Table 20.1). Perhaps the easiest way of remembering these actions is to think of the systems in terms of 'rest and digest' and 'fight/flight/fright'. If we take the sympathetic nervous system as an example, this is active in stressful situations of 'fight/flight/fright'. In evolutionary terms this meant exactly what it said – a fight/flight for life. Under these circumstances the heart rate needs to speed up in order to deliver more blood (containing oxygen and nutrients) to the body so that you can 'make a run for it'; similarly, the lungs need to dilate in order to get as much oxygen into the body as possible and the pupil needs to dilate in order to give you the requisite far vision. Under these circumstances the body has more important priorities than digestion of the last meal and elimination of waste.

However, it would be a mistake to assume that the parasympathetic and sympathetic systems have opposing effects throughout the body – there are a number of body functions which are regulated by only one of these systems.

Table 20.1   Opposing action of the parasympathetic and sympathetic nervous systems on body organs.

Organ	Parasympathetic	Sympathetic
Eye	Constriction of pupil	Dilation of pupil
Heart	Decreased heart rate and force of contraction	Increased heart rate and force of contraction
Lungs	Bronchconstriction	Bronchodilation
GI tract	Increased motility of smooth muscle	Decreased motility of smooth muscle
	Relaxation of sphincters	Constriction of sphincters
	Gastric acid secretion	
Bladder	Contraction of detrusor	Relaxation of detrusor
	Relaxation of sphincter	Constriction of sphincter

Section 3

Box 20.1   Actions of the sympathetic nervous system on body functions which are not opposed by the parasympathetic nervous system.

Blood vessels	Dilation of blood vessels in the skeletal muscle beds
	Contraction of blood vessels of skin and visceral beds
Liver	Stimulation of glycogen breakdown into glucose (glycogenolysis)
Fat	Stimulation of the breakdown of fats into ready fuel molecules (lipolysis)
Kidney	Secretion of renin
Mast cells	Inhibition of histamine release
Sweat glands	Stimulation of sweat production

Sympathetic nervous system

Box 20.1 shows the unopposed action of the sympathetic nervous system on body functions. Again, these responses make sense in terms of the 'fight/flight/fright' model.

- The regulation of blood vessel contractility allows blood to be redistributed away from the visceral beds and into the skeletal muscle beds.
- Glycogenolysis and lipolysis release fuel molecules for ready use by the body in this emergency situation.
- Inhibition of histamine release from mast cells is important as histamine acts as a bronchoconstrictor and this would impede the bronchodilation required.
- Renin acts ultimately to increase the formation of angiotensin II (Chapter 23) which enhances the contraction of peripheral blood vessels, thus supporting the redistribution of the blood to the skeletal muscle beds.
- Stimulation of sweat production helps to keep the body cool which is critical in this type of fight/flight/fright response.

 Stop and think

Why does the sympathetic nervous system increase blood flow to the skeletal muscle beds?

Parasympathetic nervous system

Box 20.2 shows the action of the parasympathetic nervous system on body function. The parasympathetic nervous system is responsible for stimulating the production of all exocrine secretions of the body, with the exception of sweat.

Section 3

> **Box 20.2   Action of the parasympathetic nervous system on body functions.**
>
> | | |
> |---|---|
> | Blood vessels | No direct innervation by the parasympathetic system; however, this system stimulates the production of nitric oxide from endothelial cells resulting in a generalised vasodilation |
> | Lacrimal gland | Stimulation of tear production |
> | Salivary gland | Stimulation of saliva production |
> | GI tract | Stimulation of gastric acid production |

Neuron structure

The autonomic nervous system is made up of nerve cells or neurons. Neurons all have a similar structure which can be divided into three main parts (Figure 20.2).

- **The cell body** – this is sometimes referred to as the 'soma' and contains the nucleus of the neuron as well as cytoplasmic organelles including mitochondria and ribosomes. It is worth remembering that even though neurons have nuclei and can synthesise proteins, they cannot divide.
- **The dendrites** – these are highly branched projections from the cell body which act as signal receivers and carry messages to the cell body.
- **The axon** – this is a long projection of the cell which carries messages away from the cell body. The axon is usually covered by a myelin sheath which prevents the message dissipating and speeds up the rate of transmission. The axon terminal may be branched to allow connection with the dendrites of a number of other neurons.

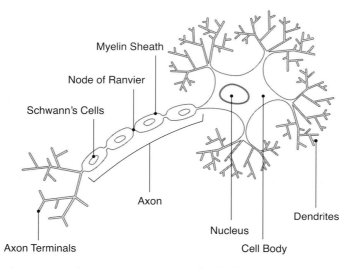

Figure 20.2   Typical structure of a neuron, or nerve cell, which is the fundamental component of the autonomic nervous system.

Neuron function

Neurons are the specialised cells which transmit signals to and from the brain at high speed. The message or signals transmitted by neurons take the form of electrical impulses which are transmitted down the axon and are known as action potentials. An action potential is generated as a result of changes in the ionic composition of both the internal environment of the neuron and the immediate external environment following the movement of sodium and potassium ions across the membrane of the neuron (Chapter 29). Although transmission down an axon is electrical, there is no physical connection between different nerves; they do not actually touch each other and so transmission of the signal from one neuron to another, or from a neuron to a muscle or gland, occurs not by electrical transmission but by chemical transmission. This process of chemical transmission is hugely important in pharmacology. The junction between two neurons or between a neuron and a tissue is called the synapse or chemical synapse (Figure 20.3).

Chemical transmitters, or neurotransmitters, are stored 'prepacked' in lipid packages called vesicles at the axon terminal. As the electrical impulse travels down the axon, it promotes the opening of calcium channels in the membrane and hence calcium enters the axon terminal. This increase in calcium stimulates the fusion of the lipid vesicles with the plasma membrane and the consequent release of neurotransmitter into the synapse. The released neurotransmitter diffuses across the synapse and binds to specific receptors on the neuron or specialised cell of the tissue, thus transmitting the message to the next cell.

Neurons in the autonomic nervous system

The autonomic nervous system (both the parasympathetic and the sympathetic branches) is made up of two neurons in sequence. The cell body of the first neuron (called the preganglionic

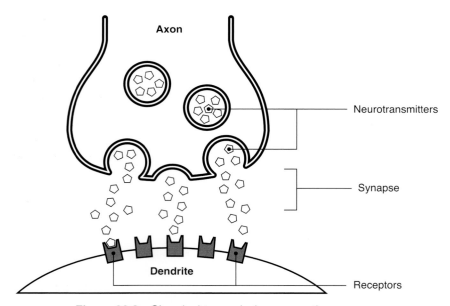

Figure 20.3 Chemical transmission across the synapse.

neuron) is always in the CNS and it is the region of the CNS in which the cell body of this neuron is located which determines whether it is parasympathetic or sympathetic. Parasympathetic nerves arise in the cranial and sacral regions of the spinal cord and sympathetic nerves arise in the thoracic and lumbar regions.

The preganglionic neuron may synapse at a single postganglionic neuron, as occurs in the parasympathetic nervous system, or it may synapse at several postganglionic neurons, as in the sympathetic nervous system.

In the parasympathetic nervous system the synapse with the postganglionic neuron is relatively close to the final intended recipient of the stimulation (muscle or gland) and so the axon of the postganglionic neuron is relatively short while in the sympathetic nervous system the axon of the postganglionic neuron is very long.

The chemical transmitter which is released from the preganglionic neuron is always acetylcholine (Ach), which diffuses across the synapse and binds to nicotinic acetylcholine receptors (nAchR) on the postganglionic neuron regardless of whether it is a parasympathetic or sympathetic nerve.

The differences between the two systems occur at the synapse of the postganglionic neuron with the cells of the organ or gland. It is here that the two systems release different neurotransmitters:

- The parasympathetic nervous system continues to use acetylcholine as its neurotransmitter at the neuroeffector junction but the receptors on the muscle/gland are muscarinic (M) receptors.
- The sympathetic nervous system uses noradrenaline (NA) as the neurotransmitter at the neuroeffector junction and the receptors to which this binds on the muscles are known as adrenergic receptors or adrenoceptors.

There are two exceptions to this rule in the sympathetic nervous system.

- **The adrenal medulla** – following acetylcholine binding to nicotinic receptors on the adrenal medulla, adrenaline is released into the bloodstream. This adrenaline can then act on adrenergic receptors in the lungs. This is extremely important as there is no direct innervation of the lungs by the sympathetic nervous system; what we mean by this is that there are no sympathetic nerves which actually go directly to the lungs. Hence the reaction of the lungs to sympathetic nervous system stimulation is entirely as a result of the release of adrenaline into the bloodstream.
- **The sweat glands** – these are similar to the lacrimal and salivary glands stimulated by the parasympathetic nervous system in that they continue to utilise acetylcholine as a neurotransmitter and this binds to muscarinic receptors on the cells of the salivary glands (Figure 20.4).

 Practice application

Drugs which mimic the effects of the autonomic nervous system are used clinically for the treatment of many different conditions including respiratory disease, myasthenia gravis, Alzheimer's disease and cardiovascular disease.

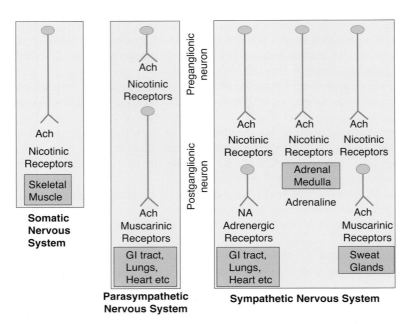

Figure 20.4 Receptor types and neurotransmitters of the autonomic nervous system (adapted from Rang *et al.*, 2007).

Cholinergic transmission

This term refers to neurotransmission which utilises acetylcholine as the neurotransmitter. Consequently cholinergic transmission is important for:

● transmission from the preganglionic to the postganglionic neuron (in both the parasympathetic and sympathetic nervous systems)
● transmission from the postganglionic neuron to the effector muscle/gland in the parasympathetic nervous system
● transmission to the sweat glands in the sympathetic nervous system
● transmission to the skeletal muscles (somatic nervous system).

Acetylcholine is stored in vesicles in the axon terminals. As the electrical signal passes down the axon, calcium channels in the terminal membranes open and calcium enters the axon terminals. This increase in calcium promotes the fusion of lipid vesicles with the plasma membrane and acetylcholine is released. Acetylcholine then diffuses across the gap and binds to either nicotinic (on neuron) or muscarinic (on muscles or glands) receptors to stimulate a response.

The body has to have a mechanism by which this response is 'turned off' otherwise acetylcholine would be continually binding and stimulating a response and this is clearly not the case. Acetylcholine is broken down at both the synapse and the neuroeffector junctions by an enzyme called acetylcholinesterase which converts it into acetate and choline. If you remember back to the beginning of the pharmacology section, we talked about the 'lock and

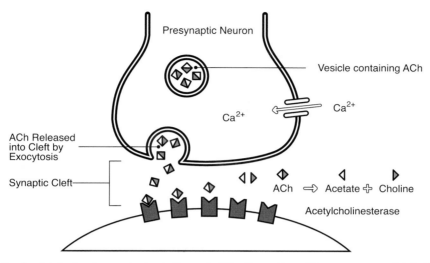

Presynaptic Neuron

Vesicle containing ACh

Ca^{2+} Ca^{2+}

ACh Released
into Cleft by
Exocytosis

Synaptic Cleft

ACh $\Rightarrow$ Acetate $+$ Choline

Acetylcholinesterase

Figure 20.5   Acetylcholine transmission is 'turned off' by the action of the enzyme acetylcholinesterase.

key' hypothesis and that ligands have to be the right shape to fit the receptor and signal a response. Neither acetate nor choline has the right shape to fit either the nicotinic or muscarinic
receptors and hence these molecules cannot generate a response – they are not the right 'key'
(Figure 20.5).

In terms of pharmacology, we can use a number of different types of drugs to either increase
or decrease cholinergic transmission in the body (Box 20.3).

Box 20.3   Drug groups which can be used clinically to modulate cholinergic transmission in the body.

Muscarinic agonists	Mimic the action of acetylcholine at muscarinic receptors in the body and hence enhance the normal response at these receptors
Muscarinic antagonists	These drugs are similar in shape to acetylcholine and so will compete with acetylcholine for muscarinic receptors. They will not, however stimulate a response and hence result in a reduced response at these receptors
Nicotinic agonists (depolarising muscle relaxants)	Mimic the action of acetylcholine at nicotinic receptors of the neuromuscular junction. However, they remain bound at these receptors for much longer than acetylcholine which results in prolonged depolarisation and muscle block
Nicotinic antagonists (non-depolarising muscle relaxants).	These drugs compete with acetylcholine for binding at nicotinic receptors
Anticholinesterase drugs	These drugs inhibit the acetylcholinesterase enzyme in the cleft or at the neuroeffector junction. This prevents acetylcholine from being broken down, increasing the amount of acetylcholine and prolonging the action of acetylcholine

Section 3

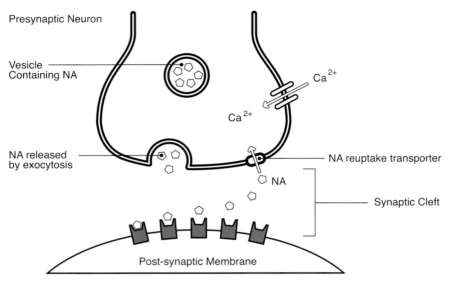

Figure 20.6 Noradrenergic transmission is 'turned off' by the reuptake of noradrenaline into the neuron.

Noradrenergic transmission

This term refers to neurotransmission which utilises noradrenaline as the neurotransmitter. Consequently noradrenergic transmission is important for transmission from the postganglionic neuron to the muscle in the sympathetic nervous system.

Just as with acetylcholine, noradrenaline is stored in vesicles in the axon terminals. As the electrical signal passes down the axon, calcium channels in the terminal membranes open and calcium enters the axon terminals. This increase in calcium promotes the fusion of lipid vesicles with the plasma membrane and noradrenaline is released. Noradrenaline then diffuses across the gap and binds to adrenergic receptors, or adrenoceptors, to stimulate a response. Unlike acetylcholine, noradrenaline is not broken down by an enzyme in the cleft. Instead, this signalling is 'turned off' by the reuptake of noradrenaline into the neuron terminal. What we mean by this is that noradrenaline in the cleft binds to a carrier molecule in the membrane of the axon terminal and this carries noradrenaline back into the nerve terminal from which it was released (Figure 20.6).

 Stop and think

Given the mechanisms of inactivation of neurotransmission in the autonomic system, how do you think drugs might act to increase this neurotransmission clinically?

The adrenoceptors to which noradrenaline binds can be subdivided into alpha- and beta-receptor subtypes

Alpha-adrenoceptors

There are two types of alpha adrenoceptor known as alpha-1 (α_1) and alpha-2 (α_2). The α_1-receptors are located on blood vessels, in the GI tract and bladder and in the eye. Stimulation of these receptors results in smooth muscle contraction. The α_2-receptors are located on nerve terminals (autoreceptors), in the brain and on platelets. Stimulation of these receptors results in termination of neurotransmitter release from the nerve terminals, inhibition of sympathetic outflow from the central nervous system and platelet aggregation.

Beta-receptors

There are three different types of beta-receptor known as beta-1 (β_1), beta-2 (β_2) and beta-3 (β_3). β_1-receptors are located mainly in the heart, with some being located in the kidney. Stimulation of these receptors increases heart rate directly and peripheral vascular resistance indirectly, through renin release from the juxtaglomerular cells of the kidney. β_3-receptors are located mainly in fat, with stimulation of these receptors resulting in lipolysis or breakdown of fat – needless to say these receptors are the subject of much drug research! β_2-receptors, on the other hand, are located throughout the rest of the body. Stimulation of these receptors results in relaxation of smooth muscle (blood vessels, bronchi, GI tract, detrusor muscle), glycogenolysis (liver), inhibition of histamine release (mast cells), tremor (skeletal muscle) and increased neurotransmitter release (nerve terminals).

The division of adrenoceptors into different subtypes is pharmacologically and clinically of enormous importance with drugs being designed to act at selective receptor subtypes.

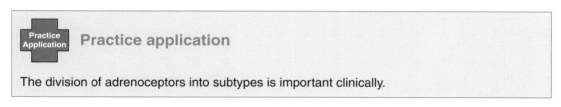

Practice application

The division of adrenoceptors into subtypes is important clinically.

The other aspect of noradrenergic transmission which needs to be considered here is the synthesis of noradrenaline (Figure 20.7). A number of drugs used clinically act by inhibiting enzymes in this pathway.

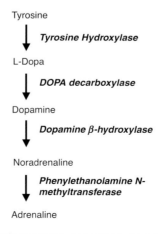

Tyrosine

Tyrosine Hydroxylase

L-Dopa

DOPA decarboxylase

Dopamine

Dopamine β-hydroxylase

Noradrenaline

Phenylethanolamine N-methyltransferase

Adrenaline

Figure 20.7   Relationship between dopamine, noradrenaline and adrenaline.

Section 3

In terms of pharmacology we can use a number of different types of drugs to either increase or decrease noradrenergic transmission in the body (Box 20.4).

Box 20.4 **Drug groups which can be used clinically to modulate noradrenergic transmission in the body.**	
Adrenoceptor agonists	Mimic the action of noradrenaline and adrenaline at adrenoceptors in the body and hence enhance the normal response at these receptors
Adrenoceptor antagonists	These drugs are similar in shape to noradrenaline and adrenaline and so will compete with these ligands for adrenoceptors. They will not, however, stimulate a response and hence result in a reduced response at these receptors
Drugs which increase noradrenaline synthesis	These drugs increase the synthesis of noradrenaline in the nerve terminal. Following electrical stimulation, more noradrenaline will be released at the neuroeffector junction, thus enhancing the response at adrenoceptors
Drugs which increase noradrenaline release	These drugs stimulate noradrenaline release from the nerve terminal. Thus they stimulate the response at adrenoceptors
Reuptake inhibitors (this mechanism is particularly important in the central nervous system)	These drugs inhibit the carrier protein which moves noradrenaline back into the nerve terminal, thus resulting in an increase in noradrenaline at the neuroeffector junction and enhancing the stimulation of adrenoceptors

Summary

- The autonomic nervous system is divided into two branches – the parasympathetic and the sympathetic – and these exert different effects on the organs of the body.
- Anatomically, the autonomic nervous system consists of two neurons: the preganglionic neuron (with its cell body in the central nervous system) and the postganglionic neuron.
- Neurotransmitters are released from the neuron by a process called exocytosis which requires high levels of calcium.
- The activity of acetylcholine is terminated by the action of the enzyme acetylcholinesterase in the synapse.
- Acetylcholinesterase breaks acetylcholine down into acetate and choline.
- The activity of noradrenaline is terminated by reuptake into the nerve terminal by a carrier molecule.
- Acetylcholine is released from all preganglionic nerves and binds to nicotinic receptors.
- Acetylcholine is released from the postganglionic nerves of the parasympathetic nervous system (and the sympathetic nerves innervating the sweat glands) and binds to muscarinic receptors.
- Noradrenaline is released from the postganglionic nerves of the sympathetic nervous system and binds to adrenoceptors.

Section 3

- Adrenaline is not a neurotransmitter but a hormone whose release into the bloodstream is stimulated by the action of the sympathetic nervous system on the adrenal glands.
- Classification of adrenceptors into different subtypes is clinically important.

✎ Activity

Please answer the following statements true or false.

1. The two main neurotransmitters which operate in the autonomic nervous system are acetylcholine and adrenaline. **True / False**
2. The sympathetic and parasympathetic nervous systems have opposing effects on GI smooth muscle motility. **True / False**
3. The sympathetic and parasympathetic nervous systems both act to stimulate sweat production. **True / False**
4. Neurotransmitters in the autonomic nervous system are released into the synapse by exocytosis. **True / False**
5. Acetylcholine is inactivated by enzymes within the synaptic cleft. **True / False**
6. Side effects of muscarinic agonists include constipation and urinary retention. **True / False**
7. Drugs which act as agonists at adrenoceptors activate the 'fight/flight/fright' response. **True / False**
8. Drugs acting at nicotinic receptors affect both the sympathetic and parasympathetic nervous systems. **True / False**
9. Drugs which act as antagonists at beta-adrenoceptors induce bronchodilation. **True / False**
10. The action of noradrenaline is curtailed by reuptake into the nerve terminal. **True / False**
11. Sympathetic nervous system stimulation to the bladder relaxes the detrusor muscle and constricts the sphincter. **True / False**
12. The parasympathetic nervous system stimulates glycogenolysis in the liver. **True / False**
13. There is direct sympathetic innervation of the lungs. **True / False**
14. Drugs which bind to beta-1-receptors modulate heart rate. **True / False**
15. Muscarinic receptors are located on the postganglionic neuron of the parasympathetic nervous system. **True / False**

Reusable learning object

Exploring the synapse. www.nottingham.ac.uk/nursing/sonet/rlos/bioproc/synapse/

Further reading

Aidley, D.J. (1998) *The Physiology of Excitable Cells*, 4th edn, Cambridge University Press, Cambridge.

Barker, R.A. (1993) *Neuroscience: An Illustrated Guide*, Ellis Horwood, New York.

Booij, L.H.D.J. (1996) *Neuromuscular Transmission*, BMJ Publishing Group, London.

Section 3

Briar, C., Lasserson, D., Gabriel, C. and Sharrack, B. (2003) *Crash Course: Nervous System*, 2nd edn, Mosby, London.

Foster, R.W. (2003) *Basic Pharmacology*, 4th edn, Arnold, London.

Kruk, Z.L. and Pycock, C.J. (1991) *Neurotransmitters and Drugs*, 3rd edn, Chapman and Hall, London.

McGavock, H. (2005) *How Drugs Work. Basic Pharmacology for Healthcare Professionals*, 2nd edn, Radcliffe Publishing, Oxford.

Page, C.P., Curtis, M.J., Sutter, M.C., *et al.* (2006) *Integrated Pharmacology*, 3rd edn, Mosby, London.

Rang, H.P., Dale, M.M., Ritter, J.M. and Flower, R. (2007) *Rang and Dale's Pharmacology*, 6th edn, Churchill Livingstone, Edinburgh.

Webster, R.A. and Jordan, C.C. (1989) *Neurotransmitters, Drugs and Disease*, Blackwell Scientific, Oxford.

Zimmerman, H. (1993) *Synaptic Transmission: Cellular and Molecular Basis*, Oxford University Press, Oxford.

21

Clinical application of the principles of the autonomic nervous system

Learning outcomes

By the end of this chapter the reader should understand:

- how drugs that target receptors within the parasympathetic nervous system can be used clinically
- why drugs that target receptors within the parasympathetic nervous system have certain cautions and contraindications
- how the hydrolysis of acetylcholine may be regulated for clinical effect
- how drugs that target receptors within the sympathetic nervous system can be used clinically
- why drugs that target receptors within the sympathetic nervous system have certain cautions and contraindications
- how the synthesis, release and reuptake of noradrenaline may be regulated for clinical effect.

This chapter describes how the autonomic nervous system can be manipulated for clinical effect. The autonomic nervous system is an ideal starting point for developing an understanding of why drugs have certain side effects and why specific cautions and contraindications are listed. The drug groups we are going to cover in this chapter are those which act through the modulation of both the parasympathetic and the sympathetic nervous systems (Box 21.1).

Section 3

The New Prescriber. Edited by J Lymn, D Bowskill, F Bath-Hextall, R Knaggs, © 2010 John Wiley & Sons.

Box 21.1 Groups of drugs used clinically which target the action of the parasympathetic and sympathetic nervous systems.

Parasympathetic nervous system	Sympathetic nervous system
Muscarinic agonists	Noradrenergic agonists
Muscarinic antagonists	Noradrenergic antagonists
Neuromuscular blockers (nicotinic antagonists)	Drugs affecting noradrenaline synthesis
Anticholinesterase drugs	Drugs affecting noradrenaline release
	Drugs affecting noradrenaline uptake

Drugs which target the parasympathetic nervous system and cholinergic transmission

Muscarinic agonists

These drugs mimic the action of acetylcholine at muscarinic receptors in the body and are sometimes referred to as parasympathomimetic. There are only two examples of this type of drug in clinical use these days: bethanechol and pilocarpine. Bethanechol is listed in the British National Formulary (BNF) for the treatment of urinary retention (although it is considered less suitable for prescribing having been superseded by catheterisation). Pilocarpine is listed for the oral treatment of dry mouth following irradiation for head and neck cancer and as eye drops for the production of miosis.

If we recap on the effect of muscarinic agonists in the body (Table 21.1), it can be seen that the parasympathetic nervous system acts to:

● promote micturation by contracting the detrusor muscle of the bladder and relaxing the bladder sphincter
● stimulate saliva production
● constrict the pupil.

Muscarinic agonists are non-selective and so will bind to and stimulate the activity of muscarinic receptors throughout the body. These drugs mimic the effects of acetylcholine, which

Table 21.1 Effect of the parasympathetic nervous system on body organs.

Organ	Effect of parasympathetic nervous system
Heart	Decreased heart rate and force of contraction
Lungs	Bronchoconstriction
GI tract	Increased motility of smooth muscle, relaxation of sphincters
Bladder	Contraction of detrusor muscle, relaxation of sphincters
Eye	Constriction of pupil
Salivary glands	Stimulate secretion
Lacrimal glands	Stimulate secretion

is the endogenous agonist, at these receptors. This explains why the same class of drugs can be used clinically to produce very different effects.

Similarly, it also explains why diarrhoea, abdominal pain and increased lacrimation are amongst the side effects listed in the BNF for both bethanechol and oral pilocarpine. Stimulation of the muscarinic receptors in the GI tract will increase the motility of the GI tract and relax the sphincters, which may lead to diarrhoea and colicky pain while stimulation of the receptors on the lacrimal glands will result in increased tear production.

 Stop and think

Why do you think these side effects are only rare when using pilocarpine eye drops?

The BNF lists asthma and COPD under cautions for oral pilpocarpine treatment. This is because stimulation of the muscarinic receptors in the lungs results in bronchoconstriction. While the level of bronchoconstriction produced may not affect healthy adults, it may be significant in patients with asthma and COPD who already have impaired lung function.

Muscarinic antagonists

These drugs compete with acetylcholine for binding to the muscarinic receptors on body organs but when bound to the receptor, they do not stimulate a response. These drugs are competitive antagonists (Chapter 14). They exhibit similar affinity for the muscarinic receptors but have reduced efficacy and consequently they reduce or inhibit the response of the parasympathetic nervous system, effectively exhibiting the opposite effect of muscarinic agonists (Table 21.2).

There are a number of these types of drugs in clinical use today including oxybutynin, tropicamide and ipratropium.

Oxybutynin

Oxybutynin hydrochloride, given orally, is indicated by the BNF for use in the treatment of urinary frequency, urgency and incontinence. As a muscarinic antagonist, oxybutynin decreases

Table 21.2 Effect of muscarinic antagonists on body organs and associated potential clinical effects.

Body organ	Effect of muscarinic antagonist	Potential side effect
Heart	Increased heart rate and force of contraction	Tachycardia
GI tract	Decreased motility of the GI tract Contraction of the sphincters	Constipation
Bladder	Relaxation of the detrusor muscle Constriction of the sphincter	Urinary retention
Salivary gland	Decreased saliva production	Dry mouth
Lacrimal gland	Decreased tear production	Dry eyes

Section 3

the contraction of the detrusor and inhibits the relaxation of the sphincter normally seen following parasympathetic stimulation, thus relaxing the bladder and allowing more urine to be stored and reducing the urge to micturate.

 Stop and think

Why are dry mouth and constipation listed as side effects of oxybutynin treatment?

Ipraropium bromide

Ipratropium bromide is an example of a muscarinic antagonist, which is used clinically in the management of chronic asthma and COPD. Ipratropium binds to the muscarinic receptors in the lungs and prevents the bronchoconstriction induced by acetylcholine.

Table 21.3 demonstrates that dry mouth, urinary retention and constipation are typical antimuscarinic side effects resulting from the fact that ipratropium can bind to muscarinic receptors in all these areas and prevent the action of acetylcholine. These side effects are only rarely experienced with ipratropium as it is given by inhalation, so is delivered directly to its site of action (a topical response). Also, the structure of ipratropium is such that it has a quaternary amine which makes it large and charged; it is not therefore absorbed very well across membranes and so rarely enters the systemic circulation.

Neuromuscular blocking drugs

Nicotinic antagonists (non-depolarising)

These drugs act as competitive antagonists at the nicotinic receptors which are located on the postganglionic nerves of both the parasympathetic and sympathetic systems and in the somatic nervous system. The main clinical action of these drugs is as a muscle relaxant in anaesthesia. Examples of these drugs are pancuronium, vecuronium and atracurium.

Table 21.3 Clinical effect of overstimulation of muscarinic receptors by anticholinesterase drugs.

Organ	Possible clinical effect of overstimulation of receptors
Heart	Bradycardia
Lungs	Shortness of breath
GI tract	Diarrhoea
Bladder	Urinary frequency
Eye	Loss of far vision
Salivary glands	Excessive saliva production
Lacrimal glands	Watery eyes

Practice application

The action of nicotinic antagonists can be overcome by increasing the levels of acetylcholine using acetylcholinesterase inhibitors.

Nicotinic agonists (depolarising)

The only nicotinic agonist used clinically is suxamethonium and this has the most rapid onset and shortest duration of action of all the neuromuscular blocking drugs. Suxamethonium competes with acetylcholine for binding at the nicotinic receptor and stimulates the same response as acetylcholine. While the activity of acetylcholine is rapidly terminated by the action of the enzyme acetylcholinesterase, suxamethonium exhibits much more prolonged activity (as it is only slowly hydrolysed in the cleft). This results in prolonged depolarisation of the membrane (Chapter 29) and short-term muscle relaxation.

Anticholinesterase drugs

These drugs inhibit the action of cholinesterase enzymes in the cleft. They reduce the breakdown of acetylcholine and increase cholinergic transmission (at both nicotinic and muscarinic receptors). Examples of these drugs are edrophonium, neostigmine and pyridostigmine and they are used clinically to:

● reverse the effects of non-depolarising neuromuscular blockers (nicotinic antagonists)
● diagnose and treat myasthenia gravis
● treat Alzheimer's disease.

Because these drugs inhibit the breakdown of acetylcholine peripherally as well as at the neuromuscular junction, they increases the stimulation of muscarinic effects throughout the body (Table 21.3) resulting in side effects such as increased salivation, diarrhoea and abdominal cramps.

Asthma is listed as a caution for the use of anticholinesterase drugs in the treatment of both myasthenia gravis and Alzheimer's disease because the reduced breakdown of acetylcholine in the lungs will result in prolonged bronchoconstriction.

Drugs which target the sympathetic nervous system and noradrenergic transmission

Adrenergic agonists

These drugs mimic the action of adrenaline and noradrenaline in the body and produce effects which are similar to stimulation of the sympathetic nervous system. These drugs are often called directly acting sympathomimetics. They are often selective for a specific receptor subgroup

Section 3

Table 21.4   Effect of the sympathetic nervous system on the body and the specific receptor subtype which is responsible for the effect.

Organ	Effect of sympathetic nervous system	Receptor subtype
Heart	Increased heart rate and force of contraction	β_1
Lungs	Bronchodilation in response to adrenaline released from the adrenal gland	β_2
GI tract	Decreased motility of smooth muscle	β_2
	Contraction of sphincter	α_1
Bladder	Relaxation of detrusor muscle	β_2
	Contraction of sphincter	α_1
Eye	Dilation of pupil (contraction of ciliary muscle)	α_1
Blood vessels	Contraction of skin and visceral beds	α_1
	Dilation of skeletal muscle beds	β_2
Liver	Glycogenolysis	β_2
Fat	Lipolysis	β_3
Kidney	Renin secretion	β_1 and β_2
Sweat	Secretion	Muscarinic
Mast cells	Inhibition of histamine release	β_2
Skeletal muscle	Tremor	β_2

(either α_1 or β_2) and hence the effects of these drugs relate to the receptor subtype they bind to (Table 21.4).

Phenylephrine

This is an α_1-specific adrenoceptor agonist currently used for eye examination because it dilates the pupil of the eye. Phenylephrine is also used in topical nasal decongestants, which can be bought over the counter. Its use in this context is due to its ability to constrict the blood vessels of the nasal mucosa, resulting in reduced oedema and easing the blockage of nasal passages. While side effects are limited because of the topical nature of phenylephrine use, systemic side effects can occur following repeated and excessive use. One such side effect is hypertension.

 Stop and think

Why is hypertension a potential systemic side effect of phenylephrine use?

Salbutamol

Salbutamol is a selective β_2-agonist which is used clinically to treat both asthma and chronic obstructive pulmonary disease. Its action in the respiratory system is to produce bronchodilation by mimicking the action of the sympathetic nervous system. It should be remembered, however, that selectivity is not the same as specificity so whilst salbutamol is more likely to bind to (has a greater affinity for) β_2-receptors, it is still able to bind to and stimulate the β_1-receptors in the heart, resulting in tachycardia being listed as a side effect.

 Stop and think

Salbutamol is generally delivered by inhalation. Can you think of two reasons why this route of administration might be preferred to the oral route?

Diabetes is also listed as a caution for salbutamol use. Table 21.5 shows that stimulation of β_2-receptors in the liver results in glycogenolysis or the breakdown of glycogen into glucose. This may lead to changes in the patient's insulin requirement and hyperglycaemia. Because this glucose cannot be taken up and used by the tissues, it can lead to fatty acids within the tissues being broken down, with the production of ketone bodies leading to ketoacidosis.

Adrenergic antagonists

These drugs act by blocking adrenaline and noradrenaline binding to adrenoceptors in the body and thus inhibit or reduce the effects of the sympathetic nervous system. These drugs are used clinically in the management of cardiovascular disease and are commonly known as beta-blockers. The side effects related to the use of these drugs vary, to a certain extent, depending on the type of adrenergic antagonist used (Table 21.5).

Labetalol, carvedilol

These drugs are non-specific adrenergic receptor antagonists and thus have affinity for both alpha- and beta-adrenoreceptors. They will therefore bind to alpha- and beta-receptors in the body, blocking the action of noradrenaline and adrenaline at both these receptor subtypes. These drugs are used clinically to treat both hypertension and angina. They reduce both cardiac output, by blocking the action of nordarenaline at the β_1-receptors in the heart and thus

Table 21.5 Some side effects of the different forms of adrenoceptor antagonists linked to the receptor subtypes they bind to.

Side effect	Non-specific adrenergic antagonists	Beta-receptor antagonists	Cardioselective beta-blockers
Bronchoconstriction	+++	+++	+
GI disturbances	++	++	+
Disturbances of micturition	+++	++	+
Visual disturbances	++	−	−
Nasal stuffiness	++	−	−

Section 3

reducing heart rate, and peripheral vascular resistance, by blocking the action of noradrenaline on the α_1-receptors in the peripheral vasculature, thus promoting vasodilation.

Stop and think

Why might the inhibition of renin production by the kidney be important in the clinical action of these drugs in treating hypertension?

Propranolol, oxprenolol, timolol

These drugs are beta-receptor antagonists, which are also used in the treatment of hypertension and angina. The difference between these drugs and labetalol and carvedilol is that propranolol, oxprenolol and timolol are solely beta-adrenoreceptor antagonists and so do not have effects on the alpha-receptors. Consequently, they do not have the extra vasodilating effect of the mixed receptor antagonists.

Atenolol, bisoprolol, metoprolol

These drugs are cardioselective beta-receptor antagonists which means that they have a greater affinity for the β_1-receptors in the heart than for the β_2-receptors elsewhere in the body.

Asthma is listed in the BNF as a contraindication for the use of beta-adrenoceptors because these drugs may block the β_2-receptors in the lungs, thus preventing the natural bronchodilation which occurs through adrenaline. While this does not present a problem in normal individuals, it can be dangerous in asthmatics. The use of beta-adrenoceptor antagonists in asthmatics would also lessen the effectiveness of treating that bronchoconstriction by β_2-agonists.

Stop and think

Why do you think uncontrolled heart failure is listed as a contraindication for the use of beta-adrenoceptor antagonists?

Some beta-adrenoceptor blocking drugs are associated with sleep disturbances and nightmares while others are not. This can be explained by the lipid solubility of the drugs. Propranolol is relatively lipid soluble and hence can cross the blood–brain barrier (BBB) resulting in central nervous system-related side effects. Atenolol, on the other hand, is much more water soluble (polar) and does not easily cross the BBB so it is associated with fewer CNS-type side effects.

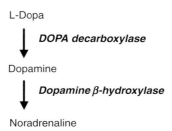

L-Dopa

DOPA decarboxylase

Dopamine

Dopamine β-hydroxylase

Noradrenaline

Figure 21.1   Production of noradrenaline from L-dopa.

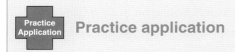 **Practice application**

The difference in lipid solubility of beta-adrenoceptor antagonists might impact on drug handling in the elderly. The more water-soluble drugs such as atenolol, celiprolol, nadolol and solatol may require dose reduction in the elderly.

Drugs affecting noradrenaline synthesis

An example of a drug which affects noradrenaline synthesis and is used clinically is carbidopa which is a DOPA decarboxylase inhibitor which prevents levodopa (L-Dopa) from being converted into dopamine (Figure 21.1).

Carbidopa is used in conjunction with levodopa in the treatment of Parkinson's disease. This results from an imbalance between the neurotransmitters dopamine and acetylcholine and is often treated by increasing dopamine levels (Chapter 30). Carbidopa prevents levodopa from being converted into dopamine in the periphery. Carbidopa does not cross the BBB while levodopa does and therefore results in higher concentrations of dopamine in the brain with lower concentrations of levodopa. It also reduces the peripheral side effects of levodopa treatment, which might include sympathomimetic effects.

Drugs affecting noradrenaline release

These drugs stimulate noradrenaline release from nerve terminals in the absence of nerve stimulation and are known as indirectly acting sympathomimetics. They are similar in shape to noradrenaline and can therefore be taken up into the nerve terminal by the reuptake carrier protein. Once in the nerve terminal, they displace noradrenaline from the vesicles in which it is stored. The increase in free noradrenaline content of the neuron results in its release into the neuroeffector junction by a carrier protein, where it can bind to and stimulate adrenoceptors. Ephedrine is an example of such a sympathomimetic drug and is used in the treatment of nasal congestion.

Drugs affecting noradrenaline uptake

These drugs decrease the reuptake of noradrenaline into the nerve terminal by inhibiting the action of the carrier protein. This increases the action of noradrenaline at the receptor.

Section 3

Imipramine is an example of a drug which affects noradrenaline uptake that is still listed clinically for the treatment of nocturnal enuresis in children. In this case, the action of imipramine relaxes the detrusor muscle and constricts the sphincter, thereby increasing the capacity of the bladder. Imipramine does not solely inhibit the carrier protein responsible for noradrenaline reuptake but also acts as an antagonist at a number of other types of receptors and it is this action which is responsible for most of the side effects of the drug. Imipramine is also used in the treatment of depression (Chapter 31).

Summary

- Drug groups which act by mimicking the action of acetylcholine on body organs are muscarinic agonists.
- Muscarinic agonists are non-selective and competitive.
- Drug groups which act by reducing the action of acetylcholine on body organs are muscarinic antagonists.
- Muscarinic antagonists are used to treat urinary frequency, asthma and COPD.
- Typical side effects of muscarinic antagonists include dry mouth, constipation and urinary retention.
- Neuromuscular blocking drugs are either nicotinic agonists (depolarising) or nicotinic antagonists (non-depolarising).
- Anticholinesterase drugs inhibit the action of acteylcholinesterase, thereby increasing the level of acetylcholine.
- Anticholinesterase drugs can be used to reverse non-depolarising neuromuscular blockade and to treat both myasthenia gravis and Alzheimer's disease.
- Drug groups which act by mimicking the action of adrenaline and noradrenaline on body organs are adrenergic agonists. Drug groups which act by reducing the action of adrenaline and noradrenaline on body organs are adrenergic antagonists.
- Division of adrenergic receptors into specific subgroups is clinically very important.
- Adrenergic antagonists can be divided into non-selective adrenergic antagonists, beta-receptor antagonists and cardioselective beta-receptor antagonists. Side effects differ between these types of antagonists.
- DOPA decarboxylase inhibitors prevent the formation of dopamine, noradrenaline and adrenaline from levodopa and are used in the treatment of Parkinson's disease.
- Drugs which stimulates the release of nordarenaline in the absence of nerve stimulation, such as ephedrine, are commonly used to treat nasal congestion.
- Inhibition of the carrier protein in the nerve terminal prevents the reuptake of noradrenaline, thus prolonging its effects. Noradrenaline reuptake inhibitors are used clinically to treat both nocturnal enuresis in children and depression.

 Activity

1. Tropicamide, a muscarinic antagonist, is used as eye drops to facilitate the examination of the fundus of the eye. Why do think tropicamide is useful in these circumstances?
2. Which of the following is not a non-depolarising neuromuscular blocking drug?

A. Pancuronium
B. Suxamethonium
C. Vecuronium
D. Rocuronium.

3. Why is bradycardia listed as a caution for the use of anticholinesterase drugs?
4. Salbutamol mimics the action of which of the following chemicals?
   A. Noradrenaline
   B. Acetylcholine
   C. Adrenaline
5. One of the most common side effects of salbutamol use is fine tremor. Can you explain why this might be the case?
6. Why would the use of beta-adrenoceptor antagonists lessen the effect of salbutamol in the lungs?
7. Why would ephedrine be useful for the treatment of nasal congestion?

Useful websites

NICE guidance for the treatment of urinary incontinence – quick reference guide. www.nice.org.uk/Guidance/CG40/QuickRefGuide/pdf/English

NICE guidance for the treatment of chronic obstructive pulmonary disease – quick reference guide. www.nice.org.uk/Guidance/CG12/QuickRefGuide/pdf/English

Further reading

Abrams, P. and Andersson, K.E. (2007) Muscarinic receptor antagonists for overactive bladder. *BJU Int*, **100**, 987–1006.

Andrus, M.R. and Loyed, J.V. (2008) Use of beta-adrenoceptor antagonists in older patients with chronic obstructive pulmonary disease and cardiovascular co-morbidity: safety issues. *Drugs Aging*, **25**, 131–144.

Barker, R.A. (1993) *Neuroscience: An Illustrated Guide*, Ellis Horwood, New York.

Barnes, P.J. (2004) Distribution of receptor targets in the lung. *Proc Am Thorac Soc*, **1**, 345–351.

British Medical Association and Royal Pharmaceutical Society of Great Britain (2010) *British National Formulary*, 59th edn, BMJ Publishing, London.

Davies, A.N. and Shorthose, K. (2007) Parasympathomimetic drugs for the treatment of salivary gland dysfunction due to radiotherapy. *Cochrane Database Syst Rev*, **3**, CD003782.

Kruk, Z.L. and Pycock, C.J. (1991) *Neurotransmitters and Drugs*, 3rd edn, Chapman and Hall, London.

Page, C.P., Curtis, M.J., Sutter, M.C., *et al.* (2006) *Integrated Pharmacology*, 3rd edn, Mosby, London.

Section 3

Rang, H.P., Dale, M.M., Ritter, J.M. and Flower, R. (2007) *Rang and Dale's Pharmacology*, 6th edn, Churchill Livingstone, Edinburgh.

Romi, F., Gilhus, N.E. and Aarli, J.A. (2005) Myasthenia gravis: clinical, immunological, and therapeutic advances. *Acta Neurol Scand*, **111**, 134–141.

Seeberger, L.C. and Hauser, R.A. (2007) Optimizing bioavailability in the treatment of Parkinson's disease. *Neuropharmacology*, **53**, 791–800.

Stafylas, P.C. and Sarafidis, P.A. (2008) Carvedilol in hypertension treatment. *Vasc Health Risk Manag*, **4**, 23–30.

Webster, R.A. and Jordan, C.C. (1989) *Neurotransmitters, Drugs and Disease*, Blackwell Scientific, Oxford.

22 The respiratory system

Learning outcomes

By the end of this chapter the reader should be able to:

- understand the nature of the regulation of the airways
- appreciate the role of inflammation in respiratory disease
- understand the mechanism of action, clinical uses and major adverse effects of the following bronchodilators:
  - beta-adrenergic receptor agonist
  - muscarinic receptor antagonists
  - methylxanthines
- understand the mechanism of action, clinical uses and major adverse effects of the following anti-inflammatory agents:
  - corticosteroids
  - leukotriene antagonists
  - cromones
  - omalizumab.

Respiratory disease

For the prescriber, the respiratory system occupies a central position. Unlike the cardiovascular system, where prescribing is very much focused on the middle-aged and elderly, respiratory disease is at least as much a problem for children and young adults. Apart from infections, pneumonias and tuberculosis (which will not be discussed here), two major inflammatory conditions dominate respiratory therapeutics: asthma and chronic obstructive pulmonary disease (COPD). Although these conditions can overlap in the same individual, there are very many differences between them in terms of pathology as well as treatment. In both cases there have been very significant advances in treatment, most particularly in asthma, but the problems are far from being solved.

The New Prescriber. Edited by J Lymn, D Bowskill, F Bath-Hextall, R Knaggs, © 2010 John Wiley & Sons.

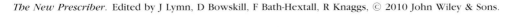
Section 3

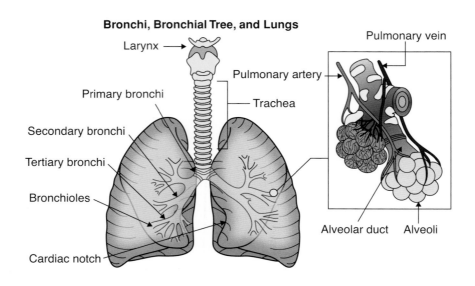

Figure 22.1 The human airways or bronchial tree.

Before considering the drugs used in these conditions, this chapter will consider the mechanisms determining the function of the airways, especially their diameter and therefore the flow of air through them. It will also summarise some current concepts of inflammation as they apply to COPD and asthma.

Regulating the airways

The human airways are often described as the bronchial tree and the reason is obvious from a diagram of their structure (Figure 22.1). There are two major influences on the flow of air through the bronchial system: smooth muscle tone (i.e. contraction versus relaxation) in the wall of the airways, and the presence or absence of inflammation in the lining of the airways, leading to mucus secretion. Of these two processes, the regulation of smooth muscle tone is certainly the more straightforward, being regulated by three mechanisms.

1. The parasympathetic nervous system, branches of the vagus (Xth cranial nerve) which innervate bronchial smooth muscle, releasing the transmitter acetylcholine and causing bronchoconstriction by acting on muscarinic receptors.
2. Circulating adrenaline which acts on beta-2 adrenergic receptors and causes bronchodilation. (Unlike most other mammalian species, human airways do not have sympathetic nerves, though sympathetic nerves do act to inhibit parasympathetic ganglia and so indirectly can promote bronchodilation.)
3. The so-called non-adrenergic non-cholinergic (NANC) nerves which are bronchodilator and where the transmitters are largely nitric oxide and vasoactive intestinal peptide (VIP).

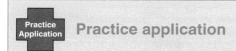

Practice application

Bronchodilator therapies are based on two mechanisms:

- activation of beta-2 adrenergic receptors in airway smooth muscle
- inhibition of muscarinic receptors.

But bronchodilation, while crucial in asthma and to a lesser extent in COPD, is not the key feature in the management of these conditions. They are basically inflammatory disorders and understanding the nature of the inflammation is vital for their safe and effective management.

Inflammation in asthma and COPD

It is now clear that the patterns and mechanism of inflammation are very different in asthma and COPD, although in severe advanced asthma the picture may begin to resemble COPD more closely. One important point is that asthma often has a strong allergic component which is completely absent in COPD. But the complexity of the inflammatory response means that antihistamines, useful in hay fever and other allergic conditions, are virtually useless in asthma. In terms of aetiology, COPD is also very different, as in the vast majority of cases there is one major underlying factor: smoking.

There has been much debate about the apparent increase in the prevalence of asthma in developed countries; one widely held hypothesis is that the absence of bacterial exposure in childhood redirects the immune system to produce the chronic inflammatory state that is the basis of asthma. But for the prescriber the primary concern must be: what can we do about asthma and COPD, once they are established?

Drug therapies in asthma and COPD

Throughout this section therapeutic recommendations will be consistent with the recommendations of the British National Formulary, with comments where appropriate. The issue of inhaler technique is of vital importance in clinical practice (spacers, breath-activated devices and so on) but will not be discussed here (see Further Reading).

Bronchodilators

There are two main types of bronchodilator:

- selective beta-2 adrenergic receptor agonists
- muscarinic receptor antagonists.

For both classes of drugs there are both short- and long-acting examples (Table 22.1) and for all these drugs when given by inhalation, paradoxical bronchospasm has been described. Bronchodilator drugs relieve symptoms and can prevent their occurrence, but have no effect

Section 3

Table 22.1 Examples of short- and long-acting bronchodilators commonly used to treat asthma and COPD.

	Selective beta-2 adrenergic receptor agonists	Muscarinic receptor antagonists
Short acting	Salbutamol Terbutaline	Ipratropium
Long acting	Salmeterol Formoterol	Tiotroprium

on the natural history of either asthma or COPD. While these drugs are mostly given by inhalation, absorption into the circulation does take place and may lead to systemic adverse effects.

A third type of bronchodilator, the methylxanthines, will also be discussed though their use has declined.

Beta-2 adrenergic receptor agonists

These drugs act predominantly on adrenergic receptors in bronchial smooth muscle, mimicking the effect of circulating adrenaline and so causing bronchodilation. To a very limited extent, they also reduce secretion from the epithelium in the bronchi. Although it is very uncommon in this country, adrenaline itself is quite frequently used for severe asthma in the United States.

Short-acting beta-2 agonists are used as 'relievers' in patients with acute exacerbations of chronic asthma, usually delivered by metered-dose inhaler. They can also be given by mouth and by subcutaneous and intravenous injection, though this leads to increased adverse effects (see below) without a clear increase in efficacy.

 Stop and think

Apart from the increase in adverse effects, what else makes the oral route less suitable for salbutamol administration?

These drugs are also used, usually delivered by nebuliser, occasionally parenterally, in the treatment of severe asthma, including life-threatening situations. The driving gas is generally oxygen in these circumstances.

Long-acting beta-2 agonists are also used as long-term bronchodilators in both chronic asthma and COPD but are not currently recommended for acute exacerbations. These drugs are usually given 12-hourly, sometimes as a single dose, particularly at bedtime, in patients with increased bronchospasm at night, and are almost always given by metered-dose inhaler or breath-activated device. In asthma (but not necessarily in COPD) long-acting beta-2 agonists must be used in conjunction with inhaled steroids (see below).

Adverse effects of beta-2-agonists (both short- and long-acting) are uncommon at normal doses, but tremor, anxiety, tachycardia and hypokalaemia may occur. Very rarely, at high doses, cardiac arrhythmias may occur.

Stop and think

Why is tachycardia a side effect of beta-2 agonist use?

Tolerance to the effects of beta-2 agonists may develop, necessitating higher doses to produce the same response, because of downregulation of beta-receptors due to chronic stimulation.

There has been controversy in the past about apparent increased mortality in patients with asthma who were receiving these drugs. Almost certainly, this was not due to any direct adverse effect but because of delays in seeking help and because patients were using the drugs without concurrent steroid therapy.

Muscarinic antagonists

These act by blocking muscarinic cholinergic receptors in bronchial smooth muscle, which are activated by the vagus nerve. They are therefore more indirect bronchodilators than the beta-agonists, in that they block the effects of a constrictor.

Short-acting muscarinic antagonists are used as maintenance treatment in chronic asthma and COPD (usually used at an earlier stage of COPD than of asthma, as it is generally considered that the cholinergic contribution is greater in COPD) and usually given 3–4 times daily. The long-acting muscarinic antagonist tiotropium, on the other hand, is currently licensed only for the maintenance therapy of COPD and at a once-daily dosage. It has been suggested that the use of long-acting muscarinic antagonists may reduce the number of exacerbations of COPD resulting in hospital admission, but this is controversial.

Muscarinic antagonists have a slower onset of action than beta-agonists and are only given by inhalation. Adverse effects of muscarinic antagonists are due to systemic absorption of the drug and are those expected from a muscarinic antagonist. Particularly important ones include acute retention in men with prostatism and raised intraocular pressure in patients with glaucoma. Blurred vision, dry mouth and constipation may all occur.

Stop and think

Why are systemic side effects of muscarinic antagonists uncommon?

There has been recent controversy regarding the cardiovascular safety of these drugs, but the best available consensus suggests that they do not increase cardiovascular risk.

Section 3

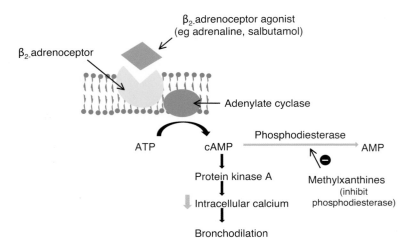

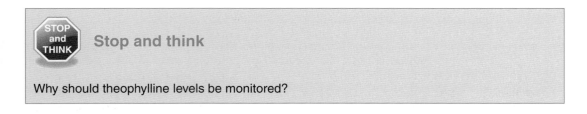

Figure 22.2 Stimulation of bronchodilation by beta-2 adrenoceptor agonists and the role of phosphodiesterase inhibition.

Methylxanthines

It goes without saying that everyone likes to know the mechanism of the drugs they prescribe. For the previous classes of bronchodilators, this was quite straightforward. There is less certainty regarding the methylxanthines, by far the best known of which is caffeine (which is no longer used in asthma!). The general view is that they inhibit enzymes called phosphodiesterases which lead to increased levels of the cellular messenger cyclic adenosine monophosphate (cAMP), which leads to relaxation of bronchial smooth muscle and bronchodilation (Figure 22.2). Other additional or alternative mechanisms have been proposed. They may have some anti-inflammatory activity.

Examples of methylxanthines still in clinical use are theophylline (given orally) and aminophylline (given IV). Theophylline, in modified-release formulations, is used in stage 4 management of chronic asthma and after beta-agonists and muscarinic blockers in COPD.

Ideally, chronic theophylline use should involve therapeutic drug monitoring, as target therapeutic plasma levels have been determined. In practice this is seldom done.

STOP and THINK — Stop and think

Why should theophylline levels be monitored?

Aminophylline is used intravenously in severe, usually life-threatening asthma. This is controversial, as there are conflicting views on the strength of evidence for this and it is not used for first-line therapy in this situation. Adverse effects of methylxanthines are frequent. Nausea and vomiting can be minimised by modified-release formulations. Central nervous system symptoms

Table 22.2 Some important potential interactions of methylxanthines with other drugs through modulation of cytochrome P450 activity.

Drug	Action on CYP450 isoform	Possible effect on plasma theophylline levels
Alcohol	Induction of CYP2E1	Decreased
Ciprofloxacin	Inhibition of CYP1A2	Increased
Clarithromycin	Inhibition of CYP3A4	Increased
Erythromycin	Inhibition of CYP3A4	Increased
Carbamazepine	Induction of CYP3A4	Decreased
Phenytoin	Induction of CYP3A4	Decreased
Cimetidine	Inhibition of CYP1A2 and CYP3A4	Increased
Disulfiram	Inhibition of CYP2E1	Increased
Rifampicin	Induction of CYP3A4	Decreased
St John's wort	Induction of CYP3A4	Decreased

are also common, with tremor and anxiety. Like beta-agonists, they can cause hypokalaemia and are more likely to cause cardiac arrhythmias. High doses can also cause convulsions.

Interactions with other drugs are of major concern, unlike the situation with beta-agonists and muscarinic receptor blockers. This is due to extensive metabolism of the methylxanthines in the liver by the cytochrome P450 system, particularly CYP1A2, CYP3A4 and CYP2E1, and can result in an increase or a decrease in the plasma concentration of methylxanthines (Table 22.2). Methylxanthines have a small therapeutic index and hence even small increases in plasma levels of methylxanthines can result in adverse effects or even toxicity.

Anti-inflammatory drugs

The transformation in the management of airways obstruction, especially in asthma, has come from the realisation that anti-inflammatory therapy alters the progression of the disease in ways that bronchodilators do not. The key drugs have been, as so often in other conditions, the corticosteroids. Fortunately, in most patients they can be delivered by inhalation, thus limiting their many adverse effects.

Corticosteroids – prednisolone, hydrocortisone, beclomethasone, fluticasone

No other class of drug even approaches the anti-inflammatory efficacy of steroids. This is because they have an unrivalled range of effects on different mechanisms within almost all types of cell involved in the inflammatory process. Like other steroid hormones (oestrogen, androgens, aldosterone and so on), the glucocorticoids bind to a receptor in the cytoplasm of the cell and then enter the nucleus. Here they selectively increase the transcription of anti-inflammatory genes while suppressing proinflammatory ones (Box 22.1). It is crucial to bear in mind that the effects of steroids take time to develop, since there is the need for changes in gene transcription and protein synthesis. The anti-inflammatory response will therefore take days rather than hours to become fully established, regardless of the route of administration of the steroid.

Section 3

Box 22.1   Some proteins whose gene expression is regulated by glucocorticoids (Adcock, Ito and Barnes, 2004).

Increased transcription	Decreased transcription
Lipocortin-1/annexin-1 (phospholipase A2 inhibitor)	Cytokines (IL-1-6, IL-9, IL-11–13, IL-16–18, TNF-alpha)
Beta-2 adrenoceptor	Chemokines (IL-8)
IL-1 receptor antagonist	Inducible nitric oxide synthase
	Cyclooxygenase 2
	Cytoplasmic phospholipase A_2
	Endothelin-1 receptors

Steroids can be given intravenously (hydrocortisone), orally (prednisolone) or by inhalation (beclomethasone, fluticasone). For both chronic asthma and COPD, the inhaled route is by far the most common. In acute severe asthma it is usual to give intravenous hydrocortisone, though for reasons already discussed, it is doubtful whether this has a faster onset of action than oral prednisolone, but one or other must be given.

 Practice application

Oral steroids should be continued for at least 5–7 days after the patient recovers from the acute episode, to reduce risk of relapse. Patients with any but the mildest symptoms of asthma must be prescribed inhaled steroids and it is vital to emphasise that treatment with these should continue even in the absence of symptoms and should not be intermittent.

The situation in relation to steroid use is less clear-cut with regard to COPD and thinking on this has changed in the last few years. It is now recommended that inhaled steroids should be prescribed for patients with moderate to severe COPD although it is recognised that not all will respond. However, there is no reliable way of identifying long-term responders and there is no long-term harm associated with inhaled steroid use. Very recent data suggest for the first time that combining inhaled steroids with a long-acting beta-agonist may actually slow the progression of the disease.

Oral prednisolone may be needed for patients with severe asthma and incomplete response to other therapies. In a small minority of patients, such treatment is indefinite and even life-long. An even smaller number of patients are steroid resistant, which presents an extremely difficult therapeutic challenge.

Adverse effects are not generally a major problem with inhaled steroids, the main ones being cough and *Candida* infection of the mucus membrane of the mouth and throat. But, as already mentioned, inhaled drugs can be absorbed to a significant extent and can have systemic side effects, including any of those listed below. However, these are rarely severe.

> **Box 22.2   Side Effects, and Associated Clinical Risks, of Long-term Systemic Steroid Therapy.**
>
> Suppression of glucocorticoid secretion from the adrenal glands.
> Immune suppression, especially cell-mediated increasing susceptibility to tuberculosis, viruses and fungi.
> Increased salt and water retention, raising blood pressure and worsening heart failure.
> Loss of potassium with hypokalaemia and muscle weakness.
> Deterioration in glucose tolerance, increasing the risk of diabetes.
> Decreased protein synthesis, with thinning of the skin.
> Increased risk of peptic ulceration.
> Increased risk of osteoporosis.
> In children, growth retardation, which is also detectable to a lesser extent with inhaled steroids.

Likewise, adverse effects are rarely troublesome with acute systemic steroid therapy, even at high doses, when given for short periods (a few days). But long-term systemic steroid therapy is a very different matter – which is why everyone would be delighted to find a viable alternative to steroids. The list of potential problems is immense (Box 22.2).

Given this alarming list, it is of course essential that any health professional caring for patients taking long-term systemic steroids should be aware of their treatment regime. All such patients must carry a steroid card (now nationally standardised) and many on indefinite treatment will also have a Medic-Alert bracelet or similar device. Sudden withdrawal of steroids (long-term therapy with doses above 5 mg prednisolone daily) can precipitate collapse and death (Addisonian crisis).

 Practice application

Patients on long-term systemic steroid therapy must receive an increased dose of steroids (usually doubled) during stressful situations such as major trauma, major surgery or myocardial infarction.

*Leukotriene antagonists (*montelukast, zafirlukast*)*

The leukotrienes are generated from arachidonic acid, a fatty acid released from the cell membrane which is also the precursor of prostaglandins and prostacyclin (Figure 22.3). They are potently pro-inflammatory, causing bronchoconstriction and oedema. It is not clear how important they are overall in asthma (probably not all in COPD) but they may be effective in patients who develop bronchoconstriction in response to aspirin and non-steroidal anti-inflammatory drugs (NSAIDs): it is thought that these patients produce large amounts of leukotrienes because the generation of prostaglandins is blocked by the NSAIDs. There is in effect diversion to the leukotrienes. However, this seems to occur only in a small minority of individuals (less than 5% of the population).

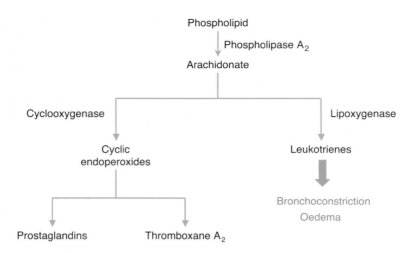

Figure 22.3 Production, and consequences of, leukotrienes in the airways.

Leukotriene antagonists are given by mouth once or twice daily and may also be particularly useful in asthma triggered by cold air or exercise. Overall, these drugs are regarded as third- or fourth-line therapy (British Thoracic Society guidelines), most asthmatic patients probably being non-responders, and should not be used in acute attacks. The effect of leukotriene antagonists may be additive with steroids.

Adverse effects of leukotriene receptor antagonists are usually minor gastrointestinal symptoms but they are, rarely, associated with the serious and potentially life-threatening Churg–Strauss syndrome (increase in asthma, sinusitis and rhinitis, high eosinophil count in the blood and vasculitis which may affect many organs). In this situation the drug must be discontinued immediately and systemic steroids given.

Cromones (Sodium cromoglycate, nedocromil sodium)

It is thought that these drugs act by preventing the release of inflammatory mediators from mast cells in the bronchi (and in the nose and conjunctiva as well). This is still not fully established, however.

These drugs are given by inhalation, usually in powder form, sometimes by nebuliser, three or four times daily.

Cromones are used only as preventive drugs, not for acute attacks. Their main use has been in allergic asthma in children but increasingly they are being replaced by inhaled steroids. They can also be used in exercise-induced asthma in both adults and children. The use of these drugs is, however, declining because of doubts about their efficacy.

Adverse effects of cromones are minor, most often cough and transient bronchospasm caused by irritation from the dry powder formulation.

Omalizumab

As mentioned earlier, in a small minority of patients with asthma the disease is not adequately controlled even with systemic steroids. In some of these individuals, where the asthma has a particularly strong allergic basis, omalizumab may be helpful. This is a monoclonal antibody against IgE, the immunoglobulin involved in allergic reactions. It has to be given by subcutaneous injection every 2–4 weeks. Hypersensitivity reactions such as rashes may occur and, more importantly, anaphylaxis. For this reason it should be given by a health professional in circumstances where there are facilities for resuscitation. Like almost all 'biologicals', omalizumab is very expensive and unlike monoclonal antibodies in some other clinical conditions, needs to be continued indefinitely. Understandably, therefore, it is used only in strictly defined circumstances.

Summary

- The conditions which dominate respiratory therapeutics are asthma and COPD.
- The major factors which restrict air flow through the bronchi are contraction of the smooth muscle and the presence of inflammation.
- Bronchial smooth muscle contraction is regulated by the parasympathetic nervous system, circulating adrenaline and the NANC nerves.
- Side effects of beta-2 agonists are uncommon at normal doses but tolerance to long-acting beta-2 agonists may occur.
- Muscarinic antagonists block the action of acetylcholine in the bronchial smooth muscle and have a slower onset of action than beta-2 agonists.
- Methylxanthines act by inhibiting the enzyme phosphodiesterase in the bronchial smooth muscle cells.
- Methylxanthines interact with other drugs through the action of the cytochrome P450 system.
- Corticosteroids increases expression of anti-inflammatory proteins and inhibit the expression of pro-inflammatory proteins.
- Because of the mechanism of action of these drugs, the therapeutic activity of steroids takes days to become established.
- Adverse effects of inhaled steroids are minimal but long-term systemic steroid use has many serious side effects.
- Leukotriene receptor antagonists are used to treat aspirin- or NSAID-induced bronchoconstriction and exercise-induced asthma, not COPD.
- Cromones prevent the release of inflammatory mediators from mast cells and are mainly used in exercise-induced asthma.
- Omalizumab is a monoclonal antibody against IgE which can be used to treat asthma in certain individuals.

 Activity

1. Human airways have extensive innervations with sympathetic nerves.   True / False
2. Long-acting beta-adrenergic agonists should not be used for management of acute asthma attacks.   True / False
3. Blurred vision may be a side effect of inhaled muscarinic antagonists such as ipratropium.   True / False

Section 3

4. Methylxanthine drugs such as aminophylline have a high therapeutic index and are therefore safe over a wide range of doses.	True / False
5. The following are recognised adverse effects of long-term systemic steroid therapy with, for instance, prednisolone:	
A. Folate deficiency	True / False
B. Hyperkalaemia	True / False
C. Increased glucose intolerance	True / False
D. Increased susceptibility to TB	True / False
E. Osteoporosis	True / False
6. Leukotrienes may be particularly effective in patients who develop bronchospasm when taking NSAIDs.	True / False
7. Cromones are very effective in the management of COPD.	True / False
8. Intravenous steroids, such as hydrocortisone, are effective in a few minutes in treating severe asthma.	True / False
9. Tolerance may develop to the bronchodilator effects of beta-adrenergic agonists such as salbutamol.	True / False
10. Omalizumab is a monoclonal antibody directed at IgG immunoglobulins.	True / False

Useful website

British Thoracic Society. www.brit-thoracic.org.uk

Reference

Adcock, A.M., Ito, K. and Barnes, P.J. (2004) Glucocorticoids. Effects on gene transcription. *Proc Am Thorac Soc*, **1**, 247–254.

Further reading

Barnes, N.C. (2007) The properties of inhaled corticosteroids: similarities and differences. *Prim Care Respir J*, **16**, 149–154.

British Medical Association and Royal Pharmaceutical Society of Great Britain (2010) *British National Formulary*, 59th edn, BMJ Publishing, London.

Cates, C.J., Crilly, J.A. and Rowe, B.H. (2006) Holding chambers (spacers) versus nebulisers for beta-agonist treatment of acute asthma. *Cochrane Database Syst Rev*, **2**, CD000052.

Cockcroft, D.W. (2006) Clinical concerns with inhaled beta2-agonists: adult asthma. *Clin Rev Allergy Immunol*, **31**, 197–208.

Guevara, J.P., Ducharme, F., Keren, R., *et al.* (2006) Inhaled corticosteroids versus sodium cromoglycate in children and adults with asthma. *Cochrane Database Syst Rev*, **2**, CD003558.

Hauser, T., Mahr, A., Metzler, C., *et al.* (2008) The leucotriene receptor antagonist montelukast and the risk of Churg-Strauss syndrome: a case-crossover study. *Thorax*, **63**, 677-682.

Lavorini, F., Magnan, A., Dubus, J.C., *et al.* (2007) Effect of incorrect use of dry powder inhalers on management of patients with asthma and COPD. *Respir Med*, **102**, 593-604.

Nauta, A.J., Engels, F., Knippels, L.M., *et al.* (2008) Mechanisms of allergy and asthma. *Eur J Pharmacol*, **585**, 354-360.

Price, D. (2008) The use of omalizumab in asthma. *Prim Care Respir J*, **17**, 62-72.

Radin, A. and Cote, C. (2008) Primary care of the patient with chronic obstructive pulmonary disease – Part 1: frontline prevention and early diagnosis. *Am J Med*, **121**, S3-S12.

Singh, S., Loke, Y.K. and Furberg, C.D. (2008) Inhaled anticholinergics and risk of major adverse cardiovascular events in patients with chronic obstructive pulmonary disease: a systematic review and meta-analysis. *JAMA*, **300**, 1439-1450.

Tashkin, D.P., Celli, B., Senn, S., *et al.*, for the UPLIFT Study Investigators. (2008) A 4-year trial of tiotropium in chronic obstructive pulmonary disease. *N Engl J Med*, **359**, 1543-1554.

Section 3

23 The cardiovascular system

Learning outcomes

By the end of this chapter the reader should be able to:

- describe the homeostatic factors involved in the regulation of blood pressure
- describe the pathophysiology of heart failure
- discuss the clinical use of drugs for the treatment of hypertension, angina and heart failure
- understand the mechanism of action and major adverse effects of:
  - calcium channel blockers
  - angiotensin-converting enzyme inhibitors/angiotensin receptor antagonists
  - beta-adrenoceptor antagonists
  - diuretics
  - digoxin
  - nitrates
  - statins.

Nature of the cardiovascular system

The cardiovascular system is composed of the heart and the blood vessels. The heart acts as an intermittent pump that supplies the body with blood while the blood vessels distribute the blood throughout the body. The concept of the heart as an intermittent, rather than a continuous, pump is important because it impacts on the structure and function of the blood vessels. Blood supply is crucial to body functioning because it is the blood which delivers oxygen and nutrients to the tissues and removes waste products such as carbon dioxide.

There are three types of blood vessels – arteries, veins and capillaries – which each have a different structure (Figure 23.1). These different structures relate specifically to the different functions of these vessel types.

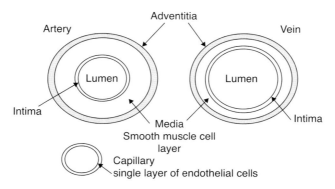

Figure 23.1   Comparison of the structure of the three types of blood vessel found in the body.

Arteries

The arteries carry oxygenated blood away from the heart to the tissues (with the exception of the pulmonary artery). The large arteries are elastic in nature and this elasticity is important as it allows these vessels to expand in order to accommodate the volume of oxygenated blood which is ejected from the left ventricle. Smaller arterioles regulate the appropriate delivery of blood to tissues; thus the arterial system acts to absorb the pulsations in cardiac output and delivers a steady flow of blood to the tissues.

This elasticity of the arteries is a function of the smooth muscle cells which make up the medial layer. It is for this reason that arteries have much larger medial layers than veins.

Veins

The role of veins is to carry deoxygenated blood back to the heart from the tissues (with the exception of the pulmonary vein) and as such these vessels are not involved in the regulation of blood flow and only require a small medial layer.

Capillaries

While both arteries and veins consist of three distinct layers – the intima (containing endothelial cells), the media (consisting of smooth muscle cells) and the adventitia (consisting of connective tissue and collagen and elastic fibres) – capillaries have only a single layer of endothelial cells. Capillaries are the vessels through which the exchange of oxygen and nutrients to the tissues and the removal of waste products from the tissues occurs. In order to ensure that these vessels can effectively carry out this function, capillaries consist only of a single layer of endothelial cells.

Cardiovascular disease

According to recent data, cardiovascular disease is responsible for the premature deaths of around 30% men and 22% of women (British Heart Foundation, 2008) and includes a multitude of conditions. However, this chapter is only going to focus on three conditions – hypertension,

Section 3

heart failure and angina – but in doing so will cover the mechanism of action of most of the major groups of cardiovascular drugs.

Hypertension

Hypertension, or persistently elevated blood pressure, is defined as a blood pressure of at least 140 mmHg systolic and/or a diastolic of 90 mmHg on three separate occasions. It is a common disorder which affects up to 30% of the developed world. However, the underlying cause of the disorder in most people is unknown and this is termed 'essential hypertension'. If hypertension is not treated it substantially increases the risk of the patient developing a number of serious conditions including coronary thrombosis, stroke and kidney failure. Sustained hypertension also leads to the hypertrophy, or growth, of the cardiac muscle of the left ventricle of the heart and the medial layer of resistance arteries which can lead to the development of heart failure and a worsening of hypertension.

Blood pressure (BP) is defined as the product of the cardiac output (CO) and the peripheral vascular resistance (PVR). So $\mathbf{BP = CO \times PVR}$.

PVR is the resistance to flow in the small arteries and is regulated by the degree of contraction of the smooth muscle cells which make up the medial layer of the vessels, CO, on the other hand, is the product of heart rate (HR) and stroke volume (SV) so $\mathbf{CO = HR \times SV}$.

Heart rate is primarily regulated by the autonomic nervous system (Chapter 20), with the sympathetic nervous system acting to increase heart rate and the parasympathetic nervous system acting to decrease heart rate. Stroke volume is regulated by the plasma volume and venous return. The larger the plasma volume and rate of venous return, the larger the stroke volume.

The two main body systems involved in the regulation of blood pressure are the:

● autonomic nervous system
● renin-angiotensin system.

Renin-angiotensin system

Renin is an enzyme produced by the juxtaglomerular cells of the kidney and its release is stimulated by:

● beta-adrenoceptor agonists
● decreased blood flow through the kidney
● reduced sodium ion concentration in the plasma.

Renin converts the inactive protein angiotensinogen to angiotensin I. Angiotensin I is then converted to angiotensin II by angiotensin-converting enzyme (ACE, Figure 23.2). Angiotensin II (AII) has significant effects on the body in relation to the regulation of blood pressure (Table 23.1).

Antihypertensive drugs

The aim of antihypertensive drugs is to decrease either CO and/or PVR, thus decreasing blood pressure. There are four main groups of antihypertensive drugs and the mechanism of action of each will be explained here.

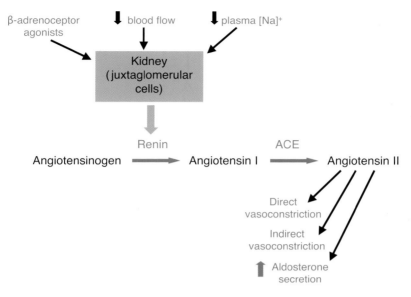

Figure 23.2 The renin-angiotensin system.

Current NICE guidelines suggest that thiazide diuretics or calcium antagonists should be first-line drugs for the treatment of hypertension in patients over 55 years of age or of African/Caribbean ethnicity. Agents affecting the renin-angiotensin system are first line for the treatment of hypertension in patients under 55 years of age. Beta-adrenoceptor antagonists are no longer recommended as first-line treatment in hypertension (NICE, 2006).

Table 23.1 Action of AII on the body and its impact on blood pressure.

Action of AII	Mechanism of action of AII	Effect on blood pressure
Direct vasoconstriction	AII binds to the angiotensin receptor (AT1) on blood vessels to produce vasoconstriction. AII is 40 times more potent than noradrenaline as a vasoconstrictor	Increases peripheral vascular resistance and therefore blood pressure
Indirect vasoconstriction	AII causes indirect vasoconstriction by promoting the release of NA from sympathetic nerves. NA then causes vasoconstriction	Increases peripheral vascular resistance and therefore blood pressure
Stimulation of aldosterone secretion	AII stimulates aldosterone release from the adrenal cortex. Aldosterone mediates retention of salt and water	Retention of salt and water increases plasma volume, therefore increasing CO and blood pressure

Section 3

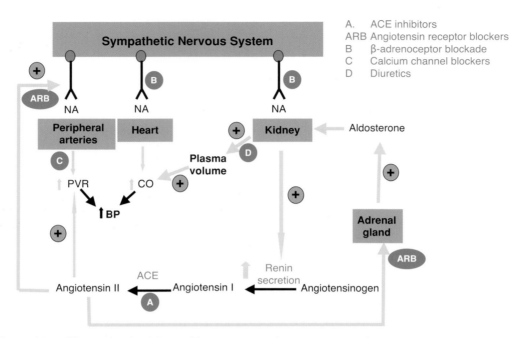

Figure 23.3 The pathophysiology of hypertension. Potential points of treatment are shown (adapted from Rang *et al.*, 2007).

Thiazide diuretics

These drugs inhibit the Na^+ and Cl^- co-transporter in the distal convoluted tubule of the kidney. This inhibits movement of Na^+ ions out of the distal convoluted tubule. If sodium ions stay in the tubule then water will also stay in the tubule, which increases salt and water excretion. This increase in water excretion reduces plasma volume, thus decreasing CO and reducing BP (Figure 23.3). While this reduction in plasma volume is responsible for the initial drop in blood pressure, the longer term effects of thiazide diuretics seem to be the result of a vasodilator effect, thus reducing PVR. The mechanism by which this vasodilation occurs is not currently known.

Thiazide diuretics are given orally and are well absorbed from the GI tract. These drugs need to be in the renal tubule in order to exert their therapeutic effect (Chapter 25); they get into the renal tubule by active tubular secretion, being carried into the tubule by the acidic carrier (Chapter 16). Increased plasma uric acid is a potential adverse effect of thiazide diuretics and occurs because it competes with uric acid for the acidic carrier in the renal tubule, therefore reducing the quantity of uric acid that can be carried into the tubule.

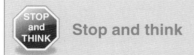 **Stop and think**

Why might diuretic drugs be ineffective in patients with reduced renal function?

Beta-adrenoceptor antagonists

These drugs block the action of noradrenaline (NA) released from sympathetic nerves on both the heart and the kidney (Figure 23.3).

Thus these drugs have a twofold mechanism of action.

- They reduce heart rate, therefore reducing cardiac output and hence blood pressure.
- They reduce renin release and therefore AII generation, leading to decreased vasoconstriction which reduces PVR, and decreased aldosterone production which reduces sodium reabsorption into plasma, reducing plasma volume and CO.

The adverse effects of these drugs are generally extensions of their pharmacological actions (Chapter 20). Although these drugs are no longer first-line treatment for hypertension, they should be considered in patients with evidence of increased sympathetic drive and those intolerant to ACE inhibitors and AII receptor antagonists.

 Practice application

If a patient's blood pressure is well controlled with a regimen containing a beta-blocker there is no absolute need to withdraw it (NICE, 2006).

Calcium channel blockers

These drugs block calcium entry into vascular smooth muscle by blocking calcium channels. A raised intracellular level of calcium is critical for stimulating contraction so preventing calcium entry into the cell results in relaxation of the smooth muscle cells of the blood vessels, thereby leading to vasodilation and a reduction in PVR and hence BP. Calcium channel blockers are given orally and are readily absorbed. The side effects are generally related to the vasodilatory activity of the drugs and include flushing, headache and reflex tachycardia.

Drugs which act on the renin-angiotensin system

These drug types prevent the vasoconstrictor effect of angiotensin II, thereby reducing PVR, and prevent the AII-stimulated production of aldosterone, thereby reducing plasma volume and cardiac output.

ACE inhibitors

These drugs prevent the production of angiotensin II. While they are very effective at lowering blood pressure, they exhibit a common side effect of a dry cough which can affect up to 35% of patients (Dicpinigaitis, 2006). This dry cough is thought to be the result of an increase in bradykinin levels in the body and occurs because, in addition to converting angiotenisn I to angiotensin II, these drugs also break down bradykinin (Figure 23.4). Bradykinin is an

Section 3

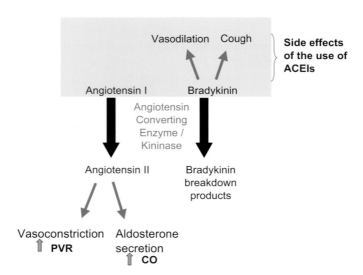

Figure 23.4 Relationship between angiotensin II and bradykinin levels as regulated by ACE.

inflammatory mediator which acts as a vasodilator, inducing tissue oedema, and stimulates the cough receptors in the airways.

Angiotensin II receptor antagonists

These drugs prevent AII binding to its receptors and generating an effect. They are useful in patients who cannot tolerate ACE inhibitors. Many of these drugs have an irreversible action at the receptor which means that despite the range of half-lives, they only need to be taken once daily.

Heart failure

Heart failure is a clinical syndrome with signs and symptoms that result from the heart's inability to maintain adequate pump function and is characterised by inadequate systemic perfusion. Despite recent advances in treating the underlying causes of the disease, such as hypertension and diabetes, the prognosis for heart failure remains poor.

Heart failure can be simply seen as a result of the heart's inability to pump sufficient cardiac output during systole – left ventricular systolic dysfunction. In the early stages of heart failure, the heart can still maintain output to match the body's metabolic demand, often through a variety of compensatory mechanisms, and the patient is asymptomatic. Indeed, as cardiac output falls, the sympathetic nervous system is activated to increase peripheral vascular resistance and blood pressure and so maintain perfusion. There is also a decrease in renal perfusion activating the renin-angiotensin and aldosterone pathways, increasing plasma volume, venous pressure and peripheral vascular resistance. While these changes are initially adaptive, acting to maintain blood pressure and cardiac output, in the long term they are maladaptive, establishing a vicious cycle of falling cardiac output, increasing peripheral vascular

Table 23.2 Heart failure (reduction in CO) initially results in compensatory measures but over time these exacerbate heart failure.

System activation	Initial response to maintain perfusion	Long-term exacerbation of heart failure
Sympathetic nervous system	Increase in PVR therefore maintaining BP Increased PVR leads to reduced renal perfusion which in turn activates the renin-angiotensin system	Increased afterload
Renin-angiotensin system	Stimulates the production of aldosterone which increases plasma volume and therefore CO	Increased preload
	Increases PVR, therefore maintaining BP	Increased afterload

resistance (afterload) and fluid retention (preload), which exacerbates the reduced ventricular function and ultimately further reduces cardiac output (Table 23.2).

Heart failure treatment

The aim of drugs used to treat heart failure is to decrease either preload and/or afterload, thus reducing the pressure on the heart and improving cardiac output (Figure 23.5). The major drug groups used in treating heart failure are as follows.

Drugs which act on the renin-angiotensin system

ACE inhibitors

Apart from being potent vasodilators, decreasing the vasoconstrictor angiotensin II and increasing the vasodilator bradykinin, these drugs reduce aldosterone release, limiting salt and water retention. Thus they reduce both preload and afterload to provide symptomatic relief. Importantly, they act directly on the heart tissue to attenuate AII-mediated remodelling and can therefore help to halt or reverse the progression of heart failure.

Angiotensin receptor blockers (ARBs)

Angiotensin receptor blockers act by inhibiting the interaction between angiotensin II and its receptors. They may be used when ACE inhibitors are not tolerated; there is also some evidence to suggest that they may provide added benefit, blocking non-ACE generated AII and having direct effects on cardiac remodelling (Burnier and Brunner, 2000).

Aldosterone antagonists

These drugs act as competitive antagonists at the aldosterone receptor in the kidney; therefore they reduce salt and water retention and thus decrease plasma volume and preload. There is also some evidence that they may have beneficial non-renal effects, improving cardiac structural remodelling and noradrenaline uptake (Zannad et al., 2000).

Section 3

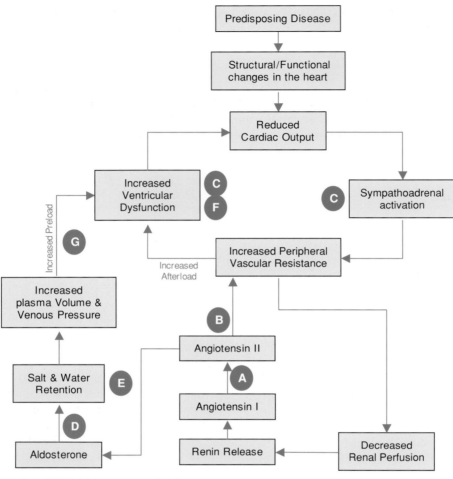

Figure 23.5 Neurohormonal activation in heart failure, initially protective but maladaptive in the long term. Potential points of treatment are shown (adapted from Rang *et al.*, 2007).

A. ACE inhibitors *e.g. enalapril*
B. Angiotensin receptor blockers (ARBs) *e.g. valsartan*
C. Beta-adrenoceptor blockade *e.g. bisoprolol*
D. Aldosterone antagonists *e.g. spironolactone*
E. Diuretics *e.g. furosemide*
F. Inotropes *e.g. digoxin*
G. *Organic Nitrates e.g. Isosorbide mononitrate*

Loop diuretics

These diuretics are much more potent than the thiazide diuretics used to treat hypertension. They act by inhibiting the $Na^+/K^+/Cl^-$ co-transporter in the loop of Henle and so reduce the Na^+ ion loss, dramatically increasing salt and water excretion in the urine. This decreases preload and congestion and improves the action of other drugs by minimising the intravascular volume. These drugs do not improve heart failure but do provide symptomatic relief. The adverse effects of these drugs are similar to those of thiazide diuretics.

Beta-adrenoceptor antagonists

It seems counterintuitive to use drugs that reduce heart rate and contractility in a failing heart, but careful use of beta-blockade can offset the maladaptive sympathoadrenal activation (Takeda *et al.*, 2004). Importantly, these drugs also improve systolic function and myocardial energetics, reduce the predisposition to arrhythmias and reverse cardiac remodelling. Therefore they not only relieve the symptoms but also ameliorate the heart failure.

 Practice application

The introduction of beta-adrenoceptor antagonists in patients whose heart failure is stabilised on a diuretic and an ACE inhibitor reduces mortality. The key to the use of these drugs is 'start low, go slow'.

Inotropes

Digoxin is the only positive inotropic drug that does not increase mortality in heart failure. Inotropes act directly on the heart itself to increase the force of contraction by inhibiting the Na^+/K^+ ATPase; they also actually reduce heart rate via an action on the vagus. While a decrease in heart rate, like the use of beta-adrenoceptor antagonists, seems counterintuitive, it actually increases the refractory period of the atrioventricular node and allows for better ventricular filling. This better ventricular filling coupled with the increase in force of contraction actually increases CO. This does not correct failure but does provide symptomatic relief and can support the heart during acute failure.

Organic nitrates

These drugs result in raised vascular nitric oxide (NO) which reduces calcium-mediated vascular contraction. NO is a potent vasodilator and hence these drugs improve coronary blood supply by dilating the coronary vasculature, reduce afterload by dilating arterial resistance vessels and, perhaps most importantly in heart failure, reduce preload by dilating venous capacitance vessels. Glyceryl trinitrate (GTN) is a commonly used short-acting nitrate which is administered sublingually or by transdermal patch. Adverse effects of nitrates include headache because of pronounced vasodilation and postural hypotension through a fall in BP.

 Stop and think

Why do you think GTN is not administered orally?

Section 3

Angina

Angina is actually the result of decreased perfusion of the myocardium itself. The pain associated with angina is actually the result of the action of chemicals released from ischaemic heart muscle on nociceptors.

The decreased perfusion of the heart muscle is most often the result of atheromatous plaque formation in the coronary arteries which reduces the lumen diameter of, and therefore the blood flow through, these vessels. One of the major problems associated with atheroma is the potential for the plaque to rupture, resulting in myocardial infarction (Trujillo and Dobesh, 2007). Interestingly, a recent systematic review suggests that women may have a slightly higher prevalence of angina than men (Hemingway *et al.*, 2008).

Antianginal drugs

The major groups of drugs used to treat angina are organic nitrates, calcium channel blockers, beta-adrenoceptor antagonists and lipid-lowering drugs. The aim of antianginal drug therapy is threefold.

To increase the perfusion of heart muscle

Organic nitrates and calcium channel blockers produce vasodilation of the coronary vessels through the production of NO and inhibition of calcium entry into cardiac cells respectively. Thus they act to increase the perfusion of the heart.

To reduce cardiac work and therefore metabolic demand

Beta-adrenoceptor antagonists decrease the sympathetic activity of the heart by blocking the action of NA and adrenaline on the beta-1-receptors. Thus they reduce cardiac work but do not have any effect on perfusion of the muscle.

The vasodilator effects of both organic nitrates and calcium channel blockers on resistance arteries and venous circulation also reduce cardiac work by reducing PVR and increasing venous return.

To prevent myocardial infarction

Lipid-lowering drugs

Cholesterol is a lipid produced in the liver which is important for normal body functioning, being a key component of the plasma membrane of all cells and the basic chemical from which a number of hormones are formed. As a lipid cholesterol cannot be transported dissolved in the bloodstream which is essentially aqueous in nature, it has to be carried around the body by special carrier proteins known as high-density lipoproteins (HDL), low-density lipoproteins (LDL) and very low-density lipoproteins (VLDL). There is an increased risk of atheromatous disease with increased serum levels of LDL cholesterol and decreased levels of HDL cholesterol. The most commonly used lipid-lowering drugs are the statins which reduce cholesterol levels in the body by inhibiting the enzyme HMG-CoA reductase (Figure 23.6).

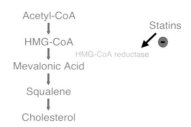

Acetyl-CoA
↓
HMG-CoA   Statins
↓   ← ●
HMG-CoA reductase
Mevalonic Acid
↓
Squalene
↓
Cholesterol

Figure 23.6 The point in the cholesterol synthesis pathway at which statins have their effect.

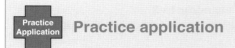 **Practice application**

Statins are used for:

- primary prevention of arterial disease in high-risk patients (elevated serum cholesterol levels), especially if other risk factors present
- secondary prevention of myocardial infarction and stroke in patients with symptomatic atherosclerotic disease (angina, transient ischaemic attacks, following acute myocardial infarction or stroke).

While there are a number of statins licensed for use in the UK, these drugs all have different pharmacokinetic properties which should be borne in mind before prescribing. All statins can be given orally and most are rapidly absorbed, being lipophilic in nature, although they may be subject to extensive first-pass metabolism. Simvastatin, probably the most commonly used statin currently, is actually a pro-drug and must be enzymatically converted to its active form in the body. Statins are predominantly metabolised by cytochrome P450 enzymes, with CYP3A4 and CYP2C9 being the most common isoforms.

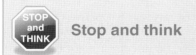 **Stop and think**

Why do you think grapefruit juice increases the possibility of adverse effects related to statins?

It is often recommended that statins are taken at night and this is because the liver makes most cholesterol at night. Different statins have different half-lives, ranging from 1 hour (fluvastatin) to 19 hours (rosuvastatin) ,and while statins with short half-lives are better taken at night, it is probably not necessary for those with long half-lives (Schachter, 2005).

Antiplatelet drugs

Like lipid-lowering drugs, antiplatelet drugs do not reduce cardiac work or increase perfusion of the heart muscle. Instead they are used to prevent myocardial infarction. The mechanism of action of these drugs will be described in Chapter 24.

Section 3

Summary

- Blood pressure = cardiac output × peripheral vascular resistance. Cardiac output = heart rate × stroke volume.
- Blood pressure is primarily controlled by the autonomic nervous system and the renin-angiotensin system.
- Renin release from the kidneys is stimulated by beta-adrenoceptor agonists, decreased blood flow through the kidney, reduced plasma sodium ion concentration.
- Angiotensin-converting enzyme converts angiotensin I to angiotensin II and breaks down bradykinin.
- Angiotensin II is the most potent vasoconstrictor produced by the body.
- The aim of antihypertensive therapy is to reduce CO and/or PVR.
- Thiazide diuretics inhibit the Na^+/Cl^- co-transporter in the distal convoluted tubule and reduce CO.
- Calcium channel blockers are vasodilators and reduce PVR.
- ACE inhibitors can produce a dry cough as a result of the build-up of bradykinin levels.
- Heart failure is the result of reduced systemic perfusion.
- The changes in the structure of the heart are initially compensatory but long term they exacerbate the reduced ventricular function.
- Afterload relates to the PVR while preload relates to fluid retention.
- Treatment of heart failure is designed to increase CO by reducing afterload and/or preload.
- Treatment of heart failure involves the use of loop diuretics and drugs which act on the renin-angiotensin-aldosterone system to reduce both preload and afterload.
- The introduction of beta-adrenoceptor antagonists in patients stabilised on diuretics and ACE inhibitors reduces mortality.
- Digoxin is a positive inotrope and acts directly on the heart to increase CO.
- Angina is the result of poorly perfused heart muscle often as a result of atheromatous disease.
- The aim of antianginal therapy is to improve myocardial perfusion, reduce cardiac work and prevent myocardial infarction.
- Organic nitrates and calcium channel blockers both increase myocardial perfusion and reduce cardiac work.
- Beta-adrenoceptor antagonists reduce cardiac work but have no effect on myocardial perfusion.
- Statins and antiplatelet drugs reduce the risk of myocardial infarction.

 Activity

1. Which of the following statements regarding hypertension are true?
   - Arteries regulate peripheral vascular resistance. True / False
   - BP = (HR × SV) × PVR. True / False
   - Hypertension does not increase the risk of stroke. True / False
   - The renin-angiotensin system is important in regulating BP. True / False
   - Plasma volume is important in regulating stroke volume. True / False

2. Which of the following statements regarding the renin-angiotensin system are true?
   - Renin release is stimulated by beta-adrenoreceptor agonists. True / False
   - Angiotensin II exerts a direct vasoconstrictor effect on peripheral vasculature. True / False
   - Angiotensin I acts as an inflammatory mediator. True / False
   - Renin acts to convert angiotensin I to angiotensin II. True / False
   - ACE inhibitors are useful in heart disease. True / False
3. Which of the following statements regarding heart failure are true?
   - In failure the heart is unable to pump enough blood to adequately meet the body's demands. True / False
   - Treatment for heart failure often aims to reduce preload and/or afterload. True / False
   - Beta-adrenoceptor antagonists are not useful in treating heart failure. True / False
   - Loop diuretics are useful for symptomatic relief in heart failure. True / False
   - Digoxin is a positive inotropic drug that does not increase mortality in heart failure. True / False
4. Which of the following statements regarding the treatment of angina are true?
   - Calcium channel blockers improve cardiac perfusion. True / False
   - Beta-adrenoceptor antagonists both reduce cardiac work and improve perfusion of the heart. True / False
   - One of the main aims of antianginal therapy is to prevent myocardial infarction. True / False
   - Organic nitrates reduce cardiac work. True / False
   - Both statins and aspirin have a role in antianginal therapy. True / False

Useful websites

British Heart Foundation. www.bhf.org.uk/

British Hypertension Society. www.bhsoc.org/

NICE guidance for the management of hypertension in adults in primary care – quick reference guide. www.nice.org.uk/Guidance/CG34/QuickRefGuide/pdf/English

NICE guidance for the management of chronic heart failure. www.nice.org.uk/Guidance/CG5/NiceGuidance/pdf/English

NICE guidance for myocardial infarction, secondary prevention – quick reference guide. www.nice.org.uk/Guidance/CG48/QuickRefGuide/pdf/English

References

British Heart Foundation Health Promotion Research Group. (2008) *Coronary Heart Disease Statistics Fact Sheet 2008/2009*, British Heart Foundation, London.

Burnier, M. and Brunner, H.R. (2000) Angiotensin II receptor antagonists. *Lancet*, **355**, 637–645.

Section 3

Dicpinigaitis, P.V. (2006) Angiotensin-converting enzyme inhibitor-induced cough. ACCP evidence-based clinical practice guidelines. *Chest*, **129**, 169S–173S.

Hemingway, H., Langenberg, C., Damant, J., *et al.* (2008) Prevalence of angina in women versus men. A systematic review and meta-analysis on international variations across 31 countries. *Circulation*, **117**, 1526–1536.

National Institute for Health and Clinical Excellence. Guidance for the management of hypertension in adults in primary care. 2006. www.nice.org.uk/Guidance/CG34/QuickRefGuide/pdf/English.

Rang, H.P., Dale, M.M., Ritter, J.M. and Flower, R. (2007) *Rang and Dale's Pharmacology*, 6th edn, Churchill Livingstone, Edinburgh.

Schachter, M. (2005) Chemical, pharmacokinetic and pharmacodynamic properties of statins: an update. *Fund Clin Pharmacol*, **19**, 117–125.

Takeda, Y., Fukutomi, T., Suzuki, S., *et al.* (2004) Effects of carvedilol on plasma B-type natriuretic peptide concentration and symptoms in patients with heart failure and preserved ejection fraction. *Am J Cardiol*, **94**, 448–453.

Trujillo, T.C. and Dobesh, P.P. (2007) Traditional management of stable angina. *Pharmacotherapy*, **27**, 1677–1692.

Zannad, F., Alla, F., Dousset, B., *et al.* (2000) Limitation of excessive extracellular matrix turnover may contribute to survival benefit of spironolactone therapy in patients with congestive heart failure: insights from the Randomized Aldactone Evaluation Study (RALES). *Circulation*, **102**, 2700–2706.

Further reading

Birkenhäger, W.H. (1990) Diuretics and blood pressure reduction: physiologic aspects. *J Hypertens*, **8**(Suppl), S3–S7.

British Medical Association and Royal Pharmaceutical Society of Great Britain (2010) *British National Formulary*, 59th edn, BMJ Publishing, London.

Page, C.P., Curtis, M.J., Sutter, M.C., *et al.* (2006) *Integrated Pharmacology*, 3rd edn, Mosby, London.

Sica, D.A. (2006) Angiotensin receptor blockers: new considerations in their mechanism of action. *J Clin Hypertens*, **8**, 381–385.

Werner, C.M. and Böhm, M. (2008) The therapeutic role of RAS blockade in chronic heart failure. *Ther Adv Cardiovasc Dis*, **2**, 167–177.

Section 3

24 Haemostasis and thrombosis

Learning outcomes

By the end of this chapter the reader should understand:

* the terms haemostasis and thrombosis and differentiate between them
* the coagulation cascade and the action of specific anticoagulant drugs within this cascade
* the process of platelet activation and the action of specific antiplatelet drugs
* the process of fibrinolysis and the action of specific fibrinolytic drugs.

Haemostasis

Haemostasis is defined as the arrest of blood loss from the body and is a normal physiological response to vascular damage. The process of haemostasis consists of three separate stages which each occur in a logical manner.

Vasoconstriction

This makes perfect sense physiologically. Haemostasis is the arrest of blood loss so the most obvious and logical step is the reduction of blood flow through the damaged vessel(s) which can be readily achieved by vasoconstriction.

Adhesion and activation of platelets

Platelets do not normally adhere to the endothelial surface of blood vessels but once endothelial damage has occurred, a number of chemicals are released which attract platelets to the damaged area. These platelets adhere to the damaged endothelial surface and in doing so become 'activated'. These activated platelets attract more platelets to the area and a 'platelet plug' is formed which 'plugs' the damaged area of the vessel, thus further reducing blood loss.

The New Prescriber. Edited by J Lymn, D Bowskill, F Bath-Hextall, R Knaggs, © 2010 John Wiley & Sons.

Fibrin formation

Fibrin formation is the end-product of the coagulation cascade and is important in solidifying and stabilising the platelet plug.

Thrombosis

Thrombosis, on the other hand, is defined as the pathological formation of a clot in the absence of bleeding. There are three key factors which predispose to thrombosis formation which were originally described by the German physician Rudolf Virchow and are still known today as Virchow's triad.

- Injury to vessel wall – such as following the rupture of an atherosclerotic plaque.
- Altered blood flow – such as in leg veins on long-haul flights.
- Abnormal coagulability of blood – such as in the latter stages of pregnancy or following the use of oral contraceptives.

Thrombi can be classified as either arterial or venous, depending on which vessel type they occur in. These different thrombi cause different clinical problems and are slightly different in their cellular make-up.

Arterial thrombi

These consist mainly of platelets and white blood cells and are generally the result of endothelial injury which itself is usually the result of underlying atherosclerotic disease. Arterial thrombi result in:

- myocardial infarction
- stroke
- peripheral ischaemia.

Venous thrombi

These consist of platelets and both white and red blood cells and are the result of blood stasis. Venous thrombi result in:

- deep vein thrombosis
- pulmonary embolism.

Role of the coagulation cascade in thrombosis and haemostasis

While it is relatively uncommon to use drugs which promote haemostasis, drugs which prevent thrombosis are commonly used clinically. This antithrombotic therapy can be divided into three separate classes which act on different aspects of thrombosis formation:

- to reduce blood coagulation (anticoagulants)
- to alter platelet function (antiplatelet drugs)
- to break down the fibrin meshwork (fibrinolytics).

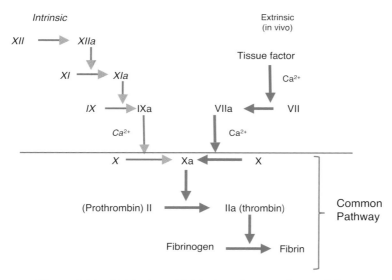

Figure 24.1 Extrinsic and intrinsic pathways of coagulation.

Before discussing exactly how these different classes of drugs act, it is important to think about the function of the coagulation cascade. There are actually two pathways of blood coagulation (Figure 24.1). The intrinsic pathway is important in the clotting of shed blood, while the extrinsic pathway is the most important coagulation pathway *in vivo*. The two pathways then converge to form a common pathway.

There are two important factors to remember in relation to the coagulation cascade.

1. The blood already contains all the necessary components for coagulation, albeit in an inactive form. These inactive precursors are activated by proteolysis, or cleavage, of the inactive form into a shorter active protein. Each active factor then cleaves the next inactive factor in the cascade. In terms of the extrinsic pathway of coagulation, it is the binding of tissue factor to factor VII in the presence of calcium that converts factor VII to VIIa which can then act on factor X to produce factor Xa, and so on.
2. Vitamin K is an important co-factor in the synthesis of functional clotting factors. Vitamin K is a fat-soluble vitamin, the name of which is derived from the German word 'Koagulation', and the action of this vitamin on clotting factors is crucial for their calcium-binding properties, and activation of clotting factors is a calcium-dependent process.

Anticoagulant drugs

These drugs prevent the production of fibrin by inhibiting the action of the clotting cascade. If fibrin is not produced then the platelet plug does not solidify and can be relatively easily disrupted by the normal flow of blood through the vessel. There are two main types of anticoagulant drugs: those which can be administered orally (e.g. warfarin) and those which can only be administered parenterally (e.g. heparin). These drugs prevent the formation of venous thrombi and are therefore used to treat and prevent deep vein thrombosis and pulmonary embolism.

Section 3

Warfarin

Pharmacodynamics

Warfarin is often referred to as a vitamin K antagonist but it is not an antagonist in the traditional sense in that it does not act on a receptor. Vitamin K needs to be activated by a reductase enzyme in order to act as a co-factor in the formation of clotting factors. In terms of the extrinsic pathway of coagulation, vitamin K is important for the production of all the components of this pathway. Warfarin actually competes with vitamin K for the reductase enzyme, thus reducing the level of activity of vitamin K and reducing the production of functional forms of all the relevant clotting factors (Figure 24.2).

The therapeutic effects of warfarin take 48–72 hours to occur because it inhibits the formation of new clotting factors. Warfarin does not have any effect on clotting factors which have already been made; hence its therapeutic action is delayed until all preformed clotting factors have been degraded. The delayed onset of action is also important in relation to the reversal of the effects of warfarin following overanticoagulation. Vitamin K can be given to reverse the effects of warfarin but this will take several hours because it will allow the formation of new functional clotting factors but will not affect the activity of preformed factors. Indeed, in an emergency it may be necessary to replace the clotting factors themselves. The major side effect associated with warfarin use is, perhaps unsurprisingly, haemorrhage. Warfarin has also been shown to be teratogenic.

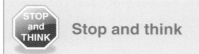
Stop and think

Why is the use of warfarin contraindicated in women in the first trimester of pregnancy?

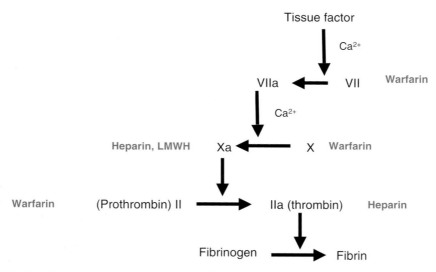

Figure 24.2   Position of action of anticoagulant drugs with the extrinsic pathway of blood coagulation.

Pharmacokinetics

Warfarin is heavily plasma protein bound, being about 99% bound to plasma albumin with a small volume of distribution. This high level of plasma protein binding has implications for co-administration with other drugs in terms of competition for the plasma protein-binding sites.

 Practice application

Aspirin and non-steroidal anti-inflammatory drugs have a high affinity for plasma albumin-binding sites and hence displace warfarin from plasma albumin. This interaction can result in an increase in the amount of free warfarin and thus increase the anticoagulant effect.

There are two stereo isomers of warfarin, the S and R forms, and these forms not only have different potencies but are metabolised by different cytochrome P450 isoenzymes. The S form is three times more potent than the R form and is metabolised by CYP2C9. The less potent R form is metabolised by CYP1A2 and CYP3A4 (Kaminsky and Zhang, 1997). This complexity in terms of activity and the number of CYP isoforms involved in metabolism makes warfarin susceptible to a significant number of drug–drug interactions (Table 24.1).

Drugs which inhibit the action of CYP isoforms will inhibit the metabolism of warfarin, resulting in an enhanced anticoagulant effect and increasing the risk of bleeding. On the other hand, drugs which induce the activity of CYP isoforms will enhance the metabolism of warfarin, reducing its anticoagulant effect and increasing the risk of clotting. Similarly, there are a number of dietary and herbal products, including leafy green vegetables, St John's wort, ginseng and gingko, which can induce CYP isoform activity and thus reduce the activity of warfarin.

Heparins

Pharmacodynamics

Unlike warfarin, heparins (unfractionated heparin and low molecular weight heparin, LMWH) have an immediate anticoagulant effect. This is because they increase the activity of antithrombin III. Antithrombin III is a naturally occurring inhibitor present in the blood as part of the normal physiological mechanisms which regulate blood coagulation. It acts by binding to

Table 24.1 Drug interactions with warfarin which occur through modulation of CYP450 enzyme activity.

Interaction with	CYP isoform affected	Effect on warfarin activity
Cimetidine	CYP1A2 and CYP3A4 inhibition	Increased warfarin activity
Erythromycin	CYP3A4 inhibition	Increased risk of bleeding
Fluconazole	CYP2C9 inhibition	
Carbamazepine	CYP3A4 induction	Reduced activity of warfarin
Phenytoin	CYP2C9 and CYP3A4 induction	Increased risk of clotting
Rifampicin	CYP2C9 and CYP3A4 induction	

Section 3

thrombin and other factors in the clotting cascade and preventing them from activating the next factor in the cascade. Heparins bind to antithrombin III, changing its three-dimensional shape and making it more likely to bind to thrombin and other clotting factors, thus increasing its activity. While both unfractionated heparin and LMWH binding to antithrombin II inhibit the action of factor Xa, only unfractionated heparin has a significant effect on thrombin (Figure 24.2). The immediate onset of action of heparin is reflected in the processes used to reverse its effects which essentially involve stopping the administration of heparin. This would then reduce the binding to, and activity of, antithrombin II. In an emergency it may be necessary to administer protamine which acts by binding to the heparin, thus preventing it from binding to antithrombin III.

Pharmacokinetics

Unfractionated heparin is very large in size and relatively polar in nature and is given either intravenously or by subcutaneous injection. It has a short half-life and can exhibit saturation kinetics such that its half-life appears to increase with increasing dose of the drug; consequently its activity requires monitoring. LMWH, on the other hand, as the name suggests, is smaller in size and has a longer half-life than unfractionated heparin. LMWH is primarily cleared via the kidneys and as such does not exhibit the same saturation kinetics as unfractionated heparin, making its activity more consistent and eliminating the need for close monitoring.

 Stop and think

Why do you think that neither unfractionated heparin nor LMWH can be given orally?

Role of platelets in thrombosis and haemostasis

Under normal healthy conditions, platelets do not adhere to the vascular endothelium but following vascular injury, platelets begin to stick to the damaged endothelium. This occurs through the binding of the glycoprotein Ia/IIb receptors on the surface of the platelets to molecules such as von Willebrand factor which are not normally exposed but become so following damage to the endothelium. Once they have started to adhere, the platelets become activated and start to secrete chemicals such as adenosine diphosphate (ADP) and thromboxane A_2 (TXA_2) which are pro-aggregatory and promote platelet aggregation. They also upregulate, or increase, the expression of glycoprotein IIb/IIIa receptors on the surface of the platelets and it is to these receptors which fibrinogen binds, causing cross-linking of the platelets and stabilising the platelet plug (Figure 24.3).

Antiplatelet drugs

Aspirin

Aspirin irreversibly inhibits the enzyme cyclooxygenase which in platelets is responsible for the production of the pro-aggregatory molecule TXA_2 (Figures 24.4 and 24.5). As platelets do

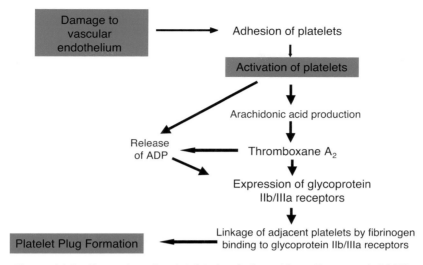

Figure 24.3 Formation of a platelet plug (adapted from Rang *et al.,* 2007).

not have a nucleus, they do not have the machinery to make new proteins and hence cannot make new cyclooxygenase enzymes to replace those which have been irreversibly inhibited. Thus the activity of this enzyme is lost for the lifetime of the platelet (around 7–10 days). Consequently, regular low-dose aspirin permanently inhibits platelet production of TXA_2 and reduces the aggregation of platelets. In terms of its antiplatelet activity, aspirin is administered orally as a single daily dose and is highly effective in the treatment and prevention of myocardial infarction and ischaemic stroke.

Adverse effects
Gastrointestinal haemorrhage
The inhibition of cyclooxygenase by aspirin prevents the formation of prostaglandins in the body. Prostaglandins reduce stomach acid secretion and promote mucus secretion, thus protecting the stomach lining from the effects of acid (Chapter 26). A reduction in prostaglandin production in the stomach can therefore leave patients susceptible to gastrointestinal bleeding.

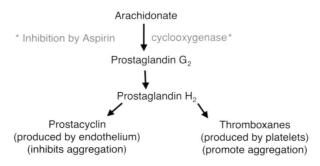

Figure 24.4 Action of aspirin to inhibit thromboxane A2.

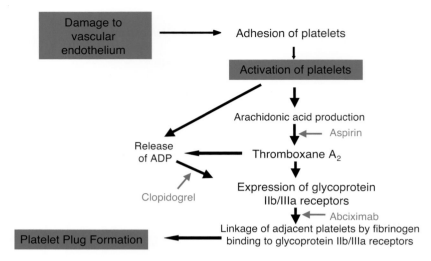

Figure 24.5   Action of antiplatelet drugs (adapted from Rang *et al.*, 2007).

Bronchospasm

The use of aspirin can also result in bronchospasm. This is because the inhibition of the enzyme cyclooxygenase by aspirin can result in a build-up of arachidonic acid in the cell membrane and this may then be converted to leukotrienes by the enzyme lipoxygenase. Leukotrienes are bronchoconstrictors (Chapter 22). This is often referred to as aspirin allergy and while present in only about 1% of the general population, it can affect around 10% of asthmatic patients. Hence the use of aspirin is cautioned in asthmatics and contraindicated in patients with a previous history of hypersensitivity to aspirin or other non-steroidal anti-inflammatory drugs.

Reye's syndrome

Aspirin is not used in children under 16 years of age due to the risk of developing Reye's syndrome which involves encephalopathy and liver disease and has a high mortality rate (Mizuguchi *et al.*, 2007). While it is often thought of as a childhood disease, it can also affect adults. It generally occurs following a viral illness and is associated with the use of aspirin (Glasgow, 2006).

Clopidogrel

Clopidogrel acts as an antiplatelet drug by inhibiting the ADP-induced aggregation of platelets. Clopidogrel binds irreversibly to ADP (P2Y12) receptors on platelets, preventing the binding of ADP itself (Figure 24.5). Clopidogrel is a pro-drug and requires metabolism by cytochrome P450 enzymes, particularly CYP3A4, in the liver to be activated. It is therefore important to consider possible interactions with other drugs. CYP3A4 inducers will speed up the activation of clopidogrel and possibly increase its therapeutic effects while CYP3A4 inhibitors will reduce the activation of clopidogrel, decreasing its therapeutic effect (Mullangi and Srinivas, 2009).

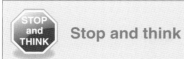

Stop and think

How might rifampicin and erythromycin alter the activity of clopidogrel?

Practice application

Clopidogrel is the drug of choice in aspirin-sensitive patients and can also be used in conjunction with aspirin for additive effects. While dual antiplatelet therapy with aspirin is associated with a lower risk of thromboembolic events, it has a higher risk of major bleeding.

Abciximab

This is a monoclonal antibody (signified by the ending 'mab' which stands for monoclonal antibody) to the glycoprotein IIb/IIIa receptors. Abciximab binds to these receptors, preventing the binding of fibrin and hence the stabilisation of the platelet plug (Figure 24.5).

Fibrinolytic cascade

Activation of the coagulation cascade automatically leads to activation of the fibrinolytic cascade. This cascade leads to the formation of plasmin which digests fibrin. Thus, activation of the fibrinolytic cascade acts to break down thrombi.

Fibrinolytic (thrombolytic) drugs

These drugs have a dynamic action resulting in the breakdown of thrombi. Examples of these drugs are streptokinase and alteplase, both of which act as plasminogen activators converting plasminogen to plasmin (Figure 24.6) which then acts to break down fibrin. Fibrinolytic drugs are principally used in the treatment of acute myocardial infarction because their ability to break down thrombi means that the artery is unblocked, allowing reperfusion of the tissue and limiting damage.

Streptokinase

Streptokinase is actually derived from beta-haemolytic streptococci and consequently it is antigenic. The presence of antibodies can reduce the effectiveness of streptokinase and hence it should only be used once within a 12-month period.

Section 3

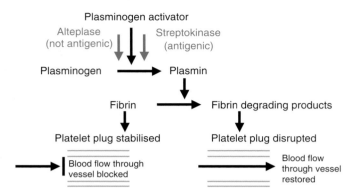

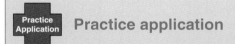

Figure 24.6   Fibrinolytic cascade and the action of fibrinolytic drugs (adapted from Winstanley and Walley, 2002).

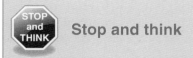 **Practice application**

Streptokinase may be less effective in patients who have recently suffered from a severe streptococcal infection due to the presence of antibodies.

Alteplase

Alteplase is a recombinant protein of the naturally occurring activator of plasminogen and as such it is not antigenic. It can therefore be used in patients with antibodies to streptokinase.

Adverse effects of fibrinolytic drugs

The main adverse effect of fibrinolytic drugs is bleeding. Fibrinolytic drugs act by breaking down blood clots and cannot differentiate between pathological thrombi and normal haemostatic clots. Consequently the use of fibrinolytic drugs is contraindicated in patients with active bleeding ulcers and those who have undergone recent surgery or trauma.

Some patients may exhibit an allergy to streptokinase (Betancourt *et al.*, 2005).

Stop and think

What type of adverse drug reaction (A or B) is allergy to streptokinase likely to be?

Section 3

Summary

- Haemostasis is the body's normal physiological response to vascular damage.
- Thrombosis is the pathological formation of a blood clot in the absence of bleeding.
- The extrinsic pathway of coagulation is the most important pathway *in vivo*.
- All components of the coagulation cascade are present in the blood in an inactive form and are activated by proteolysis.
- Vitamin K is an important co-factor in the synthesis of functional clotting factors.
- Anticoagulants act to prevent the formation of fibrin.
- Warfarin competes with vitamin K and reduces the formation of new functional clotting factors.
- Heparin binds to antithrombin III to have an immediate anticoagulant effect.
- Platelets bind to damaged endothelium and become activated. These activated platelets aggregate to form a platelet plug.
- Aspirin inhibits the activity of cyclooxygenase for the lifetime of the platelet.
- Clopidogrel binds irreversibly to P2Y12 receptors to prevent ADP-induced platelet aggregation.
- The fibrinolytic cascade produces plasmin which acts to break down fibrin.
- Streptokinase is antigenic.

✏ Activity

1.	Warfarin is administered intravenously.	True / False
2.	The effects of warfarin can be reversed by vitamin K.	True / False
3.	Warfarin exerts its pharmacological effects within an hour.	True / False
4.	Heparin prevents the formation of functional clotting factors.	True / False
5.	Heparin anticoagulation can be reversed with protamine.	True / False
6.	LMWH exerts its effects equally on thrombin and factor Xa.	True / False
7.	Both aspirin and clopidogrel act irreversibly.	True / False
8.	Aspirin can cause bronchoconstriction in susceptible patients.	True / False
9.	Streptokinase activity can be diminished by previous streptococcal infection.	True / False
10.	Streptokinase and alteplase prevent fibrin formation.	True / False
11.	Alteplase is antigenic.	True / False
12.	Thrombosis is a normal physiological response to vascular injury.	True / False

References

Betancourt, B.Y., Marrero-Miragaya, M.A., Jiménez-López, G., *et al.* (2005) Pharmacovigilance program to monitor adverse reactions of recombinant streptokinase in acute myocardial infarction. *BMC Clin Pharmacol*, **5**, 5.

Glasgow, J.F. (2006) Reye's syndrome: the case for a causal link with aspirin. *Drug Saf*, **29**, 1111–1121.

Section 3

Kaminsky, L.S. and Zhang, Z.Y. (1997) Human P450 metabolism of warfarin. *Pharmacol Ther*, **73**, 67-74.

Mizuguchi, M., Yamanouchi, H., Ichiyama, T. and Shiomi, M. (2007) Acute encephalopathy associated with influenza and other viral infections. *Acta Neurol Scand*, **115** (Suppl 186), 45-56.

Mullangi, R. and Srinivas, N.R. (2009) Clopidogrel: review of bioanalytical methods, pharmacokinetics/pharmacodynamics, and update on recent trends in drug–drug interaction studies. *Biomed Cromatogr*, **23**, 26-41.

Rang, H.P., Dale, M.M., Ritter, J.M. and Flower, R. (2007) *Rang and Dale's Pharmacology*, 6th edn, Churchill Livingstone, Edinburgh.

Winstanley, P. and Walley, T. (2002) *Medical Pharmacology*, 2nd edn, Churchill Livingstone, Edinburgh.

Further reading

Ageno, W., Crotti, S. and Turpie, A.G. (2004) The safety of antithrombotic therapy during pregnancy. *Expert Opin Drug Saf*, **3**, 113-118.

British Medical Association and Royal Pharmaceutical Society of Great Britain (2010) *British National Formulary*, 59th edn, BMJ Publishing, London.

Jenkins, C., Costello, J. and Hodge, L. (2004) Systematic review of prevalence of aspirin induced asthma and its implications for clinical practice. *BMJ*, **328**(7437), 434.

Keller, T.T., Squizzato, A. and Middeldorp, S. (2007) Clopidogrel plus aspirin versus aspirin alone for preventing cardiovascular disease. *Cochrane Database Syst Rev*, 3, CD005158.

Nutescu, E.A., Shapiro, N.L., Ibrahim, S. and West, P. (2006) Warfarin and its interactions with foods, herbs and other dietary supplements. *Expert Opin Drug Saf*, **5**, 433-451.

Page, C.P., Curtis, M.J., Sutter, M.C., *et al.* (2006) *Integrated Pharmacology*, 3rd edn, Mosby, London.

25 The renal system

Learning outcomes

By the end of this chapter the reader should be able to:

- describe the basic structure and list the functions of the kidneys
- describe the basic principles of glomerular filtration
- assess an individual's renal function using common biochemical measures and grade the severity of renal failure
- describe the effects of renal failure on drug kinetics
- safely adjust drug doses for a patient with renal failure, utilising standard reference materials
- give examples of drugs which require careful dose adjustment in renal failure
- be aware of drugs that should be used with caution or should be avoided in patients with renal impairment
- explain the modes of action of commonly used diuretics and the implications for their use in patients with renal failure
- explain the classification of nephrotoxicity into predictable and idiosyncratic reactions.

Structure and function of the kidneys

Structure of the kidneys

The kidneys are situated at the back of the abdomen behind the peritoneum, one on either side of the aorta. Each kidney is 10–12 cm in length and is surrounded by a fibrous capsule. Each capsule is surrounded further by fat (perinephric fat) and by another layer of fibrous tissue (perinephric fascia). An adrenal gland sits on top of each kidney enclosed by the perinephric fascia. The outer zone of the kidney is called the renal cortex and the inner zone is called the renal medulla. Figure 25.1 shows the kidney in cross-section.

The basic functional unit of the kidney is called the nephron (Figure 25.2). Each kidney has between 400,000 and 800,000 nephrons. This number declines with increasing age. Each nephron is composed of a glomerulus, which is a ball of highly porous capillaries, and an associated tubule that leads to the collecting duct. Blood is filtered by the glomerulus to

The New Prescriber. Edited by J Lymn, D Bowskill, F Bath-Hextall, R Knaggs, © 2010 John Wiley & Sons.

Frontal section through the Kidney

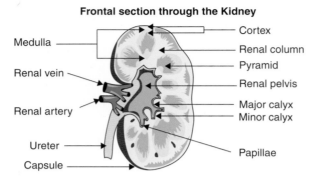

Medulla

Renal vein

Renal artery

Ureter

Capsule

Cortex

Renal column

Pyramid

Renal pelvis

Major calyx

Minor calyx

Papillae

Figure 25.1 Cross-section of the human kidney (www.commons.wikimedia.org/wiki/Image:Illu_kidney2.jpg).

form urine in the Bowman's capsule, which is the start of the tubule. The composition of the urine is continually modified along the length of the tubule by the reabsorption and secretion of substances. A large amount of blood passes through the glomeruli every minute (approximately 25% of the total cardiac output), and approximately 180 litres of glomerular filtrate are produced over a 24-hour period (more than 30 times the average circulating total blood volume!). All but 1–2 litres of this filtrate are reabsorbed by the tubules of the nephrons back into the bloodstream. The whole process allows the plasma to be adequately filtered, but the very efficient reabsorptive processes prevent volume and electrolyte depletion.

A ureter drains the urine from each kidney into the bladder. The ureter arises from the renal pelvis. Each renal pelvis divides into two or three major calyces which in turn subdivide into two or three minor calyces. The collecting duct of each nephron flows into a papillary duct which opens out on a renal papilla into a minor calyx.

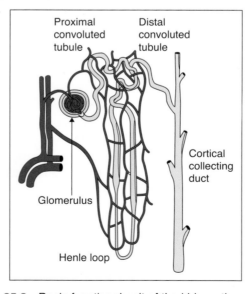

Proximal convoluted tubule

Distal convoluted tubule

Cortical collecting duct

Glomerulus

Henle loop

Figure 25.2 Basic functional unit of the kidney, the nephron.

Table 25.1   Functions of the kidneys.

Function type	Description of function
Regulatory	Control of body fluid volume and composition.
	Regulation of water, sodium, potassium, chloride, magnesium and phosphate excretion.
	Regulation of acid–base balance through the reabsorption of bicarbonate and the excretion of hydrogen ions.
Excretory	Excretion of waste products and drugs.
Endocrine	Production of hormones, for example erythropoietin (stimulates red blood cell production), renin (converts angiotensinogen to angiotensin I) and prostaglandins (powerful vasodilatory agents in the kidney).
Metabolic	Metabolism of vitamin D to the potent active form, and of small molecular weight proteins.

Functions of the kidneys

The kidneys have a number of very important functions (Table 25.1). Their principal role is the regulation of the volume and composition of body fluid to maintain a stable extracellular environment and the elimination of waste material.

Risk factors for kidney disease

There are a number of factors which make the chances of a person having kidney disease more likely. If you are considering prescribing medication for a patient in one of these groups it would be sensible to check their renal function first.

- Increasing age (kidney function declines with increasing age).
- Ethnic group – kidney disease is more common amongst the Asian population.
- Diabetes (type 1 and type 2, especially if longstanding).
- Hypertension.
- Vascular disease, for example heart disease and stroke.

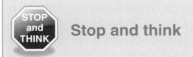 **Stop and think**

Think about the patients you see in your day-to-day work. Are they at risk of kidney disease? How are you going to determine those individuals in whom you need to take kidney function into account when prescribing?

Section 3

The principles of glomerular filtration

Blood enters the glomerulus via an afferent arteriole and leaves via an efferent arteriole. The high hydrostatic pressure in the glomerular capillaries exceeds the opposing pressures within them and the Bowman's capsule, resulting in water, ions and small molecules being driven across the filtration barrier into the Bowman's capsule. Pressure changes within the afferent and efferent arterioles affect glomerular filtration. Pressure in the glomerular capillaries is reduced by afferent arteriolar constriction and increased by efferent arteriolar constriction.

The molecular size of a substance and its electrical charge, protein binding, configuration and rigidity determine whether it crosses the filtration barrier and enters the filtrate or remains in the blood (Box 25.1). The filtration barrier has a net negative electrical charge, meaning that the movement of negatively charged molecules is restricted relative to those molecules with a positive or neutral charge.

Box 25.1   Examples of substances 'filtered' and 'not filtered' by the kidneys.

Filtered	Not filtered
Water	Plasma proteins
Electrolytes	Red blood cells
Urea	White blood cells
Creatinine	

The glomerular filtration rate (GFR) is a measure of the rate at which the blood is filtered by the kidneys. The GFR is therefore an important indicator of kidney function. The normal GFR depends on age, sex and body size, but is approximately 120 ml/min. There are a number of ways of estimating the GFR, each of which has its own limitations, and these are discussed in more detail below.

Assessing kidney function

Serum urea and creatinine

Serum urea and creatinine have commonly been used to estimate kidney function. Both are substances produced by the body and excreted by the kidney which can be measured easily in the laboratory. Urea (measured in mmol/l) is a small molecule produced by the liver which is the waste product of protein metabolism. Creatinine (measured in μmol/l) is derived from creatine which is a component of muscle cells. The blood levels of both can be affected by a number of factors. Urea levels are raised, for example in dehydration and in gastrointestinal bleeding, and tend to be low if someone is malnourished, or in liver disease. Creatinine levels are affected by muscle mass and values tend to be higher in people with a large muscle bulk.

When kidney function is impaired, urea and creatinine accumulate in the blood. However, due to the physiological reserve of the kidneys, the level of neither substance rises substantially until the level of renal function has deteriorated significantly; that is, when the GFR has fallen to around 30 ml/min. This limits their usefulness in assessing kidney function.

Clearance methods

Clearance (CL) is defined as the volume of plasma from which a substance is completely removed or cleared by the kidneys per unit time. The ideal marker for measuring clearance is freely filtered by the glomerulus and is neither reabsorbed, secreted, synthesised or metabolised by the tubules. For such substances, the amount filtered by the glomerulus is equal to the amount excreted in the urine.

There is no naturally occurring ideal marker to measure clearance, so creatinine has traditionally been used for this method to estimate the GFR. Creatinine is used because its rate of production is typically very constant and serum levels and urinary output therefore vary very little throughout a 24-hour period. However, because a small amount of creatinine is secreted by the tubules, GFR measured by creatinine clearance can be overestimated. This is more pronounced when the GFR is low as tubular secretion of creatinine increases. Urine is collected over a 24-hour period and the urinary creatinine level is measured. A 24-hour urinary collection also indicates urine flow in millilitres per minute. A plasma creatinine level is measured at some point in the 24-hour period. Using the formula below, the creatinine clearance can be calculated.

$$\text{Creatinine clearance} = \frac{U \times V}{P}$$

where
     V is the rate of urine flow
     U is the urine concentration of creatinine
     P is the plasma concentration of creatinine
    Normal range: men 90–140 ml/min
                 women 80–125 ml/min.

Estimation equations

Glomerular filtration rate and creatinine clearance can also be predicted from estimation equations using the plasma creatinine. These are the methods commonly used in everyday practice.

The Cockcroft–Gault equation allows rapid estimation of the creatinine clearance from the plasma creatinine in a patient with a stable creatinine. This formula incorporates the patient's weight.

$$C_{cr} \text{ (ml/min)} = \frac{(140\text{-age}) \times \text{weight (kg)} \times f}{\text{Plasma creatinine (}\mu\text{mol/l)}} \qquad \begin{array}{l} f = 1.23 \text{ (males)} \\ 1.04 \text{ (females)} \end{array}$$

where C_{cr} = estimated creatinine clearance.

The Cockcroft–Gault equation takes into account the increasing creatinine production with increasing weight, and the decline in creatinine production with age. However, the equation does not adjust for body surface area.

More recently, an equation to predict the GFR from the plasma creatinine concentration has been developed from data obtained in the Modification of Diet in Renal Disease (MDRD) study. The formula, which takes into account body surface area, calculates the estimated GFR (eGFR) using the patient's age, sex and creatinine levels, and also makes an adjustment if the patient is

Table 25.2 Five stages of chronic kidney disease, classified according to the level of the eGFR.

Stage of CKD	eGFR (ml/min/1.73 m^2)
1	90* *with underlying structural kidney disease
2	60–90* *with underlying structural kidney disease
3	30–60
4	15–30
5	<15

Afro-Caribbean. It is becoming increasingly common in the UK for the serum creatinine result to be accompanied by a value for the eGFR.

In 2002, the National Kidney Foundation in its Kidney Disease Outcome Initiative Guidelines (K/DOQI) proposed five stages of chronic kidney disease (CKD), classified according to the level of the eGFR, which is given in ml/min/1.73 m^2 and approximately equates to the percentage function of the kidneys. These stages of CKD are now universally used by the renal community (Table 25.2).

There are limitations to both of these estimation equations. They are less accurate in certain populations, including individuals with a normal GFR, children, pregnant women, elderly patients, specific ethnic groups and those with an unusual body shape and/or weight, for example morbid obesity and amputees. Neither of the equations is validated in acute kidney injury (acute renal failure). In these situations, alternative methods for calculating the GFR should be considered, for example clearance methods.

Drug use in patients with renal impairment

Drug prescribing for patients with renal impairment is problematic for a number of reasons. People with impaired renal function usually have other medical problems, for example diabetes, are often elderly and take many different types of medication. This in itself predisposes them to increased adverse effects from medicines. However, in renal impairment, the body often handles drugs differently, leading to further increased risk of drug toxicity. These combined effects mean that patients with impaired kidney function are a high-risk group for drug management. Many of the adverse effects, however, are predictable and can be avoided or minimised by careful medicine prescribing and use.

 Stop and think

Think about drugs that you might prescribe in practice. Which drugs may require dose reduction in renal impairment? Where are you going to find out the necessary information to recommend altered doses for these drugs?

Section 3

Renal impairment can affect all four pharmacokinetic parameters: absorption, distribution, metabolism and excretion.

Absorption

Generally of little clinical significance, with notable exceptions. For example, the intestinal absorption of both dietary and supplemental iron is significantly reduced in CKD.

Distribution

Volumes of distribution may be altered due to fluid overload, reduced albumin and altered protein binding. This can impact significantly on drug distribution. For example, phenytoin is ordinarily 90% protein bound with the unbound 10% being the active drug. In renal impairment, low albumin levels and high levels of urea (molecules of which may bind to albumin) leave fewer binding sites for drugs. Thus a much smaller proportion of the drug is protein bound. Care needs to be taken when interpreting phenytoin levels (low levels may not necessarily be subtherapeutic). Ideally, a free fraction serum level should be taken but, as this is often not available, a total serum level can be interpreted bearing in mind albumin and urea levels.

Metabolism

The kidney is a site of drug metabolism but in most cases this is minimal compared to the liver. However, there are examples where the loss of renal metabolism can be seen clinically. For example, patients with renal impairment may need smaller doses of insulin as insulin is partially metabolised by the kidney.

Excretion

The kidney is the major organ involved in drug elimination from the body. Drugs and/or their metabolites that are excreted by the renal route are excreted more slowly in patients with kidney disease and if this is not taken into account, this can lead to accumulation in the body (Figure 25.3).

It is therefore necessary to adjust dosing of drugs cleared by the kidneys and this can be done either by increasing the dosage interval (Figure 25.4) or by reducing the dose (Figure 25.5).

Drug dosing in renal impairment

Now that you are aware of the effect that renal failure may have on the kinetics of a drug, it is important to be able to apply this in practice. The extent to which the kinetics is altered depends on:

- the properties of the drug
- the severity of the patient's renal impairment.

The recent introduction of eGFR has a valuable role to play in highlighting patients with CKD who may require dose adjustment. However, the MDRD formula differs from the

Section 3

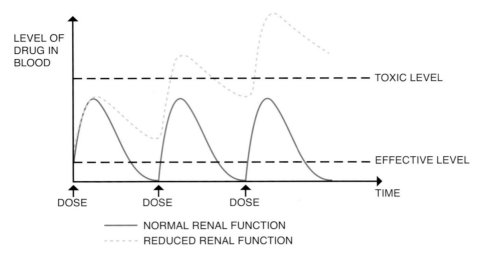

Figure 25.3 Accumulation of drug in renal failure.

Cockcroft–Gault equation because it gives a GFR estimate normalised for a body surface area of 1.73 m^2 whereas Cockcroft–Gault estimates individual creatinine clearances. Most drug dosage recommendations in the literature are based upon Cockcroft–Gault estimates of creatinine clearance. In patients of an average height and build, there is good correlation between the two equations and for the majority of drugs in patients of average weight, either calculation can be used to determine drug dosing. However, eGFR should not be used for calculating drug doses in patients at extremes of weight nor for potentially toxic drugs of a narrow therapeutic index. In these circumstances the difference between the two equations may be clinically significant and Cockcroft–Gault estimates should be used to avoid potential drug over/underdoses.

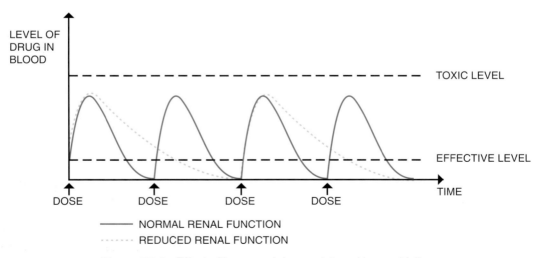

Figure 25.4 Effect of increased dosage interval in renal failure.

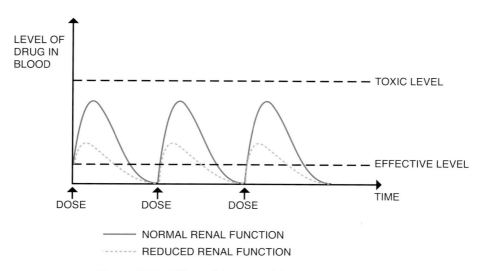

NORMAL RENAL FUNCTION
REDUCED RENAL FUNCTION

Figure 25.5   Effect of decreased dose in renal failure.

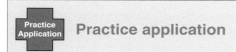 **Practice application**

It is important to remember the limitations of both the eGFR and Cockcroft–Gault estimation equations that we discussed earlier. When using either equation, creatinine levels should be stable and the clinical picture should always be taken into account.

Once you have an estimate of the patient's renal function, there are a number of reference sources that can guide you on whether or not you need to adjust the dose of the drug you wish to prescribe. The most readily available source for most will be the British National Formulary (BNF) in which guidance on the use and dosing of drugs in renal failure are provided. Where possible, values for eGFR, creatinine clearance or other measure of renal function are included.

For example, for cefalexin (BNF, 2010):

eGFR 40–50 ml/min/1.73 m^2	max 3 g daily
eGFR 10–40 ml/min/1.73 m^2	max 1.5 g daily
eGFR <10 ml/min/1.73 m^2	max 750 mg daily

Sometimes the BNF may indicate that a dose reduction is necessary but refers the prescriber to specialist information for more details. For example, with gabapentin – reduce dose if eGFR less than 80 ml/min/1.73 m^2; consult product literature.

Manufacturers often provide information on dosing in renal impairment in their Summary of Product Characteristics. These are available free online at emc.medicines.org.uk which is a very useful website when further information is required.

Section 3

Further specialist reference sources may be available at specialist renal units or medicines information centres.

Drug dosing in dialysis

Prescribing for patients on dialysis is further complicated as many drugs are cleared from the body by dialysis. When prescribing drugs for patients in this situation, consult specialist literature or seek advice from your local renal unit.

Examples of drugs that may need dose adjusting in renal impairment

Not all drugs will need dose adjusting for patients with chronic kidney disease. Whether or not dose reduction is required depends on what proportion of the drug is excreted by the kidney in an active form and how toxic the drug is if it accumulates. For example, a drug that is largely metabolised in the liver, with minimal dose-related side effects, is likely to need no dose reduction and careful monitoring of side effects is sufficient. Conversely, drugs that are cleared by the kidneys with a narrow therapeutic index may need very precise dose adjustment and monitoring of both efficacy and side effects (Box 25.2).

Monitoring

Sensitivity to some drugs is increased in renal impairment even if accumulation does not occur and patients with CKD can be extremely sensitive to the side effects of drugs. Therefore, even when guidance on dosing is followed, it is imperative that the patient is monitored for signs of drug toxicity and doses adjusted/alternative drugs used as appropriate.

Nephrotoxicity

There are a number of drugs which should be avoided completely or used with great caution in people with impaired kidney function. This is because they may themselves cause a further deterioration in kidney function or can be directly harmful to the kidneys if they accumulate should their excretion be impaired. This is called nephrotoxicity, which can be either predictable or idiosyncratic.

Box 25.2 **Examples of drugs that need careful dose adjustment in renal failure**

Antibiotics, for example gentamicin, vancomycin, levofloxacin, co-amoxiclav
Gabapentin
Low molecular weight heparins
Digoxin
Opioids

Table 25.3   Drugs causing predictable nephrotoxicity.

Drug group	Mechanism
Non-steroidal anti-inflammatory drugs (NSAIDs) For example, ibuprofen and diclofenac	By inhibiting prostaglandin production, they can cause a critical reduction in glomerular perfusion.
ACE inhibitors and angiotensin II receptor blockers (ARBs) For example, ramipril, lisinopril, candesartan, losartan	These drugs can cause acute kidney injury by altering renal blood flow in patients with renovascular disease.
Aminoglycoside antibiotics For example, gentamicin	These drugs are directly toxic to the kidneys if the serum levels are high because of reduced clearance.
Ciclosporin	Causes chronic glomerular damage and scarring in the kidney.

 Practice application

Patients with impaired renal function excrete drugs more slowly and are highly susceptible to the effects of nephrotoxic drugs.

Predictable

This is where the harmful effect of the drug on the kidneys can be predicted (often this is dose or level related). Examples of drugs causing predictable nephrotoxicity and which therefore which should be avoided or used with caution are shown in Table 25.3.

Idiosyncratic

The harmful effect of the drug on the kidney is unexpected. These are rare events which occur in susceptible individuals. Examples of drugs causing idiosyncratic nephrotoxicity include:

- antibiotics, for example penicillins
- NSAIDs
- diuretics
- proton pump inhibitors, for example lansoprazole.

Other drugs which should be avoided

Metformin, used in the treatment of type 2 diabetes, can provoke lactic acidosis, the risk of which is greater in patients with impaired kidney function. It should be discontinued when the eGFR falls below 30 ml/min/1.73 m^2 (BNF and NICE guidelines).

Stop and think

Are any of the drugs that you might prescribe in practice nephrotoxic? What factors will you need to consider before prescribing these drugs and what parameters might you need to monitor?

Use of diuretics in renal failure

Diuretics are drugs that cause a net loss of sodium and water from the body by an action on the kidney. They are commonly used in chronic kidney disease to treat hypertension, increase urine output and prevent fluid accumulation.

Diuretics can be split into three families: loop diuretics, thiazide diuretics and potassium-sparing diuretics (Table 25.4). All three classes of diuretic (with the exception of spironolactone) act from within the tubular lumen and therefore must reach their site of action by being secreted into the proximal tubule. This secretion is lessened in the failing kidney and so the response to diuretics is reduced in CKD.

In practice, this means that thiazides are generally ineffective if the creatinine clearance is less than 30 ml/min unless used in combination with a loop diuretic, so the former are rarely used in patients with moderate to severe renal impairment. Use of loop diuretics is widespread but the doses required are often much higher than those used in the general population (e.g. furosemide doses of up to 500 mg daily).

The use of potassium-sparing diuretics is limited in kidney disease as patients often cannot tolerate the increased potassium levels they cause and so potassium should be monitored extremely closely if these diuretics are required.

Renal patients on diuretic therapy must not be allowed to become dehydrated as this may worsen existing renal failure.

Table 25.4 Action of the three classes of diuretic drugs.

	Loop	Thiazide	Potassium sparing
Examples	Furosemide, bumetanide	Bendroflumethiazide, metolozone	Spironolactone, amiloride
Site of action	Thick segment of loop of Henle	Distal convoluted tubule	Collecting duct
Mechanism of action	Inhibits Na reabsorption	Inhibits Na reabsorption	Spironolactone is an aldosterone antagonist, amiloride blocks Na channels
Effect on plasma K	Decreased	Decreased	Increased

Section 3

Summary

- The nephron is the basic functional unit of the kidney and consists of a glomerulus and an associated tubule which leads to the collecting duct.
- The main role of the kidney is regulating body fluid volume and composition.
- Glomerular filtration rate (GFR) is an important indicator of kidney function.
- Creatinine clearance can be predicted from the Cockcroft-Gault equation.
- Kidney disease can be divided into five stages according to the eGFR.
- Renal impairment does not generally affect drug absorption or metabolism.
- Drug distribution can be altered in renal impairment due to fluid overload and reduced plasma albumin concentration.
- Many drugs are excreted more slowly in renal impairment and drug dosages may need to be adjusted accordingly.
- Drugs which need careful dose adjustment in renal impairment include some antibiotics, gabapentin, digoxin, opioids and low molecular weight heparins.
- Drugs which cause nephrotoxicity should be avoided or used with great caution in people with impaired kidney function.
- Diuretics exert their pharmacological action from within the lumen of the tubule.
- Doses of diuretics may need to be higher in patients with renal impairment.
- It is important to identify patients at risk of kidney disease before you start prescribing.
- Check whether careful dose adjustment or caution is required for the drug you wish to prescribe. If you find that dose adjustment is necessary, use eGFR or Cockcroft-Gault where appropriate to estimate the degree of renal function and follow dosage guidance in the available reference sources.

Activity

1. In addition to its regulatory and excretory roles, the kidney is also a synthetic and metabolic organ. **True / False**
2. Kidney disease is more common amongst Caucasian populations. **True / False**
3. The molecular weight and electronic charge of a molecule partly determine if it is filtered by the kidney. **True / False**
4. Creatinine is a substance produced by the body that is both filtered and actively secreted by the kidneys. **True / False**
5. The Cockcroft–Gault equation gives an estimation of creatinine clearance normalised for body surface area. **True / False**
6. Renal impairment can affect all four ADME pharmacokinetic parameters. **True / False**
7. The MDRD equation is the recommended method of estimating renal function for use in modifying drug doses in patients at extremes of weight. **True / False**
8. Dosing of opiates should be adjusted in renal impairment due to their narrow therapeutic index and method of elimination from the body. **True / False**
9. Potassium-sparing diuretics are the diuretic of choice in patients with renal impairment. **True / False**
10. A reduction in kidney function due to ramipril could be described as an idiosyncratic reaction. **True / False**

Section 3

References

British Medical Association and Royal Pharmaceutical Society of Great Britain (2010) *British National Formulary*, 59th edn, BMJ Publishing, London.

National Kidney Foundation (2002) K/DOQI clinical practice guidelines for chronic kidney disease: evaluation, classification and stratification. *Am J Kidney Dis*, **39**(Suppl 1), S1–S266.

Useful websites

Electronic Medicines Compendium. emc.medicines.org.uk

NICE guidance CG87 Type 2 diabetes – newer agents (a partial update of CG66) – quick reference guide. www.nice.org.uk/nicemedia/live/12165/44322/44322.pdf

Reusable learning objects

Kidney anatomy. www.nottingham.ac.uk/nursing/sonet/rlos/bioproc/kidneyanatomy/index.html

Physiology of the kidneys. www.nottingham.ac.uk/nursing/sonet/rlos/bioproc/kidneyphysiology/index.html

Further reading

Ashley, C. and Currie, A. (eds) (2009) *The Renal Drug Handbook*, 3rd edn, Radcliffe Publishing, Oxford.

Department of Health Management of Medicines (2004) *A Resource Document for Aspects Specific to the National Service Framework for Renal Services*, Department of Health, London.

Devaney, A. and Thompson, C. (2006) Chronic kidney disease – new approaches to classification. *Hosp Pharm*, **13**, 406–410.

Levey, A.S., Bosch, J.P., Breyer-Lewis, J.B., *et al.* (1999) A more accurate method to estimate the glomerular filtration rate from serum creatinine: a new prediction equation. *Ann Intern Med*, **130**: 461–470.

Pannu, N. and Nadim, M.K. (2008) An overview of drug-induced acute kidney injury. *Crit Care Med*, **36**(4 Suppl), S216–S223.

Taber, S.S. and Pasko, D.A. (2008) The epidemiology of drug-induced disorders: the kidney. *Expert Opin Drug Saf*, **7**, 679–690.

Section 3

26 The gastrointestinal system

Learning outcomes

By the end of this chapter the reader should be able to:

- explain the physiological control of gastric acid secretion
- describe the mechanism of action, pharmacokinetics, unwanted effects and clinical uses of:
  - antacids
  - histamine (H_2) receptor antagonists
  - Proton pump inhibitors
  - misoprostil
  - sucralfate
- understand in broad terms the control of the vomiting reflex
- identify the four main receptor types involved in the vomiting process and their location
- describe the mechanism of action, pharmacokinetics, unwanted effects and clinical uses of:
  - histamine H_1 receptor antagonists
  - muscarinic receptor antagonists
  - $5HT_3$ receptor antagonists
  - D_2 receptor antagonists
- describe the mechanism of action, pharmacokinetics, unwanted effects and clinical uses of laxative agents
- understand the mechanism of action, pharmacokinetics, unwanted effects and clinical uses of antimotility agents.

The New Prescriber. Edited by J Lymn, D Bowskill, F Bath-Hextall, R Knaggs, © 2010 John Wiley & Sons.

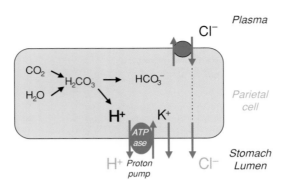

Figure 26.1 Acid secretion by the parietal cell.

Dyspepsia and peptic ulcer disease

Nervous system intervention

The gastrointestinal (GI) tract has its own intrinsic nervous system that is responsible for GI tract movements and secretions. This intrinsic nervous system receives messages from the autonomic nervous system which influences the activity of the GI tract (Chapter 20).

Physiological control of acid secretion

Essentially chloride (Cl^-) ions and potassium (K^+) ions are actively secreted from parietal cells into the lumen. The K^+ is then exchanged for hydrogen ions (H^+) generated within the cell. The H^+ is actively pumped out by the proton pump (a K^+/H^+ ATP-ase pump), leaving us with H^+ and Cl^- ions in the lumen of the stomach to make hydrochloric acid (HCl) (Figure 26.1).

Factors which affect acid secretion (Figure 26.2)

Both acetylcholine, from vagal efferents, and gastrin, secreted from G cells, stimulate acid secretion directly and indirectly via histamine release. Histamine from enterochromaffin-like (ECL) cells acts on histamine H_2 receptors to stimulate acid secretion directly.

Prostaglandins E_2 (PGE_2) and I_2 (PGI_2, also known as prostacyclin) are local hormones which act directly on parietal cells to decrease acid secretion. They also increase bicarbonate and mucus secretion, in addition to causing vasodilation of mucosal blood vessels to increase local blood flow, all of which protects the stomach from the harmful effects of acid.

Pharmacological suppression of acid secretion

Antacids

Antacids do not alter or reduce gastric acid secretion; instead, they act by neutralising gastric acid (raising gastric pH). Antacids provide a rapid onset of symptom relief in milder forms of dyspepsia but can impair the absorption of other drugs by raising gastric pH or by combining with other drugs to form complexes.

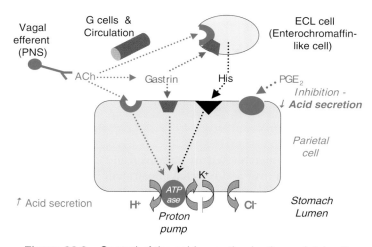

Figure 26.2   Control of the acid secretion by the parietal cell.

Alginates (e.g. gaviscon)

These contain alginic acid which combines with saliva to produce a foam raft. This then floats on the top of the gastric contents to protect the oesophagus.

Histamine H_2 receptor antagonists (e.g. cimetidine, ranitidine, nizatidine)

H_2 receptor antagonists competitively inhibit the action of histamine at the H_2 receptors (Figure 26.3) and decrease both basal (continuous) and food-stimulated acid secretion. H_2 receptor antagonists do not fully inhibit acid secretion, however, as they do not block the direct stimulatory action of acetylcholine and gastrin on the muscarinic and G receptors respectively.

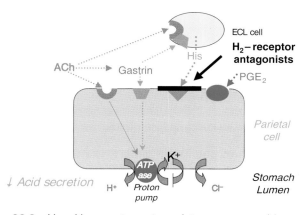

Figure 26.3   How H_2 receptor antagonists suppress acid secretion.

Section 3

Practice application

H$_2$ receptor antagonists are more effective than antacids at controlling signs and symptoms of indigestion and dyspepsia as they actually suppress gastric acid secretion rather than just manage the symptoms.

H$_2$ receptor antagonists are metabolised by the liver and excreted by the kidneys. Dose adjustments may be necessary if liver and/or renal impairment is present. Common side effects of H$_2$ receptor antagonists include diarrhoea, headache, dizziness and rashes. Cimetidine can also cause gynaecomastia (breast enlargement) due to an affinity for androgen receptors, which can be quite painful in men. In women it can cause galactorrhoea (secretion of breast milk) as it inhibits the metabolism and breakdown of the female hormone oestradiol.

While there is little to choose between available H$_2$ receptor antagonists in terms of efficacy and side effects, there are differences in the potential for drug interactions. Cimetidine inhibits the cytochrome P450 (CYP450) system and can therefore interact with other drugs metabolised by this enzyme system. This is an important consideration for drugs with a narrow therapeutic window, including warfarin and theophylline (increasing their effect along with the potential for adverse effects and toxicity).

Stop and think

Why would ranitidine or nizatidine be better options than cimetidine in patients taking amitriptyline?

Proton pump inhibitors (e.g. lansoprazole, omeprazole, pantoprazole and rabeprazole)

Proton pump inhibitors (PPIs) inhibit the proton pump directly and hence the secretion of acid (Figure 26.4). They only inhibit actively acid-secreting proton pumps. However, this inhibition is irreversible and so the parietal cells need to produce new pumps or activate resting pumps before they can secrete more acid. As this takes time, PPIs have a long duration of action. PPIs markedly inhibit both basal and stimulated gastric acid secretion (dose related) and provide the most rapid and effective acid suppression.

Practice application

PPIs are more effective than H$_2$ receptor antagonists both in terms of controlling indigestion and dyspeptic symptoms, but also in healing rates of oesphagitis and peptic ulcer disease. They are cost-effective.

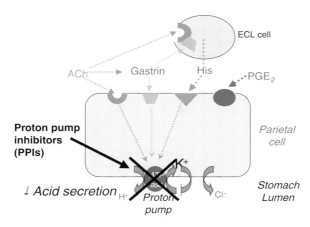

Figure 26.4   How proton pump inhibitors suppress acid secretion.

Although no dose adjustment is required in the elderly or individuals with impaired renal function, doses may need to be reviewed in patients with severely impaired liver function. Generally PPIs are well tolerated. Common side effects experienced are diarrhoea, nausea and abdominal pain. The diarrhoea is thought to be related to the profound acid suppression which can alter the bacterial content of the gut, resulting in diarrhoea. This effect is possibly dose and age related.

All PPIs increase gastric pH which can alter the absorption of drugs that require an acid environment, for example iron salts. Differences between PPIs do exist, however, in the degree to which they are metabolised by the CYP450 enzyme system, and subsequently their potential to affect the metabolism of other drugs. Omeprazole affects the CYP450 enzyme system the most and has a greater potential for drug interactions. Rabeprazole and pantoprazole have fewer drug interactions.

Another important consideration is patient ethnicity. PPIs are metabolised in the liver by an isoenzyme of the cytochrome P450 enzyme system. There are genetic differences in the activity of this enzyme which influence the pharmacokinetics and pharmacodynamics and hence the effectiveness of PPI therapy (Chapter 16). Inter-ethnic differences in enzyme activity should be considered in PPI selection in different population groups.

Prostaglandin analogues (e.g. misoprostil)

These drugs mimic the action of the naturally synthesised prostaglandins, directly inhibiting gastric acid secretion by the parietal cell. They also enhance the secretion of mucus and bicarbonate, and increase mucosal blood flow via vasodilation. Unfortunately, misoprostil is poorly tolerated and its use is limited by its side effects of secretary diarrhoea and abdominal cramps.

Sucralfate

Sucralfate is a complex substance containing aluminium which in the acid environment of the stomach forms a gel with mucus. This reduces the degradation of mucus by the enzyme pepsin, and so limits the ability of acid to damage the lining of the stomach. In addition, sucralfate also has a physical protective action as it stimulates mucus and bicarbonate secretion and prostaglandin production.

Section 3

Table 26.1   Drugs associated with adverse gastrointestinal effects.

Mode of adverse GI effect	Examples
Pharmacological mode of action – reduce lower oesophageal sphincter tone and increase acid exposure	Alcohol, antimuscarinics (e.g. antidepressants), calcium channel blockers, progesterone (surge in first trimester of pregnancy)
Impair GI defences	Aspirin and NSAIDs inhibit prostaglandin synthesis – increase acid secretion and reduce cytoprotection
Direct injury to the GI tract	Oesophageal damage by bisphosphonates, local irritation with alcohol, aspirin, iron salts

Sucralfate requires an acid environment to work and so concurrent administration of antacids should be avoided. More importantly, it reduces the absorption of some drugs (due to adsorption where sucralfate binds to other drugs, preventing their absorption), including digoxin and theophylline and certain antibiotics. These drugs need to be administered either 1 hour before or 4 hours after sucralfate to avoid reduced absorption.

Prokinetics (e.g. metoclopramide, domperidone)

In certain patients prokinetic agents may be of benefit, especially as an adjunct to acid suppression as they enhance co-ordinated contraction, increase gastric emptying, relieve gastric stasis, reduce reflux and regurgitation and emesis. Metoclopramide and domperidone are dopamine receptor antagonists. Aside from their antiemetic action (discussed later), they have a peripheral action in the GI tract and act as prokinetics. Dopamine, a natural neurotransmitter in the body, acts on dopamine receptors in the GI tract to inhibit the release of acetylcholine, reducing GI motility. Dopamine antagonists such as metoclopramide block this inhibitory effect and therefore increase motility.

Other considerations

It is important to remember that almost any drug can affect the GI tract and result in drug-induced GI disorders (Table 26.1). It is therefore important to review a patient's current medication for potential causes (as well as diet and lifestyle causes), as part of a management strategy. Where possible, these agents should be reviewed and if appropriate/safe to do so, discontinued.

Nausea and vomiting

Nausea and vomiting is a protective response to poisonous substances but can also be caused by other stimuli, particularly medical interventions. In the healthy population, however, the most common cause of nausea and vomiting is alcohol!

How is the vomiting reflex controlled?

Nausea is an unpleasant sensation that precedes vomiting. Typical signs and symptoms include pallor, tachycardia and salivation. Retroperistalsis often accompanies nausea with reflux of

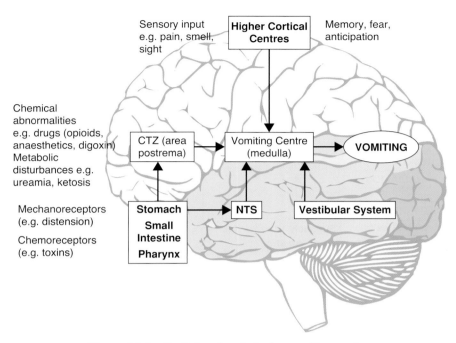

Figure 26.5   Excitatory inputs to the vomiting centre.

intestinal contents. Retching follows, and may or may not progress to vomiting. Vomiting is not under voluntary control but is a reflex action.

The vomiting centre (VC) controls the vomiting process in the brain. It receives excitatory messages from numerous sources including the chemoreceptor trigger zone (CTZ). The CTZ is found outside the blood–brain barrier (BBB) and so can be stimulated by chemicals in both the blood and the cerebrospinal fluid (Figure 26.5). Hence there are a number of different causes of nausea and vomiting (Figure 26.6). Once the cause of nausea and vomiting is known, the receptor types involved can be determined and this influences the class of drug we select. Other additional factors that influence drug choice include side-effect profile, concurrent disease states and relative cost.

There are four main neurotransmitters involved in the vomiting process: histamine (His), acetylcholine (ACh), serotonin (5HT) and dopamine (DA). These agonists act on H_1, muscarinic, $5HT_3$ and D_2 receptors respectively (Figure 26.7). Drugs used in the management of nausea and vomiting act by targeting one or more of these receptors.

Mechanism of action of antiemetics

Histamine H_1 receptor antagonists/antihistamines (e.g. cinnarizine, cyclizine, promethazine)

The H_1 receptors are located in the vestibular system and in the VC itself (Figure 26.7). The management of nausea and vomiting involves using an antihistamine with antagonist activity at H_1 receptors and with central activity. Remember, H_2 receptors are involved in gastric acid secretion and H_2 receptor antagonists are not effective in the management of nausea and vomiting.

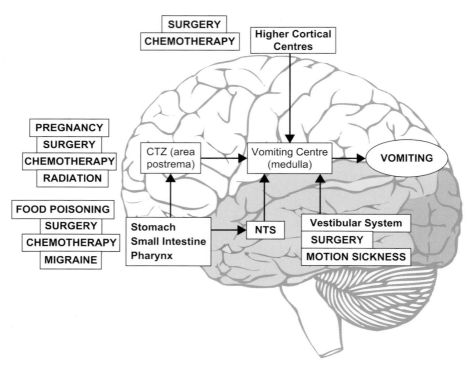

Figure 26.6 Common causes of nausea and how they influence the vomiting process.

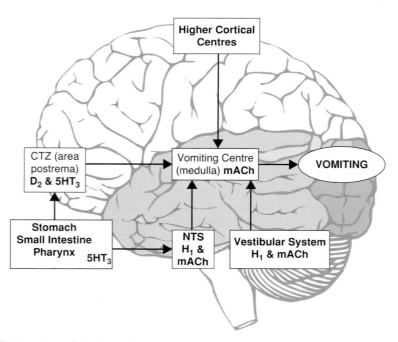

Figure 26.7 The four main receptor types involved in the vomiting process.

As well as acting on H_1 receptors, antihistamines also have a degree of antimuscarinic activity, which impacts on their side-effect profile. The combined sites of action on both H_1 and muscarinic receptors mean that antihistamines are particularly effective against vestibular causes (e.g. motion sickness, postoperative nausea and vomiting (PONV) or increased vestibular sensitivity following opioid administration). Antihistamines are effective against most causes of nausea and vomiting due to their effect on the VC (as well as the nucleus tractus solitarius, NTS) via their action on the muscarinic receptors located here.

Stop and think

Why do you think the side effects of H_1 antagonists include dry mouth, urinary retention, blurred vision, dizziness, drowsiness and sedation?

Muscarinic receptor antagonists (e.g. hyoscine)

The main antimuscarinic drug used is hyoscine. It is a non-selective, competitive muscarinic antagonist but also antagonises H_1 receptors in the VC and vestibular system. It is more effective than antihistamines in the management of motion sickness and is less sedating but causes similar adverse effects and is generally less well tolerated. For this reason, this class of drug should also be used with caution in the elderly.

$5HT_3$ receptor antagonists (e.g. ondansetron, granisetron)

The $5HT_3$ receptor antagonists block the receptors in the GI tract (~80% of $5HT_3$ receptors can be found in the GI tract), the CTZ and the NTS. They are therefore highly effective against nausea and vomiting due to drugs/toxins such as chemotherapy and PONV. Any side effects experienced by the $5HT_3$ receptor antagonists are mild and tend to be limited to headaches, dizziness and GI upset (diarrhoea and constipation). Their main limitation for use is their cost as they are expensive in comparison to other agents.

D_2 receptor antagonists (e.g. metoclopamide, domperidone, prochlorperazine, levomepromazine and haloperidol)

There are many different types of agents that act as non-selective dopamine receptor antagonists. While they have slightly different profiles, they all have a central dopamine antagonist action, along with a peripheral action in the GI tract. Dopamine receptors are the most abundant receptor type in the CTZ and so these are effective agents to use in the management of nausea and vomiting due to chemical and metabolic disturbances (e.g. uraemia, ketosis) and drugs (e.g. opioids). As metoclopramide also has weak $5HT_3$ receptor antagonist activity at higher doses, it can also be used in chemotherapy-induced nausea and vomiting.

The prokinetic effect of metoclopramide and domperidone means that they are particularly effective in the management of migraine, when gastric stasis is thought to be a cause of nausea

Section 3

and vomiting. In contrast, this prokinetic effect also means that they are best avoided after bowel surgery.

Metoclopramide can cross the BBB and hence the side-effect profile is due to its effect on dopamine receptors elsewhere in the central nervous system. In particular, it can cause extrapyramidal side effects including movement disorders and parkinsonian-like features. Metoclopramide can also stimulate prolactin release and cause galactorrhoea and menstrual disorders with prolonged use, due to non-specific dopamine receptor antagonism.

Stop and think

Why would domperidone be a more appropriate antiemetic than metoclopramide for a patient with Parkinson's disease?

Some antipsychotic agents (prochlorperazine, levomepromazine, haloperidol) can also be used in the management of nausea and vomiting due to their antagonism of dopamine receptors. These agents also have weak antagonistic activity against H_1 and muscarinic receptors, in addition to dopamine and $5HT_3$ receptor antagonism. Hence they are also effective in treating nausea and vomiting caused by stimulation of the vestibular system and the VC.

Practice application

- Antihistamines/antimuscarinics are good for vestibular disturbances and PONV.
- D_2 receptor antagonists are good for drug-induced nausea and vomiting and PONV.
- $5HT_3$ receptor antagonists are good for chemotherapy and PONV.

What about combinations of antiemetics?

A combination of antiemetics may often be required and so it is important to think about which agents are acting where so that you can prescribe a logical combination of drugs that act on different receptor types. Remember that antiemetics often have more than one mode of action. Figure 26.8 summarises the main sites of action of the different antiemetics discussed.

Constipation

The prevalence of constipation increases with age, is more common in women and is a common complaint during pregnancy. Constipation can seriously affect a person's quality of life, causing abdominal pain and distension, nausea, anorexia, malaise, overflow diarrhoea in faecal impaction, halitosis and confusion. Predisposing factors include poor dietary fibre intake,

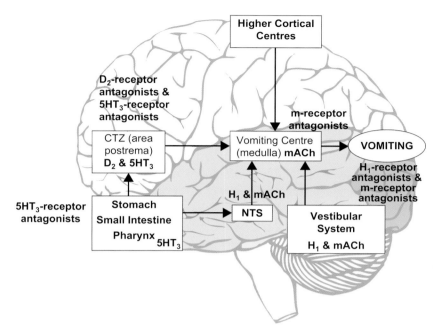

Figure 26.8   Sites of action of the four main classes of antiemetic agents.

poor fluid intake, reduced mobility, underlying conditions (e.g. depression, hypothyroidism, Parkinson's and hypercalcaemia) and drugs.

The most common drug-related causes are opioids and drugs with antimuscarinic side effects (e.g. tricyclic antidepressants). Opiates act on opioid receptors to inhibit the release of acetylcholine presynaptically while antimuscarinics antagonise the muscarinic receptors postsynaptically. Both therefore inhibit parasympathetic activity, reducing tone and peristaltic movements in the GI tract, resulting in constipation.

Laxatives

The main aim of treatment is to avoid complications of constipation and improve quality of life. Good-quality evidence of effectiveness of laxatives is limited, with little clinical evidence regarding whether one class of laxatives is superior to another. Choice is therefore based on patient preference, cause and type of constipation, time to take effect, concurrent disease states, fluid status/intake, adverse effects and cost.

Bulk-forming laxatives (e.g. methylcellulose, bran, ispaghula husk)

These agents consist of indigestible polysaccharides which are not broken down by normal gut processes. They therefore retain fluid within the stool and gut lumen, increasing the faecal mass. This stimulates the stretch receptors in the lower GI tract and promotes peristalsis. Unfortunately, these agents take several days to work and so are not suitable for acute management but are a good option for long-term control.

Section 3

It is essential to ensure that individuals maintain an adequate intake of fluid to avoid intestinal obstruction. Avoid using bulk-forming laxatives in people with intestinal obstruction, faecal impaction or severe dehydration.

There are no serious side effects but bulk-forming laxatives can cause flatulence, abdominal distension and bloating, although these tend to settle with continued use.

Osmotic laxatives (e.g. lactulose, macrogols)

This class of agents consist of poorly dissolved solutes, with lactulose being the most common. These agents are not absorbed and remain in the GI tract where they draw fluid from the body into the bowel by osmosis, increasing the volume of stool. This accelerates the movement of the material through the small intestine and when the increased amount reaches the colon, distension results in purgation.

Lactulose takes several days to exert its effect and so, like bulk laxatives, is not appropriate for acute management of constipation. It also needs to be taken regularly for it to work fully, with a good fluid intake. High doses can cause flatulence, bloating and cramps. In large doses it can cause diarrhoea and electrolyte disturbances.

Faecal softeners (e.g. docusate sodium, glycerol, arachis oil)

Docusate sodium has a surfactant action which reduces surface tension, allowing water and intestinal fluids to penetrate into the faecal mass, promoting softening. Docusate sodium also has stimulant properties at higher doses. These agents are generally well tolerated but at higher doses, docusate sodium can cause similar side effects to stimulant laxatives.

Stimulant laxatives (e.g. senna, bisacodyl, sodium picosulphate)

Stimulant laxatives directly stimulate the colonic nerves to induce peristalsis. They also affect fluid balance, increasing the water and electrolyte content in the stool, promoting an increase in faecal motility. Stimulant laxatives produce a laxative effect within 8–12 hours and so will usually have an effect the next morning when taken orally prior to going to bed at night.

Prolonged high doses should be used with caution as tjey can lead to diarrhoea and significant fluid and electrolyte imbalance. Prolonged use can also result in colonic atony and tolerance, resulting in the need for further laxative use and potential laxative dependency.

 Stop and think

Which class of laxative would be most appropriate for the acute management of constipation?

Diarrhoea

There are many causes of diarrhoea (infection, secondary to antibiotics, adverse drug effects) and the first step in the management of diarrhoea is to review potential causes. Examples of drugs that can cause diarrhoea include magnesium-containing antacids, PPIs, misoprostil, metoclopramide, iron salts, digoxin toxicity, antibiotics and of course laxatives!

Often diarrhoea is transient and self-limiting. If the diarrhoea is drug related, then manage this as appropriate (e.g. reduce dose, switch to an alternative agent, discontinue). If an infective cause is suspected, remember antibiotics will be of no value for viral infections. It is best to let an infection run its course in these situations to allow the infective agent to leave the body naturally.

Where treatment with antimotility agents is considered necessary, then codeine (a weak opioid) and loperamide (a synthetic opioid) can be prescribed. Opiates reduce motility of the GI tract, allowing reabsorption of fluid and reducing the passage of watery stool. As loperamide does not cross the BBB, it does not cause the central side effects such as sedation and confusion associated with codeine use and so may be preferable in the management of diarrhoea.

Summary

- Parietal cells pump hydrogen ions into the stomach lumen via a K^+/H^+ ATPase or proton pump.
- Gastic acid secretion is increased by the action of histamine (on H_2 receptors), acetylcholine (on muscarinic receptors) and gastrin (on G-receptors).
- Gastric acid secretion is reduced by the action of prostaglandins.
- Antacids do not alter gastric acid secretion but neutralise gastric acid.
- H_2 receptor antagonists do not completely inhibit gastric acid secretion.
- The H_2 receptor antagonist cimetidine inhibits cytochrome P450 activity.
- PPIs have an irreversible effect on the proton pump and hence have a long duration of action.
- Knowledge of the possible causes of nausea and vomiting along with the receptor types involved will help influence the class of drug selected for individual patients.
- The four main neurotransmitters involved in stimulating nausea and vomiting are histamine (on H_1 receptors), acetylcholine (on muscarinic receptors), 5HT (on $5HT_3$ receptors) and dopamine (on D_2 receptors).
- The D_2 receptor antagonist metoclopramide can cross the BBB and cause extrapyramidal side effects.
- Constipation can be the result of lifestyle and/or pharmacological factors.
- There are four main classes of laxatives available for use. Choice is based on patient preference, cause and type of constipation, time to take effect, concurrent disease states, fluid status/intake, adverse effects and cost.
- Diarrhoea is generally transient and self-limiting and as such may not require pharmacological intervention.

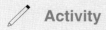 **Activity**

1. Select the agent that will provide the most rapid and effective gastric acid suppression in the management of peptic ulcer disease.
   A. Gaviscon
   B. Metoclopramide

C. Omeprazole

D. Ranitidine

2. A 65-year-old man has a history of atrial fibrillation (AF) and is on long-term anticoagulation with warfarin. Choose the H_2 receptor antagonist which can interact with and enhance the anticoagulant effect of warfarin when prescribed concurrently.

A. Cimetidine

B. Famotidine

C. Nizatidine

D. Ranitidine

3. A 60-year-old man has an extensive past medical history and is managed with an extensive list of medications. Which PPI has the greater potential for drug interactions due to its effect on the cytochrome P450 enzyme system and the metabolism of certain drugs such as warfarin?

A. Lansoprazole

B. Omeprazole

C. Pantoprazole

D. Rabeprazole

4. A 35-year-old female migraine sufferer experiences nausea and vomiting at the onset of an attack. Which of the following will be the most effective drug to manage her nausea and vomiting?

A. Cyclizine

B. Lorazepam

C. Metoclopramide

D. Ondansetron

5. A 55-year-old woman presents with nausea and vomiting due to labyrinthitis. Which of the following will be the most effective drug to prescribe in the management of her nausea and vomiting?

A. Cyclizine

B. Lorazepam

C. Metoclopramide

D. Ondansetron

6. A 70-year-old patient presents complaining of constipation. Which of the following medications is the most likely to cause constipation as a side effect?

A. Bendroflumethiazide

B. Codeine phosphate

C. Ibuprofen

D. Omeprazole

7. Which of the following laxatives used in the management of constipation has the quickest onset of action?

A. Fybogel

B. Lactulose

C. Movicol

D. Senna

Useful website

NICE guidance on dyspepsia – quick reference guide. www.nice.org.uk/Guidance/CG17/QuickRefGuide/pdf/English.

Further reading

Fock, K.M., Ang, T.L., Bee, L.C. and Lee, E.J. (2008) Proton pump inhibitors: do differences in pharmacokinetics translate into differences in clinical outcomes? *Clin Pharmacokinet*, **47**, 1-6.

Ford, A.C., Delaney, B., Forman, D. and Moayyedi, P. (2006) Eradication therapy for peptic ulcer disease in Helicobacter pylori positive patients. *Cochrane Database Syst Rev*, 2, CD003840).

Gan, T.J. (2007) Mechanisms underlying postoperative nausea and vomiting and neurotransmitter receptor antagonist-based pharmacotherapy. *CNS Drugs*, **21**, 813-833.

Humphries, T.J. and Merritt, G.J. (1999) Review article: drug interactions with agents used to treat acid-related diseases. *Aliment Pharmacol Ther*, **13** (Suppl 3), 18-26.

Jordan, K., Sippel, C. and Schmoll, H.J. (2007) Guidelines for antiemetic treatment of chemotherapy-induced nausea and vomiting: past, present, and future recommendations. *Oncologist*, **12**, 1143-1150.

Schubert, M.L. and Peura, D.A. (2008) Control of gastric acid secretion in health and disease. *Gastroenterology*, **134**, 1842-1860.

Shi, S. and Klotz, U. (2008) Proton pump inhibitors: an update of their clinical use and pharmacokinetics. *Eur J Clin Pharmacol*, **64**, 935-951.

Vanderhoff, B.T. and Tahboub, R.M. (2002) Proton pump inhibitors: an update. *Am Fam Physician*, **66**, 273-280.

Wald, A. (2007) Appropriate use of laxatives in the management of constipation. *Curr Gastroenterol Rep*, **9**, 410-414.

Wallace, J.L. (2008) Prostaglandins, NSAIDs, and gastric mucosal protection: why doesn't the stomach digest itself? *Physiol Rev*, **88**, 1547-1565.

Section 3

27 The endocrine system

Learning outcomes

By the end of this chapter the reader should be able to:

- identify the location of the main glands and hormones of the endocrine system
- describe how glucose homeostasis is maintained by the hormones insulin and glucagon
- describe the differences between type 1 and type 2 diabetes
- describe, using named examples, the mechanism of action of drugs used to treat diabetes
- describe the regulation of thyroxine (T_4) and tri-iodothyronine (T_3) release by the hypothalamic-pituitary-thyroid axis
- describe the physiological functions of T_3 and T_4 and relate these to the symptoms of hypo- and hyperthyroidism
- describe, using named examples, the mechanism of action of drugs used to treat hypo- and hyperthyroidism.

The endocrine system

The endocrine system is composed of a diverse range of organs, tissues and cells which regulate most of our body systems (Figure 27.1). The signalling molecules released from endocrine organs are hormones and they act upon target cells which contain receptors specific for that hormone. Hormones may be classified as either circulating or local. A circulating hormone travels via the circulation to reach distant target cells (Figure 27.2); insulin and follicle-stimulating hormone are examples of circulating hormones. Local hormones can either paracrine or autocrine. Paracrine hormones act upon neighbouring cells, therefore negating the need to enter the bloodstream; the term *para* means 'beside'. Autocrine hormones, as the name suggests, act upon the same endocrine cell from which they were released (Figure 27.2).

The New Prescriber. Edited by J Lymn, D Bowskill, F Bath-Hextall, R Knaggs, © 2010 John Wiley & Sons.

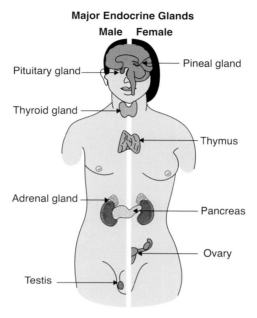

Major Endocrine Glands

Male   Female

Pituitary gland

Thyroid gland

Adrenal gland

Testis

Pineal gland

Thymus

Pancreas

Ovary

Figure 27.1   Location of the major glands and endocrine hormones (www.commons.wikimedia.org/wiki/Image:Illu_endocrine_system.jpg).

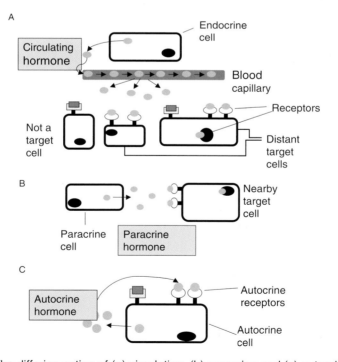

A

Circulating hormone

Endocrine cell

Blood capillary

Not a target cell

Receptors

Distant target cells

B

Paracrine cell

Paracrine hormone

Nearby target cell

C

Autocrine hormone

Autocrine receptors

Autocrine cell

Figure 27.2   The differing action of (a) circulating, (b) paracrine and (c) autocrine hormones.

Section 3

Stop and think

Classify the following list of hormones as autocrine, paracrine or endocrine: adrenaline, oestrogen, gastrin, insulin, growth hormone.

Mechanisms of hormone action

Hormones act upon specific receptors on target cells, which can be classified by their location within the target cell as either membrane bound or intracellular.

Membrane-bound receptors (e.g. insulin receptor) are located within the plasma membrane of the target cell; this provides easy access for hormones within the interstitial fluid. Generally, these receptors initiate a cellular effect by utilising components which already exist within the cell, eliciting a fast response.

Intracellular receptors may be located within the cytoplasm (the glucocorticoid receptor) or nucleus (thyroid hormone receptor) of the target cell; hormones must cross the plasma membrane and enter the target cell in order to interact with intracellular receptors. Activated intracellular receptors then initiate the production or inhibition of cellular proteins. This effect takes several hours as new cellular components have to be produced or existing components degraded before cellular changes become apparent.

Glucose homeostasis and diabetes mellitus

The endocrine pancreas

Plasma glucose concentrations are tightly regulated by the hormones insulin and glucagon. The organ responsible for the maintenance of normal plasma glucose is the pancreas. The pancreas consists of both non-endocrine cells, which are responsible for the production of digestive juices (the exocrine pancreas), and endocrine cells (the endocrine pancreas); the endocrine pancreas accounts for only 1–1.5% of the mass of the whole pancreas. Within the endocrine pancreas are 0.7–1 million clusters of cells named pancreatic islets or islets of Langerhans. There are three main cell types located within the endocrine pancreas (Table 27.1); these cells manufacture and secrete the hormones insulin, glucagon and somatostatin.

The most potent stimulator of insulin secretion is glucose; after ingestion of a meal, glucose stimulates insulin secretion from beta-cells. Insulin circulates in the blood and acts upon insulin

Table 27.1 The function of each of the three cell types located in the endocrine pancreas.

Cell type	Hormone	Function
Alpha-cells	Glucagon	Raises blood glucose concentrations.
Beta-cells	Insulin	Lowers blood glucose concentrations.
Delta-cells	Somatostatin	Acts as a paracrine hormone to inhibit both insulin and glucagon.

Section 3

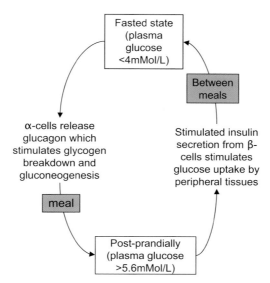

Figure 27.3   Regulation of blood glucose by the endocrine pancreas.

receptors in target tissues in order to promote glucose uptake and reduce plasma glucose levels. The release of insulin from beta-cells, just like the release of neurotransmitters from nerve cells, occurs through the process of calcium-mediated exocytosis. Glucose has an inhibitory effect on glucagon secretion, therefore between meals, when plasma glucose concentrations are low, this inhibitory effect of glucose is removed. Glucagon is released from alpha-cells and promotes the breakdown of stored glycogen and stimulates gluconeogenesis. This increases the available energy for tissues (Figure 27.3). The effects of insulin in the body can be described as endocrine, paracrine and cellular effects and these are described below.

Endocrine (peripheral) effects of insulin

Insulin promotes the storage of nutrients in most of the organs and tissues of the body. However, there are three organs and tissues which are particularly specialised for the purpose of energy storage: skeletal muscle, adipose tissue and the liver.

The first organ reached by insulin via the bloodstream is the liver. Insulin acts upon the liver in two ways: by promoting glycogen synthesis and storage and inhibiting both the production of new glucose (gluconeogenesis) and the breakdown of glycogen stores into glucose (glycogenolysis). In skeletal muscle, insulin promotes protein and glycogen synthesis and increases glucose transport into muscle cells. Adipose tissue responds to insulin signalling by promoting triglyceride storage, inhibiting lipolysis or breakdown of stored triglycerides and increasing glucose transport into adipocytes.

Paracrine effects of insulin

As well as regulating metabolism in distant organs, insulin has a paracrine role in the pancreas. Insulin has an inhibitory effect on the alpha-cells within the pancreatic islets, which reduces glucagon secretion.

Section 3

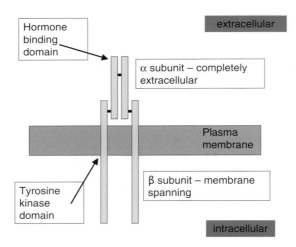

Figure 27.4 The structure of the insulin receptor.

Cellular actions of insulin

The biological effects of insulin are mediated through the insulin receptor (Figure 27.4) which is located within the plasma membrane of the cell. The insulin receptor consists of four subunits – two alpha- and two beta-subunits. The alpha-subunits are completely extracellular, whereas the beta-subunits are membrane spanning. The alpha-subunits contain the binding site for the insulin hormone while the beta-subunits initiate many of the intracellular changes regulated by insulin.

Insulin binding causes the receptor to be activated and initiates the biological changes which lead to the reduction of plasma glucose levels. One group of cellular proteins stimulated by the activated insulin receptor are the insulin receptor substrates (IRS), which initiate a cascade of cellular events which culminate in the reduction of plasma glucose (Figure 27.5). The IRS-stimulated pathway is known to mediate many metabolic changes within the cell, including glycogenesis and decreased gluconeogenesis.

Insulin binding also stimulates the recruitment of glucose transporter 4 (GLUT4) to the cell membrane. When insulin is not bound to its receptor, GLUT4 remains in intracellular vesicles; upon insulin receptor activation, these vesicles relocate to the membrane and fuse with it, allowing glucose to flow into the cell (Figure 27.5). Not all tissue types require GLUT4 to take up glucose; the brain and liver utilise insulin-independent transporters.

A number of other cellular pathways exist to facilitate insulin-stimulated protein synthesis, glycogenesis, antilipolysis and decreased glycolysis and gluconeogenesis. All these systems act together to reduce plasma glucose concentrations.

Diabetes mellitus

Diabetes mellitus is a disorder characterised by hyperglycaemia (elevated blood glucose). There are two distinct types of diabetes: insulin dependent (type 1) and non-insulin dependent (type 2).

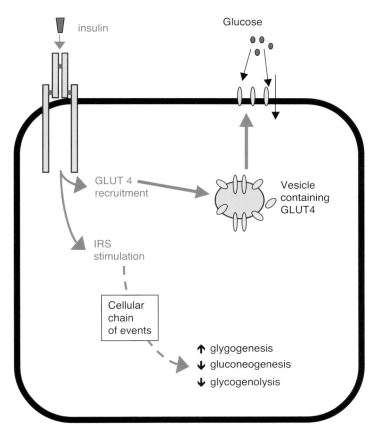

Figure 27.5 Mechanism of insulin action at a cellular level.

Insulin-dependent diabetes mellitus (IDDM or type 1) is often referred to as juvenile onset because a diagnosis is often made during childhood. One study in the UK gave the average age of diagnosis of type 1 diabetes as 20.6 in 2005 (Sharp, Brown and Qureshi, 2008). An autoimmune reaction destroys pancreatic beta-cells so no insulin is produced. This type of diabetes must be treated with insulin replacement therapy.

Insulin-independent diabetes (non-insulin dependent diabetes mellitus (NIDDM or type 2), on the other hand, may be described as age-onset diabetes, although this terminology may now be outdated, as more and more young people are being diagnosed. Indeed, the age of diagnosis of type 2 diabetes decreased between 1992 and 2005 from 57.1 to 54 (Sharp, Harvey and Williams, 2008). Data from the USA show that 2.5 million people below the age of 44 were suffering from type 2 diabetes in 2005 and these figures are set to increase over the coming years (Sharp, Harvey and Williams, 2008). Individuals with NIDDM often produce insulin, sometimes at lower concentrations than normal, but their cells do not respond to insulin signalling. This means that insulin is not always required to treat NIDDM.

The word *diabetes* actually means 'a siphoning of water through the body' which refers to the frequent need to urinate experienced by diabetics. This polyuria is caused by osmotic diuresis. Under normal conditions, very little glucose reaches the proximal tubules of the kidney

Section 3

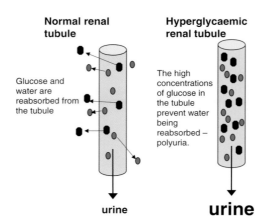

Figure 27.6   Demonstration of glycosuria.

as it is taken up for storage in tissues. Any glucose which does reach the proximal tubule is normally reabsorbed into the bloodstream. If blood glucose level exceeds the capacity of the tubules to reabsorb all the glucose present in the glomerular filtrate, the renal threshold is reached and glucose spills into the urine (glycosuria) (Figure 27.6). Osmotic diuresis occurs as the osmotic pressure of the glucose 'holds' water molecules in the tubule; this large volume of urine leads to polyuria.

Ketoacidosis results when cells of the body become deficient in glucose, which happens as insulin is not stimulating the uptake of glucose into cells. As a result, the cells start to utilise other energy sources, including metabolising fatty acids. A byproduct of fatty acid metabolism is ketones, which are harmful to the body and the kidney will attempt to remove them via the urine. The build-up of ketones in the blood is called ketoacidosis.

Treatment of diabetes

Insulin

Insulin replacement therapy is always used to treat insulin-dependent (type 1) and some cases of non-insulin dependent (type 2) diabetes. Many of the insulins used today are human analogues, made by recombinant DNA technology, rather than being extracted and purified from the pancreas of animals.

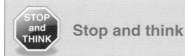 **Stop and think**

As insulin is a protein, it is destroyed by the juices of the GI tract. This limits the possible routes of administration of insulin. Which of the following routes of administration would be suitable: oral, intravenous, subcutaneous injection?

Table 27.2 Different formulations of insulin available.

Insulin type	Pharmacokinetics
Rapid-acting insulins (insulin lispro)	Designed to work in the same way as the insulin normally produced to cope with a meal. Onset of action of approximately 15 minutes. Duration of action of between 2 and 5 hours.
Short-acting insulin or soluble insulin	Rapid onset of action, 30–60 minutes. Duration of up to 8 hours.
Intermediate-acting insulins (isophane insulin, insulin zinc suspension)	Intermediate action. Onset of action of approximately 1–2 hours. Duration of action of 16–35 hours.
Long-acting insulins (insulin glargine)	Normally used once a day. They achieve a steady-state level after 2–4 days.

Many different formulations of insulin exist, but they can be broadly classified as being rapid, short, intermediate or long acting (Table 27.2). A regimen using these preparations will be devised to match an individual's requirements. NICE has some excellent guidelines which should be used when making clinical decisions.

Regular human insulin is crystalline zinc insulin dissolved in a clear solution at pH 3.5. However, insulin is more physiologically active at a neutral pH so is mixed with a buffer to achieve this. Regular insulin produces a rapid and short-lived effect. The chemical and pharmacokinetic properties of regular insulin can be altered by attaching other molecules onto it or changing the amino acid sequence. This can alter the onset and/or duration of action; for example, three amino acids have been altered in the insulin molecule to produce the long-acting insulin glargine. Insulin glargine is soluble at pH 4 and becomes neutral when injected subcutaneously; this forms a precipitate which slowly releases insulin glargine into the plasma.

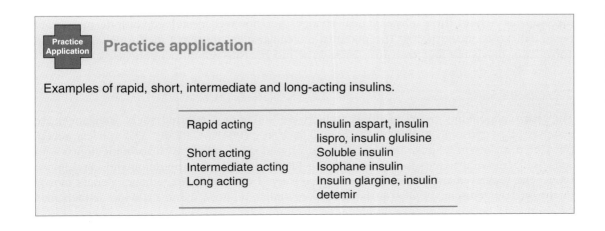

Practice application

Examples of rapid, short, intermediate and long-acting insulins.

Rapid acting	Insulin aspart, insulin lispro, insulin glulisine
Short acting	Soluble insulin
Intermediate acting	Isophane insulin
Long acting	Insulin glargine, insulin detemir

Section 3

Table 27.3   The main groups of antidiabetic drugs.

Group	Drug examples	Physiological mechanism
Sulphonylureas	Glicazide Glibenclamide Tolbutamide	Increase insulin secretion from the beta-cells of the pancreas.
Biguanides	Metformin	Reduce glucose production in the liver and increase peripheral glucose uptake.
Thiazolidinediones	Pioglitazone Rosiglitazone	Sensitise peripheral tissues to insulin. Stimulate glucose and fatty acids uptake into adipocytes. Stimulate transcription of genes involved in insulin signalling.

Oral antidiabetic agents

Oral antidiabetic agents are used to treat type 2 diabetes, sometimes in combination with insulin. There are three main groups of antidiabetic drugs: sulphonylureas, biguanides and thiazolidinediones (Table 27.3).

Sulphonylureas

Sulphonylureas are the only group of oral antidiabetic agents which increase insulin secretion from the pancreas; in this respect, some beta-cell functionality is required. As described previously, calcium ions are required to stimulate insulin release from beta-cells. Under resting conditions, K^+ ions exit beta-cells via a specific channel, maintaining cellular polarisation. The sulphonylurea drugs bind to a receptor on this K^+ channel, causing it to close and allowing the beta-cell to become depolarised. This depolarisation allows the entry of Ca^{2+} into the beta-cell; the Ca^{2+} ions stimulate the release of insulin by exocytosis (Figure 27.7).

Biguanides

Metformin is the only biguanide drug available in the UK; it does not increase insulin secretion but decreases hepatic gluconeogenesis and increases peripheral glucose uptake. The molecular mechanisms behind these physiological changes are not well described, despite metformin being developed in the 1950s. The potential molecular mechanisms of metformin are listed in Table 27.4; this is not an exhaustive list and the mechanisms are not all conclusive.

Thiazolidinediones

The thiazolidinedione group of drugs (which are sometimes referred to as glitazones) are agonists of peroxisome proliferator activated receptor (PPAR)γ. PPARγ is a nuclear receptor, found mainly in adipose tissue. The main physiological action of thiazolidinediones is to sensitise peripheral tissues to insulin. Despite PPARγ being found predominantly in adipose tissue, the improvement in insulin sensitivity observed with thiazolidinediones occurs mostly in the skeletal muscle. PPARγ is thought to modulate adipose tissue cytokines which may communicate between adipose tissue and skeletal muscle.

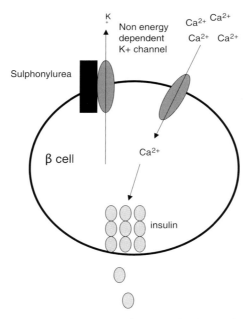

Figure 27.7   Mechanism of action of sulphonylureas.

As well as improving insulin sensitivity, the thiazolidinediones also promote redistribution of lipid within the body. Extra-adipocyte lipid storage, for example in the liver and skeletal muscle, is thought to play a role in insulin resistance; by redistributing these stores of lipid to adipose tissue, insulin sensitivity can be improved.

Other oral antidiabetic drugs exist, such as acarbose and repaglinide, but sulphonylureas, biguanides and thiazolidinediones are by far the most commonly prescribed.

Table 27.4   Potential molecular mechanisms of metformin action.

Mechanism	Outcome
Enhanced muscle uptake of insulin	Improved signalling of insulin.
Restoration of enzyme activity in the insulin-signalling cascade (Figure 27.7)	Increased stimulation of insulin-dependent cellular events, for example increased GLUT4 translocation to the membrane.
Inhibition of enzymes in the gluconeogenic pathway in the liver	Reduction of gluconeogenesis.
Reduction of the uptake of gluconeogenic substrates in the liver	Reduction of gluconeogenesis.
Reduction of hepatic mitochondrial respiration	Reduced energy supply to the liver resulting in reduced gluconeogenic ability.
Stimulation of adenosine monophosphate-activated protein kinase	Inhibition of hepatic glucose production and increased glucose uptake in skeletal muscle.

Section 3

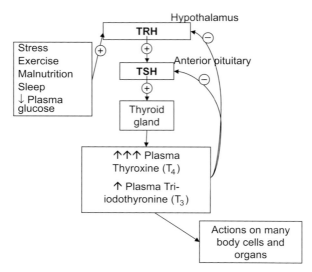

Figure 27.8 Feedback regulation of thyroid hormones.

The thyroid gland

Thyroid function

The thyroid gland is located in the neck in front of the larynx and trachea. The primary hormone secreted from the thyroid gland is thyroxine (T_4); tri-iodothyronine (T_3) is secreted in smaller concentrations. In the periphery, T_4 is transformed into T_3 by the enzyme 5′deiodinase. As the name 'tri-*iodo*thyronine' suggests, iodine is an essential component in these hormones.

Release of the thyroid hormones from the thyroid gland is regulated via the hypothalamic-pituitary-thyroid axis. A number of stimuli, such as decreased plasma glucose or exercise, promote the hypothalamus to release thyrotrophin-releasing hormone (TRH). Once released, TRH acts on the anterior pituitary gland to stimulate the secretion of thyroid-stimulating hormone (TSH or thyrotrophin). TSH stimulates the release of T_4 and T_3 from the thyroid gland (Figure 27.8) as well as iodine metabolism and cell growth. Once secreted, T_3 and T_4 circulate widely in the body, affecting many different organ systems. Thyroid hormones travel bound to a thyroid-binding globulin which facilitates their transport. In order to maintain thyroid function homeostasis, T_3 can negatively feedback to the hypothalamus and pituitary to 'switch off' TRH and TSH secretion, respectively.

Practice application

Laboratory blood results contain information on 'free' and 'total' thyroid hormones. The free T_4 (FT_4) is the T_4 in the blood which is not bound to thyroid-binding globulins and is therefore freely available to bind to thyroid receptors. Total T_4, as the name suggests, is the total concentration of T_4 in the blood and includes free and bound T_4.

Table 27.5 Summary of thyroid effects within the body.

Metabolism	Growth	Development
↑ Basal metabolic rate	Necessary for growth in children	Essential for the growth and development of the foetal an neonatal brain
↑ Body heat production ↑ Fat mobilisation ↑ Insulin-dependent entry of glucose into cells ↑ Gluconeogenesis and glycogenolysis ↑ Sympathetic activation in the heart, skeletal and adipose tissue		

Thyroid hormones exert the majority of their biological effects via a nuclear receptor. Once T_4 reaches its target cell, it is converted into the more active T_3 which then interacts with the thyroid receptor. As described previously, biological effects exerted via nuclear receptors take some time to occur, up to days; this is due to the transcriptional changes that must take place in the cell.

Thyroid hormones regulate a number of biological processes (Table 27.5), which can be grouped into metabolic effects and regulation of growth and development. Thyroid hormones have a key role in regulating growth and development in the foetus and neonate. The foetus begins to produce its own thyroid hormones after about 3 months, but in early gestation relies on transfer of thyroid hormones across the placenta from the mother. A lack of dietary iodine during foetal and neonatal development or genetic impairment of the genes which produce thyroid hormones causes a disorder known as cretinism which is associated with muscle weakness and metal impairment.

Hypothyroidism

Insufficient thyroid hormone secretion is known as hypothyroidism. There are many potential causes including:

● autoimmune disease – causing a failure of the thyroid gland to produce thyroid hormones in sufficient quantities (most common cause)
● congenital lack of thyroid gland – born with no thyroid gland
● deficiency of TRH (hypothalamus) or TSH (pituitary) secretion
● surgical removal
● lack of iodine in the diet (rare in the UK).

Considering the 'normal' effects of thyroid hormones (Table 27.5), the potential symptoms of hypothyroidism can be readily determined. There is a slow-down of metabolism which leads to weight gain, sensitivity to the cold, lethargy due to impaired nutrient metabolism, puffy skin due to polysaccharide and fluid deposition, abnormally slow reflexes and decreased alertness. There may also be goitre.

Section 3

When there is a deficiency of thyroid hormones, the normal negative feedback of T_3 and T_4 to the hypothalamus and pituitary (Figure 27.8) is halted. With the 'brakes' removed from the pituitary, increased TSH is released and continues to stimulate the thyroid gland in an attempt to increase plasma T_3 and T_4. TSH promotes cell growth in the thyroid gland and this may produce goitre.

Hypothyroidism can be treated pharmacologically by replacing the deficient hormones. Most commonly, T_4 is administered in the form of levothyroxine sodium. T_4 can be transformed into T_3 in the tissues by the enzyme 5'deiodinase; the pharmacodynamics of levothyroxine are the same as the endogenous hormone. Liothyronine (T_3) can also be used, but has a much shorter duration of action and is usually reserved for hypothyroid emergencies. Drugs for the treatment of hypothyroidism do not alter the synthesis or release of hormones from the thyroid gland; they simply provide an exogenous source of hormone.

Hyperthyroidism

Overproduction of thyroid hormones is termed hyperthyroidism; the clinical result of a high plasma concentration of thyroid hormones is referred to as thyrotoxicosis. The most common cause of hyperthyroidism is an autoimmune disease (Graves' disease).

Again, considering the 'normal' effects of thyroid hormones (Table 27.5), the potential symptoms of hyperthyroidism can be determined. There is an increase in metabolism which leads to weight loss, excessive sweating and poor tolerance of warm temperatures, fatigue due to muscle weakness as muscle proteins are broken down, abnormally fast heart rate/palpitations, and abnormally acute alertness making the individual irritable, tense or anxious.

When there is an oversecretion of thyroid hormones, the normal negative feedback of T_3 and T_4 to the hypothalamus and pituitary (Figure 27.8) is enhanced. This decreases TSH and TRH secretion from the hypothalamus and pituitary in an attempt to decrease plasma T_3 and T_4. However, the thyroid does not respond to the reduced signals and continues to produce T_3 and T_4.

Hyperthyroidism may be treated pharmacologically with a group of drugs known as thioureylenes (carbamizole and propylthiouracil) which:

• prevent the incorporation of iodine into the structure of the thyroid hormone
• block the peripheral conversion of T_4 to (more active) T_3.

These drugs do not act upon preformed thyroid hormones. The thyroid gland stores large amounts of preformed hormone so thioureylenes may take 2–3 weeks to be clinically effective. If the thyroid continues to overproduce thyroid hormones, alternative treatments such as radio-iodine or surgical removal of the thyroid gland may be required.

Some of the symptoms of hyperthyroidism are caused by increased adrenoceptor stimulation, such as tachycardia and palpitations. Symptomatic relief from these symptoms can be provided with beta-adrenergic receptor blockers (e.g. propranolol).

Summary

• The endocrine system regulates a diverse range of physiological and biochemical functions within the body.

- Glucose homeostasis is regulated by the hormones insulin and glucagon which are secreted from the pancreas.
- Insulin is not secreted from the pancreas in individuals with insulin-dependent diabetes.
- Exogenous insulin treatments are used in type 1 diabetes; a range of short-, medium- and long-acting insulins are available.
- Insulin acts upon a membrane-bound receptor to facilitate the storage of glucose, thereby reducing plasma concentrations.
- Non-insulin dependent diabetes mellitus (type 2 diabetes) is characterised by insulin resistance.
- A number of drugs, including sulphonylureas, which improve insulin secretion, and biguanides, which improve peripheral responsiveness to insulin, are used to treat type 2 diabetes.
- The thyroid gland regulates growth and metabolism via secretion of thyroxine (T_4) and tri-iodothyronine (T_3).
- T_4 is enzymatically transformed to T_3 (the active form of the hormone) which acts primarily upon a nuclear receptor.
- Hypo- and hyperactive thyroid states can be treated pharmacologically with levothyroxine and thioureylenes respectively.

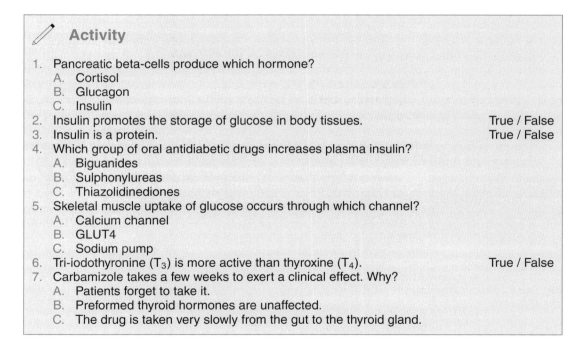

✏ Activity

1. Pancreatic beta-cells produce which hormone?
   A. Cortisol
   B. Glucagon
   C. Insulin
2. Insulin promotes the storage of glucose in body tissues.   True / False
3. Insulin is a protein.   True / False
4. Which group of oral antidiabetic drugs increases plasma insulin?
   A. Biguanides
   B. Sulphonylureas
   C. Thiazolidinediones
5. Skeletal muscle uptake of glucose occurs through which channel?
   A. Calcium channel
   B. GLUT4
   C. Sodium pump
6. Tri-iodothyronine (T_3) is more active than thyroxine (T_4).   True / False
7. Carbamizole takes a few weeks to exert a clinical effect. Why?
   A. Patients forget to take it.
   B. Preformed thyroid hormones are unaffected.
   C. The drug is taken very slowly from the gut to the thyroid gland.

Useful website

Diabetes UK. www.diabetes.org.uk

Thyroid Disease Manager. www.thyroidmanager.org/thyroidbook.htm

Section 3

NICE guidance on type 2 diabetes – full guideline. www.nice.org.uk/nicemedia/pdf/CG66diabetesfullguideline.pdf

NICE guidance on type 1 diabetes in adults – quick reference guide. www.nice.org.uk/Guidance/CG15/QuickRefGuide/pdf/English

NICE guidance on type 1 diabetes in children and young people – quick reference guide. www.nice.org.uk/guidance/index.jsp?action=download&o=29392

Reference

Sharp, P.S., Brown, B. and Qureshi, A. (2008) Age at diagnosis of diabetes in a secondary care population: 1992-2005. *Br J Diabetes Vasc Dis*, **8**, 92-95.

Further reading

Bassett, J.H., Harvey, C.B. and Williams, G.R. (2003) Mechanisms of thyroid hormone receptor-specific nuclear and extra nuclear actions. *Mol Cell Endocrinol*, **213**, 1-11.

British Medical Association and Royal Pharmaceutical Society of Great Britain (2010) *British National Formulary*, 59th edn, BMJ Publishing, London.

Brunton, S.A. (2008) The changing shape of type 2 diabetes. *Medscape J Med*, **10**, 143.

Delange, F. (2007) Iodine requirements during pregnancy, lactation and the neonatal period and indicators of optimal iodine nutrition. *Public Health Nutr*, **10**, 1571-1580.

Devdhar, M., Ousman, Y.H. and Burman, K.D. (2007) Hypothyroidism. *Endocrinol Metab Clin North Am*, **36**, 595-615.

Gardner, D.G. and Shoback, D. (2007) *Greenspan's Basic and Clinical Endocrinology*, McGraw-Hill Medical, New York.

Lepore, M., Pampanelli, S., Fanelli, C., *et al.* (2000) Pharmacokinetics and pharmacodynamics of subcutaneous injection of long-acting human insulin analog glargine, NPH insulin, and ultralente human insulin and continuous subcutaneous infusion of insulin lispro. *Diabetes*, **49**, 2142-2148.

Page, C.P., Curtis, M.J., Sutter, M.C., *et al.* (2006) *Integrated Pharmacology*, 3rd edn, Mosby, London.

Rang, H.P., Dale, M.M., Ritter, J.M. and Flower, R. (2007) *Rang and Dale's Pharmacology*, 6th edn, Churchill Livingstone, Edinburgh.

Rossetti, P., Porcellati, F., Fanelli, C.G., *et al.* (2008) Superiority of insulin analogues versus human insulin in the treatment of diabetes mellitus. *Arch Physiol Biochem*, **114**, 3-10.

28 Contraception

Learning outcomes

By the end of this chapter the reader should be able to:

- describe the endocrine regulation of ovulation in relation to the mechanism of action of oral contraceptives
- list the actions of oestrogens and progestogens on the body
- describe the clinical uses, mechanism of action, pharmacokinetics and unwanted effects of oestrogens
- describe the clinical uses, mechanism of action, pharmacokinetics and unwanted effects of progestogens
- understand the potential drug–drug interactions associated with contraceptive failure.

Endocrine regulation of the female reproductive system

Like many body systems, the female reproductive system is tightly regulated by hormones which begins in the hypothalamus with the secretion of gonadotrophin-releasing hormone (GnRH). GnRH travels along the hypophyseal portal vessels to the anterior pituitary gland where it stimulates the release of both follicle-stimulating hormone (FSH) and luteinising hormone (LH). FSH and LH travel to target organs to exert their biological effects, which include stimulating the ovaries (and testes in the male) to secrete oestrogen, progesterone and testosterone (Figure 28.1). Oestrogen, progesterone and testosterone exert a number of effects around the body and eventually plasma levels will reach a high enough concentration to cause negative feedback to the pituitary and hypothalamus.

Follicle-stimulating hormone causes one oocyte in each ovarian cycle to mature and become the dominant follicle which will be released at ovulation. LH concentrations peak midcycle and promote ovulation.

Oestrogen and progesterone are the body's own sex hormones; they are steroid hormones and derived from cholesterol (Figure 28.2). The main oestrogen found in the human body is oestradiol. The majority of oestrogens are secreted from the ovary and placenta. Oestrogens have a wide range of effects on the body (Box 28.1). As well as their reproductive, metabolic

The New Prescriber. Edited by J Lymn, D Bowskill, F Bath-Hextall, R Knaggs, © 2010 John Wiley & Sons.

Section 3

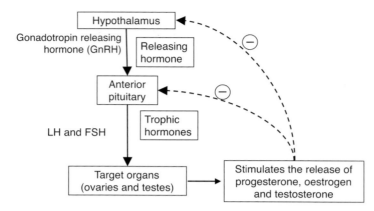

Figure 28.1   Endocrine regulation of the female reproductive system.

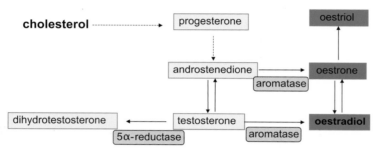

Figure 28.2   Production of oestrogens, progesterone and testosterone from cholesterol (adapted from Rang *et al.*, 2007).

Box 28.1   **Summary of the main effects of oestrogens.**

Reproductive system	Metabolic effects	Somatic effects
Stimulates growth and maturation of the internal and external genitalia and breasts at puberty.	Anabolic effects	Stimulates lengthening of long bones and feminisation of the skeleton (pelvis).
Promotes proliferative phase of the uterine cycle.	Stimulates Na+ reabsorption by the renal tubule (inhibits diuresis).	Inhibits bone resorption.
Promotes oogenesis and ovulation.	Increases HDL (reduces LDL) blood levels.	Promotes hydration of the skin.
Stimulates capacitation of sperm.	Enhanced coagulability of the blood.	Stimulates the female pattern of fat deposition. Appearance of axillary and pubic hair.

Section 3

Box 28.2 **Physiological functions of progestogens.**

Reproductive system	Other effects
Glandular development of the breasts.	Increased insulin levels.
Cyclic glandular development of the endometrium.	Competes with aldosterone at the renal tubule, causing decreased Na^+ reabsorption.
Critical for successful reproduction.	Increases body temperature.

and somatic (affecting cells other than sperm and ova) effects, oestrogens also have neural effects including feminisation of the brain.

Progesterone, the body's natural 'progestogen', is secreted by the corpus luteum and the placenta. Small amounts are also secreted by the testes and adrenal cortex. Synthetic steroids that mimic the actions of endogenous progesterone are called progestins. Progestogens have a role in a number of physiological functions (Box 28.2).

Mechanism of action of oestrogen and progesterone

Oestrogen and progesterone, like most steroid hormones, act primarily upon intracellular receptors. The mechanism of action (Figure 28.3) is very similar to that of tri-iodothyronine (Chapter 27). The oestrogen receptors (ERs) and progesterone receptors (PRs) act as transcription regulators involved in diverse physiological functions, including regulation of the female reproductive system, mammary gland development, metabolism and bone density. ERs and PRs can interact directly with specific target sequences of DNA known as oestrogen or progesterone response elements.

Oestrogen receptors and PRs are not restricted to the reproductive system and are located throughout the body. Oestrogen binding to receptors outside the reproductive system, for

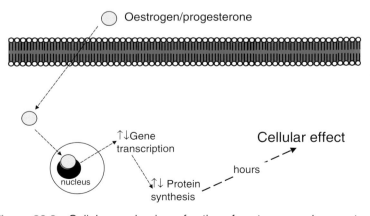

Figure 28.3   Cellular mechanism of action of oestrogen and progesterone.

example in the gastrointestinal tract, is responsible for some of the side effects seen with contraceptive drugs.

Once activated, response elements modulate transcription of a target gene. This modulation can be to either increase protein production or repress transcription, which will decrease the production of the associated protein. One must remember that increasing or decreasing proteins takes time (hours), so the clinical effect is not immediate. For example, pre-existing proteins must first be 'used up' before an effect is observed.

As well as binding to receptors, the sex hormones bind to transport proteins in the blood to facilitate their movement through the circulation. The sex hormone-binding globulin (SHBG) carries mostly oestradiol, corticosteroid-binding globulin (CBG) carries mostly progesterone and albumin can carry both hormones.

Non-contraceptive uses of oestrogen and progesterone

Oestrogens can be used to treat primary ovarian failure in order to stimulate secondary sexual characteristics and menstruation. The treatment of secondary ovarian failure with oestrogens and progesterone (HRT) is more controversial as links with some types of cancer have been suggested. A study in 2007 published data demonstrating an increased risk of ovarian cancer in UK women using HRT (Beral, 2007). HRT may provide short-term relief of some symptoms (hot flushes/sweating), promote calcium uptake into bone, which is useful in women at risk of osteoporosis, and reduce the risk of cardiovascular disease.

Progesterone alone is used in the treatment of endometriosis and as a second- or third-line treatment of breast cancer, endometrial or renal carcinoma.

Formulations of oestrogens and progesterones

Natural (oestradiol and oestriol) and synthetic oestrogens (mestranol, ethinylestradiol (EE)) are available in many different preparations for a wide range of indications. Natural and synthetic oestrogens are absorbed well from the GI tract. Natural oestrogens are rapidly metabolised in the liver by the CYP450 system, synthetic oestrogens less so. This means that synthetic oestrogens are more potent and more likely to affect liver function. Oestrogens undergo a variable amount of enterohepatic cycling and this is the basis for some drug interactions.

There are two main types of progestogen: the naturally occurring hormone and its derivatives (for example, medroxyprogesterone acetate and levonorgestrel) and the testosterone derivatives (for example, norethisterone, ethinodiol and norgestrel). Naturally occurring progesterone is virtually inactive due to first-pass metabolism; medroxyprogesterone is an injectable formulation. The testosterone derivatives can be administered orally. Some have androgenic activity and are metabolised to oestrogenic products. Newer products such as desogestrel and gestodene are being used in contraception. Progestogens are also metabolised by the CYP450 system and are excreted in urine after conjugation, but do not undergo enterohepatic recycling.

 Stop and think

What does the ability to utilise transdermal administration tell us about the chemical composition of oestrogen?

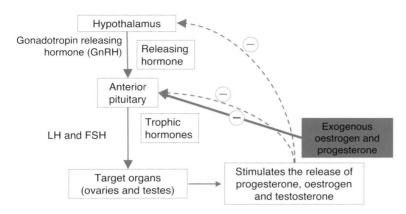

Figure 28.4 Mechanism of action of the oral contraceptives. By providing an extra exogenous source of oestrogens and or progestogen, the negative feedback to the pituitary is enhanced.

Hormonal contraception

There are two main types of oral contraceptive available in the UK: the combined oral contraceptive (COC) and the progesterone-only pill (POP).

Combined oral contraceptive

The COC is a highly effective method of contraception in the absence of intercurrent illness and potential drug interactions. The COC contains an oestrogen and a progestogen. The oestrogen in most modern COC pills is EE while the progestogen may be norethisterone, levonorgestrel or gestodene. Gestodene is more potent and has less androgenic activity but may be linked to increased risk of thromboembolism (Farmer *et al.*, 1997).

In order to understand the mechanism of action of the COC, we must return to the hormonal control of the ovarian and uterine cycles (Figure 28.4). Oestrogen and progesterone provide negative feedback to the pituitary to modulate the secretion of LH and FSH. By administering extra oestrogen and progesterone, we increase the negative feedback to the pituitary. Oestrogen specifically inhibits FSH secretion; this suppresses development of the primary follicle. Progestogens inhibit secretion of LH which prevents the LH surge mid-cycle, therefore inhibiting ovulation. This inhibition of FSH and LH is the primary mechanism of the COC; one must remember that these effects are generated by the molecular activity of oestrogens and progestogens at their nuclear receptors (Figure 28.4).

The COC also causes changes to the reproductive tract – the secondary mechanism. The progestogen makes the cervical mucus more hostile to sperm penetration and the endometrial lining becomes more resistant to implantation. However, there is little good-quality evidence regarding the biochemical/cellular changes that prevent implantation.

Progesterone-only contraceptive

The POP is less effective than the COC as it only causes partial inhibition of ovulation. The amount of progestogen in POPs is less than that in COCs – they do not prevent ovulation consistently and approximately 40% of women using POP ovulate. The progestogen also makes the cervical mucus more hostile to sperm penetration; the volume of mucus decreases and the viscosity and cell content increase, resulting in little or no sperm penetration. Endometrial changes that reduce the likelihood of implantation are also thought to occur, but are not supported with rigorous evidence.

Practice application

The POP is a suitable alternative for women in whom oestrogen is contraindicated, for example, those with a risk of venous thrombosis, smokers and older women.

Parenteral progesterone-only contraceptives

Parenteral forms of progestogens are also available; these come in the form of injectables and implants. Medroxyprogesterone acetate as an intramuscular injection is as effective as the COC, causes suppression of ovulation and makes cervical mucus less hospitable to sperm. The progestogen-only implant has equivalent efficacy to the POP by causing partial suppression of ovulation. Evidence of ovulation is observed in 10% of cycles of women using the progestogen-only implant in the first year; by 5 years 30-75% of cycles are ovulatory.

Drug interactions

There are a number of significant drug–drug interactions and adverse drug reactions which can reduce the efficacy of the hormonal contraceptives. Many of the effects of the drug–drug interactions involve EE, the oestrogen in many COC. The interactions can be divided by the stage of pharmacokinetics which is affected. As the potential outcome of contraceptive failure is an unwanted pregnancy, all drug interactions must be taken seriously. As well as drug interaction where the hormonal contraceptive is the 'victim', EE can also alter the pharmacokinetics of co-administered drugs; that is, as a 'perpetrator'.

Absorption

Oral contraceptives are absorbed across the wall of the small intestine so if vomiting or diarrhoea occurs within 2 hours of taking the COC or POP, the efficacy of the drug may be reduced due to incomplete absorption. Vomiting can be caused by many factors, including certain drugs such as antitumour agents and even the oral contraceptive pill!

Metabolism

Ethinylestradiol and progestogens undergo extensive first-pass metabolism.

The enzyme CYP3A4 is the most abundant subtype of cytochrome P450 found in adult hepatocytes and is responsible for phase I metabolism of EE in the liver and also the small intestine. EE also undergoes extensive phase II metabolism comprising conjugation via sulphation and glucuronidation.

Box 28.3   Drugs which induce the metabolism of EE.

Antiepileptic drugs	Carbemazepine, phenytoin, phenobarbital, primidone
Antifungal drugs	Griseofulvin
Antiretroviral drugs	Ritonavir, amprenavir
Enzyme-inducing antibiotics	Rifampicin, rifabutin
Immunosuppressant	Tacrolimus
GI drugs	Lansoprazole (very weak effect)
Herbal supplements	St John's wort (not much good-quality evidence)

 Stop and think

Which route of administration allows EE and progestogens to be absorbed directly into the bloodstream, thus bypassing first-pass metabolism?

Enzyme inhibition and induction

The CYP450 enzymes may be induced or inhibited by certain drugs. Inhibition of CYP450, for example by fluconazole or grapefruit juice, produces a reduction in the metabolism of hormonal contraceptives. While toxicity is thought to be rare, one must be conscious of the potential side effects of high doses of EE, such as venous thromboembolism.

Induction of CYP450 by co-administered drugs is a much more serious consideration in contraceptive pharmacology. A range of drugs (Box 28.3) are known to induce (or speed up) the activity of CYP450 and therefore increase the metabolism of EE and progestogens. The potential consequence of co-administration of the COC or POP with a CYP450 inducer is contraceptive failure.

The progestogen-only injectable contraceptive is, however, unaffected by enzyme-inducing drugs. The Faculty of Family Planning and Reproductive Health Care provides guidance on the management of women taking enzyme-inducing drugs.

 Stop and think

Is your patient taking any other medication, prescribed or otherwise, which may affect the efficacy of oral contraception? Is oral contraception the best choice for this patient? Would another route of administration be more suitable?

Section 3

Box 28.4   Effect of COC on co-administered drugs.

Decreased clinical effect	Increased clinical effect
Warfarin	Cyclosporin
Tricyclic antidepressant	Theophylline
Lamotrigine	Ropinirole

Non-enzyme inducing drugs

Once conjugated, EE and progestogens are excreted into the gut via bile. EE conjugates are broken down by commensal (or 'friendly') bacteria in the gut into active forms which can be reabsorbed back into the bloodstream (enterohepatic recycling), providing an extra source of EE. This extra source of EE is thought to be clinically important in only a very small number of women (<1%). Progestogens do not undergo enterohepatic recycling.

Bacteria involved in enterohepatic recycling are vulnerable to attack from broad-spectrum antibiotics. Non-enzyme inducing antibiotics can temporarily reduce these bacteria, potentially reducing the amount of EE available for clinical effect.

Oestrogen's effects on co-administered drugs

Hormonal contraceptives may also affect the metabolism of certain co-administered drugs (Box 28.4), depending on the nature of these drugs; there may be significant clinical effects.

Combined oral contraceptives induce glucuronosyltransferase (an enzyme which promotes glucoronidation during phase II metabolism) activity which may increase the excretion of drugs which are metabolised by this pathway. The co-prescription of lamotrigine (an antiepileptic drug) with the COC is particularly problematic as COCs can reduce the plasma levels of lamotrigine (40–60%) if the patient is not already on an enzyme-inducing antiepileptic drug.

The COC may also inhibit CYP3A4, thus increasing the plasma concentration of other drugs which utilise this method of metabolism. An example of a drug whose concentration is increased with co-administration of COCs is cyclosporin.

 Practice application

Contraception may be compromised pharmacologically if:

- vomiting occurs <2 hours post oral dose
- non-enzyme inducing antibiotics interfere with enterohepatic recirculation
- liver enzyme-inducing drugs are taken concurrently.

Emergency contraception

Trials on emergency contraception (also termed postcoital contraceptive (PCC)) were first described in the 1930s. Yuzpe *et al.* (1974) developed a regimen using 0.1 mg EE and 0.5 mg levonorgestrel within 72 hours of unprotected intercourse and repeated 12 hours later. More recently, levonorgestrel (1.5 mg) has emerged as the most effective method with fewer side effects and higher efficacy than the Yuzpe regimen.

The mechanism of levonorgestrel as a PCC remains unclear but may involve effects on sperm, the endometrium and/or follicle development. Once implantation takes place, however, emergency contraception is no longer effective. The effects of PCC can be influenced by enzyme-inducing drugs by the same mechanism as the COC and POP.

Summary

- The female reproductive system is regulated primarily by the hormones oestrogen and progesterone.
- Oestrogen and progesterone are secreted from the ovaries following stimulation by FSH and LH. Negative feedback by oestrogen and progesterone provides fine tuning of FSH and LH secretion.
- Contraceptive drugs mimic these oestrogens and progesterone in order to provide exogenous negative feedback to the pituitary gland, thereby reducing release of LH and FSH; this is the primary mechanism of action.
- Oestrogen and progesterone also have direct contraceptive effects on the reproductive system which are classified as secondary mechanisms of action.
- The POP is less effective than the COC as ~40% of women taking the POP ovulate.
- Drug–drug interactions with the hormonal contraceptives include liver enzyme-inducing effects and non-liver enzyme-inducing effects.
- Postcoital contraceptives contain a progestogen and work by impairing ovulation.

Activity

1. Luteinising hormone is secreted from which endocrine gland?
   A. Hypothalamus
   B. Pituitary
   C. Ovary
2. Negative feedback of oestrogen to the pituitary reduces secretion of FSH. True / False
3. Progesterone acts primarily via membrane-bound receptors. True / False
4. The POP is most suitable for young women at low risk of thromboembolism. True / False
5. Liver enzyme-inducing drugs may affect the efficacy of the COC and emergency contraceptive by:
   A. increasing enterohepatic recycling
   B. amplifying the rate of metabolism of oestrogen
   C. binding to the ovaries.

Section 3

Useful website

NICE guidance on epilepsy in adults and children.
www.nice.org.uk/Guidance/CG20/Guidance/pdf/English

References

Beral, V. (2007) Ovarian cancer and hormone replacement therapy in the Million Women Study. *Lancet*, **369**, 1703–1710.

Farmer, R.D.T., Lawrenson, R.A., Thompson, C.R., *et al.* (1997) Population-based study of risk of venous thromboembolism associated with various oral contraceptives. *Lancet*, **349**, 83–88.

Rang, H.P., Dale, M.M., Ritter, J.M. and Flower, R. (2007) *Rang and Dale's Pharmacology*, 6th edn, Churchill Livingstone, Edinburgh.

Yuzpe, A.A., Thurlow, H.J., Ramzy, I. and Leyshon, J.I. (1974) Post coital contraception – a pilot study. *J Reprod Med*, **13**, 53–58.

Further reading

British Medical Association and Royal Pharmaceutical Society of Great Britain (2010) *British National Formulary*, 59th edn, BMJ Publishing, London.

Burkman, R., Schlesselman, J.J. and Zieman, M. (2004) Safety concerns and health benefits associated with oral contraception. *Am J Obstet Gynaecol*, **190**, S5–S22.

Canderelli, R., Leccesse, L.A., Miller, N.L. and Davidson, J.U. (2007) Benefits of hormone replacement therapy in postmenopausal women. *J Am Acad Nurse Pract*, **19**, 635–641.

Collins, J. and Crosignani, P.G. (2003) Hormonal contraception without estrogens. *Hum Reprod Update*, **9**, 373–386.

Enmark, E. and Gustafsson, J.A. (1999) Oestrogen receptors – an overview. *J Intern Med*, **246**, 133–138.

Faculty of Family Planning and Reproductive Health Care Clinical Effectiveness Unit (2005) Drug interactions with hormonal contraceptives. *J Fam Plann Reprod Health Care*, **31**, 139–151.

Glasier, A. (2006) Emergency contraception. *BMJ*, **333**(7568), 560–561.

Leonhardt, S.A., Boonyaratanakornkit, V. and Edwards, D.P. (2003) Progesterone receptor transcription and non-transcription signaling mechanisms. *Steroids*, **68**(10–13), 761–770.

Sitruk-Ware, R. (2006) New progestagens for contraceptive use. *Hum Reprod Update*, **12**, 169–178.

Spitz, I.M. (2003) Progesterone antagonists and progesterone receptor modulators: an overview. *Steroids*, **68**(10–13), 981–993.

Section 3

29 Introduction to the central nervous system

Learning outcomes

By the end of this chapter the reader should be able to:

- describe the major areas of the brain and their associated functions
- demonstrate an understanding of the basic properties of nerve cells such as the action potential, graded potential and the chemical synapse
- identify the principal neurotransmitters in the central nervous system and their physiological effects
- identify examples of illnesses that are based on alterations in these neurotransmitters.

Central nervous system

The nervous system can be divided into two components, namely the peripheral nervous system and the central nervous system (CNS). The central nervous system can be further divided into the spinal cord and the brain. The spinal cord conducts signals to and from the brain; sensory information is conducted from the peripheral nervous system to the brain while motor information is transferred from the brain to effector systems throughout the body. The brain receives sensory input from the spinal cord as well as from its own nerves, which are the olfactory and optic nerves. Most of the power of the brain is devoted to processing these sensory inputs and initiating and co-ordinating the appropriate motor outputs.

The New Prescriber. Edited by J Lymn, D Bowskill, F Bath-Hextall, R Knaggs, © 2010 John Wiley & Sons.

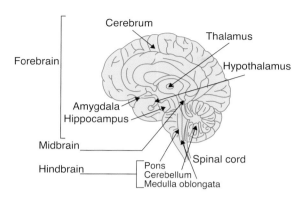

Figure 29.1   Major anatomical areas of the brain.

Parts of the brain

The brain can be divided into three major areas known as the hindbrain, midbrain and forebrain which are themselves divided into different regions (Figure 29.1) and are all responsible for regulating different functions.

The hindbrain

The hindbrain is at the top of the spinal cord and it consists of three separate structures.

● **Medulla oblongata** – responsible for maintaining basic homeostatic functions such as breathing and heart rate.
● **Pons** – involved in movement control, sensory analysis and arousal.
● **Cerebellum** –involved in movement regulation and balance.

The midbrain

The midbrain is the smallest processing region of the brain but it has a vital role in relaying sensory information and connects the hindbrain to the forebrain. The key anatomical regions are as follow.

● **Tectum** – involved with visual and auditory processing.
● **Cerebral peduncle** – contains the large axon bundles involved in voluntary movement.
● **Substantia nigra** – neural pathways associated with initiation of movement. Dysfunction of these pathways occurs in Parkinson's disease.

The forebrain

The forebrain is the largest part of the brain and where conscious thought and action are initiated. Anatomically it is made up of the following parts.

● **Cerebrum** – the outer layers forming the cerebral cortex are responsible for the control of perception, memory and all higher cognitive functions.
● **Thalamus** – relays sensory information to the cerebral cortex.
● **Hypothalamus** – involved in the regulation of homeostatic function of the body.
● **Limbic system** – important in memory, emotion and decision making.

Section 3

This neuroanatomy has fascinated scientists and clinicians for generations and there are many online resources for this topic should you need to refer to it as you work through this chapter (see Useful Website).

Neuronal structure and function

The basic structural unit of the brain and spinal cord is the nerve cell or neuron. However, in order for these nerve cells to function normally, the support of glial cells is required.

Glial cells

These cells do not directly take part in the electrical communication in the CNS but are nonetheless critically important because they provide the neurons with nutrients, form the myelin insulation around neurons, provide anatomical support for brain structures, destroy pathogens and recycle dead neurons. Taking this together, glia can modulate neuronal function. Motor neuron disease is an example of a glial disorder that leads to a dysfunction of the control of voluntary muscles.

Anatomy and physiology of nerve cells

The neuron is one of the cornerstone concepts of neurophysiology, so much so that it is worth extending your knowledge of its function a bit further. In Chapter 20 we looked at the basic structure of the neuron and discussed its function; it is important here to think about this in more detail (Figure 29.2).

The principal communication medium of the nervous system is electrical charge. In our journey from input to output of a neuron, we will look at these events and by reviewing

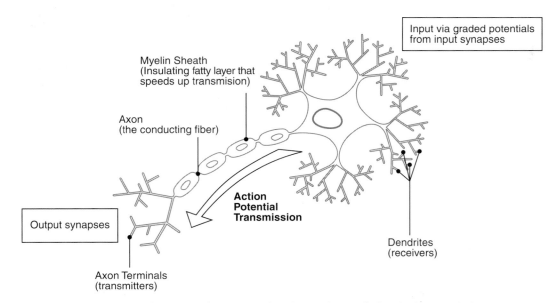

Figure 29.2 Anatomy of a neuron showing pathway of electrical transmission.

the function of the neuron, you can learn a great deal about how the whole nervous system functions.

Integration of inputs via the dendrites

The electrical events at the input end of the neuron are small and termed graded potentials. These graded potentials can be excitatory (EPSP) or inhibitory (IPSP). It is the addition of these postsynaptic potentials (PSP) that determines what information the neuron will transmit.

Excitatory postsynaptic potential (EPSP)

An EPSP is a local depolarisation of the membrane of the receiving neuron (the postsynaptic neuron) due to release of transmitters from the input neuron (presynaptic). This transmitter binds to receptors on the membrane of the postsynaptic neuron, opening sodium (Na^+) and/or calcium (Ca^{2+}) channels as well as closing chloride (Cl^-) and/or potassium (K^+) channels.

Inhibitory postsynaptic potential (IPSP)

An IPSP is a local hyperpolarisation of the membrane of a postsynaptic neuron due to release of transmitter from the presynaptic terminal. This transmitter binds to receptors on the membrane of the postsynaptic neuron, closing sodium (Na^+) and/or calcium (Ca^{2+}) channels as well as opening chloride (Cl^-) and/or potassium (K^+) channels.

The combination of IPSPs and EPSPs provides the electrical stimulation to the neuron in order for it to filter stray information and add together (summate) the information that needs to be transmitted. There are two categories of summation: one to do with the frequency of stimulation (temporal) and the other to do with the anatomical position of the input synapses (spatial).

- **Temporal summation** – adding together of EPSPs generated by firing of the same presynaptic terminal at high frequency to generate an action potential in the postsynaptic neuron (Figure 29.3b).
- **Spatial summation** – adding together of EPSPs generated by firing of two or more presynaptic neurons simultaneously to generate the action potential in the postsynaptic neuron (Figure 29.3c).

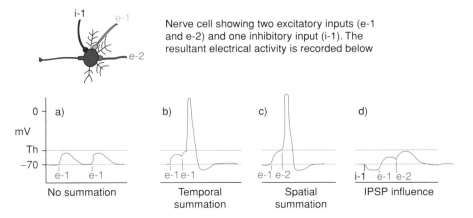

Figure 29.3 The influence of excitatory and inhibitory inputs onto a nerve cell as measured by electrodes in nerve cells. Th, threshold for action potential generation; mV, millivolt (membrane potential).

Action potential transmission

The combination of EPSPs and IPSPs when summed at the axon hillock (the site where the axon meets the cell body) can produce a depolarising threshold electrical stimulus that generates the propagating 'all or none' electrical signal for transmission over distance. The evoked spike of electrical activity is the action potential (Figure 29.4) and it is this that is propagated along the axon to the output synapse. The speed at which the action potential travels is dependent on the size of the axon (larger diameter is faster) and amount of myelin insulation (longer nerves have more myelin wrapped around the axon). In some of the very long nerves involved in controlling skeletal muscle function, the speed of transmission can be as much as 25 m/s. The properties of the myelin insulation produce an effect called 'saltatory' conduction, where the electrical signal jumps along the nerve following the path of least resistance (gaps in the myelin). This transmission can be effectively blocked by local anaesthetic agents as they disrupt nerve membrane channel function. The failure of this insulation is a component of several neuromuscular disorders including motor neuron disease.

Output synapses

This is a physical gap between neurons and their target cells (e.g. neurons, muscles and glands) which promotes a primarily unidirectional flow of information (pre to post). In the next section, we will look at the chemical transmitters produced by the body in order to cross this gap.

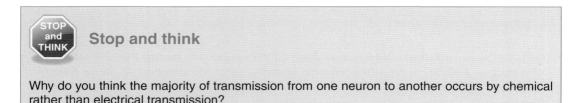

Stop and think

Why do you think the majority of transmission from one neuron to another occurs by chemical rather than electrical transmission?

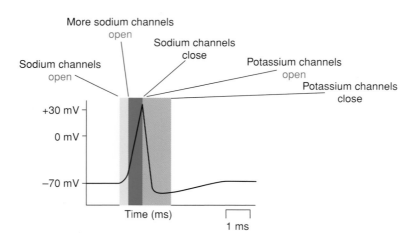

Figure 29.4   Ionic components of the action potential showing the roles of sodium (Na^+) and potassium (K^+) in its formation.

Table 29.1 Principal neurotransmitters in the central nervous system and the receptor classes they interact with in order to produce an excitatory or inhibitory response.

Neurotransmitter	Postsynaptic excitation (receptor labels)	Postsynaptic inhibition (receptor labels)
Acetylcholine	nAChR, M_1, M_3, M_5	M_2, M_4
Noradrenaline	Alpha-1, beta	Alpha-2
Dopamine	D_1	D_2
Serotonin (5HT)	$5HT_2$, $5HT_3$, $5HT_4$, $5HT_6$, $5HT_7$	$5HT_1$, $5HT_5$
Gamma-amino butyric acid (GABA)		GABA-A, GABA-B, GABA-C
Glutamate	AMPA, kainate, NMDA	
Opioids		Mu, delta, kappa, ORL

Principal neurotransmitters of the CNS

Understanding the basic functions of these neurotransmitters in the CNS allows you to apply that knowledge to drugs that interact with these systems. An agonist will mimic or enhance the 'normal' physiological response and an antagonist will stop or reduce the 'normal' response and may even promote the opposite effect. The following brief overview of the neurotransmitters listed in Table 29.1 highlights their main effects (primarily within the CNS).

Acetylcholine

There are two receptor subtypes associated with acetylcholine (ACh) and these are the nicotinic (nAChR) and the muscarininc (M) receptors. Both subtypes are found in the CNS and just as is seen in the autonomic nervous system, acetylcholine is broken down in the synaptic cleft by the enzyme acetylcholinesterase. In the CNS, acetylcholine is involved with:

- motor co-ordination pathways
- arousal
- short-term memory and cognition
- central pain perception
- central breathing control.

The link between acetylcholine and the motor co-ordination pathways suggests a link between acetylcholine signalling and Parkinson's disease while the association with short-term memory and cognition suggests a link to Alzheimer's disease (Chapter 30).

Noradrenaline

Noradrenaline (called norepinephrine in North America and most of Europe) is a monoamine neurotransmitter which has a similar synthesis pathway to dopamine. This means that drugs affecting dopamine synthesis (e.g. L-dopa) will also modify noradrenaline production. There are two receptor subtypes associated with noradrenaline: alpha- and beta-receptors. The actions of noradrenaline in the synaptic cleft are ended by reuptake mechanisms (noradrenaline

Section 3

transporters), and subsequent cellular metabolism by monoamine oxidase (MAO) enzymes (MAO-A). Noradrenaline is associated with the following:

- ascending tracts involved with mood, behaviour, stress, depression, reward reinforcement
- blood pressure and sympathetic tone in the brainstem
- control of sleep/wake cycle and levels of arousal in the locus coeruleus
- temperature regulation, sleep and arousal in the hypothalamus
- 'fight and flight' reactions and anxiety.

The link between noradrenaline and mood, behaviour and sleep/wake cycle points to the involvement of this neurotransmitter in depression and anxiety.

Dopamine

Dopamine (DA), also a monoamine neurotransmitter, has a similar synthetic pathway to noradrenaline. There are two dopamine receptor subtypes, namely D_1 and D_2 receptors. Drugs affecting the autonomic nervous system may modulate actions of the dopaminergic system. As is seen with noradrenaline, the action of dopamine in the synaptic cleft is ended by the removal of dopamine by reuptake mechanisms (dopamine transporters), and subsequent cellular metabolism by MAO-B. It is worth noting that the monoamine oxidase involved in the breakdown of dopamine is not the same isoform as that involved in the breakdown of noradrenaline. In the brain dopamine is involved in:

- ascending tracts from the ventral tegmental area to the mesolimbic/mesocortical regions, controlling mood, behaviour and stress
- ascending tracts from the substantia nigra to the corpus striatum associated with control of movement
- communication between the hypothalamus and the pituitary gland. As a consequence, a side effect of some antipsychotics is prolactin-induced subfertility.

It is the involvement of dopamine pathways in the mesolimbic/mesocortical regions of the brain which suggest that alteration to dopamine transmission may be important in depression, addiction and schizophrenia. Similarly, the involvement of dopamine pathways in the substantia nigra which is associated with movement control suggests a major role for dopamine in Parkinson's disease (Chapter 30).

 Practice application

Drugs of abuse, including heroin, amphetamines, cocaine, marijuana, alcohol, nicotine and caffeine, trigger release and/or increase the effective levels of dopamine in the CNS.

Section 3

Serotonin (5-Hydroxytryptamine or 5HT)

Serotonin is widely distributed both within and outside the CNS (including mast cells, platelets, enterochromafin cells of the digestive tract). In fact, more serotonergic cells are located in the digestive tract (98%) than the brain. The action of serotonin in the synapse is curtailed by the reuptake of serotonin into the presynaptic neuron and the subsequent cellular metabolism by monoamine oxidase enzymes. The monoamine oxidase involved in the breakdown of serotonin is MAO-A, the same isoform involved in the breakdown of noradrenaline.

Within the CNS, serotonin:

- suppresses appetite: drugs that increase 5HT levels are appetite suppressants (e.g. D-fenfluramine)
- interacts with hormonal systems and the CNS: for example, oestrogen can modify presynaptic 5HT levels
- is found at low levels in depressed and aggressive people and is linked with the aetiology of many mental health disorders such as depression, anxiety, schizophrenia, eating disorders, obsessive compulsive disorder and panic disorders.

Outside the CNS, 5HT is a potent vasoconstrictor and modulates the clotting cascade.

 Practice application

Serotonin syndrome is a potentially fatal effect that can be precipitated by a combination of serotonergic agents (such as an SSRI with an MAO inhibitor) that may produce: euphoria, drowsiness, sustained rapid eye movement, over-reaction of reflexes, rapid muscle contraction, shivering, diarrhoea, loss of consciousness and death.

Gamma-amino butyric acid (GABA)

Gamma-amino butyric acid is the primary inhibitory neurotransmitter of the CNS with cell bodies being widespread throughout the CNS. There are a substantial number of short projections and local pathways in the CNS and spinal cord. One of the most well-described effects of GABA receptor function is the desensitisation that occurs with prolonged exposure to GABA or GABA stimulants (such as barbiturates or benzodiazepines). These drugs become less effective with prolonged exposure in a dose-dependent way.

Within the CNS, GABA is involved with:

- motor control, vision, sensory processing, epilepsy, arousal, Huntington's disease, Alzheimer's disease, psychoses, endocrine regulation, catatonia, memory loss, brown adipose tissue regulation, analgesia, anaesthesia and gastric motility
- sedation, which can be useful in a variety of mental health conditions.

Section 3

Stop and think

Why do you think the GABAergic system is the drug target for some hypnotic and anxiolytic medications?

Glutamate

Glutamate is the major fast-acting neuroexcitatory agent in the CNS and its effects may be linked to its widespread distribution in the CNS. Glutamate is involved with:

- cell death processes (necrosis and apoptosis), either as a causative agent or promoter of the effect. Hence glutamate plays an important role in neurodegenerative disorders, including Alzheimer's disease, stroke and amyotrophic lateral sclerosis
- reflex pathways in the spinal cord
- long-term potentiation (memory) in the hippocampus
- sensory processing, motor co-ordination and movement disorders.

Endogenous opioids

All currently recognised opioid receptors (four classes: mu, kappa, delta and ORL) are found both in opioid-specific pathways and scattered throughout the CNS. Analysis of the distribution of neurons that contain or respond to opioids in the CNS suggests that these neurotransmitters are involved with:

- analgesia: reduces intensity of pain by inhibiting the release of pain-signalling transmitters
- euphoria, addiction and drug reinforcement
- sedation
- respiratory depression: respiration is reduced with all doses, with the respiratory centers in the brainstem becoming less sensitive to higher levels of CO_2
- cough suppression (antitussive)
- nausea and vomiting: stimulates receptors in the area postrema
- reduced GI motility.

Via their activation of mu receptors in the mesolimbic dopamine system, opioids reduce the inhibition exerted by GABAergic neurons on dopaminergic neurons in the ventrotegmental area, releasing more DA and reinforcing this pathway. The presence of opioid receptors in the hypothalamus means that they have an effect on temperature regulation and hormone secretion

Further information on the clinical use of opioids as analgesics can be found in Chapter 34.

Summary

- The brain can be divided into three major areas known as the hindbrain, midbrain and forebrain.
- The basic structural unit of the brain and spinal cord is the nerve cell or neuron.
- The combination of IPSPs and EPSPs provides the electrical stimulation to the neuron in order for it to filter stray information and add together (summate) the information that needs to be transmitted.
- There are two categories of summation, one concerned with the frequency of stimulation (temporal) and the other concerned with the anatomical position of the input synapses (spatial).
- Transmission across the synapse is chemical rather than electrical.
- Acetylcholine is broken down in the synaptic cleft by the enzyme acetylcholinesterase.
- Acetylcholine is associated with both motor co-ordination and short-term memory and cognition.
- The actions of monoamines in the synaptic cleft are ended by their removal by uptake mechanisms and subsequent cellular metabolism by monoamine oxidase enzymes.
- Alterations in dopamine are associated with neurodegenerative disorders.
- GABA is the primary inhibitory neurotransmitter of the CNS.
- Glutamate is the major fast-acting neuroexcitatory agent in the CNS.

Activity

1. The brain is divided into three major areas (hindbrain, midbrain and forebrain). True / False
2. The tectum is only involved with auditory processing. True / False
3. The limbic system is important in emotion and decision making. True / False
4. Glial cells take no direct part in electrical communication in the CNS. True / False
5. An EPSP is a local hyperpolarisation of the membrane of the receiving neuron. True / False
6. A small-diameter axon has the fastest transmission of action potentials. True / False
7. Noradrenaline and dopamine have different synthesis pathways. True / False
8. Serotonin is more prevalent in the CNS than in any other part of the body. True / False
9. Dopamine and serotonin are broken down by the same monoamine oxidase enzyme. True / False
10. Glutamate is the major excitatory neurotransmitter in the CNS. True / False

Useful website

CNS Forum. www.cnsforum.com/educationalresources/imagebank

Further reading

Aidley, D.J. (1998) *The Physiology of Excitable Cells*, 4th edn, Cambridge University Press, Cambridge.

Barker, R.A. (1993) *Neuroscience: An Illustrated Guide*, Ellis Horwood, New York.

Section 3

Briar, C., Lasserson, D., Gabriel, C. and Sharrack, B. (2003) *Crash Course: Nervous System*, 2nd edn, Mosby, London.

Kruk, Z.L. and Pycock, C.J. (1991) *Neurotransmitters and Drugs*, 3rd edn, Chapman and Hall, London.

Page, C.P., Curtis, M.J., Sutter, M.C., *et al.* (2006) *Integrated Pharmacology*, 3rd edn, Mosby, London.

Rang, H.P., Dale, M.M., Ritter, J.M. and Flower, R. (2007) *Rang and Dale's Pharmacology*, 6th edn, Churchill Livingstone, Edinburgh.

Webster, R.A. and Jordan, C.C. (1989) *Neurotransmitters, Drugs and Disease*, Blackwell Scientific, Oxford.

Zimmerman, H. (1993) *Synaptic Transmission: Cellular and Molecular Basis*, Oxford University Press, Oxford.

Section 3

30 Neurodegenerative disorders

Learning outcomes

By the end of this chapter the reader should be able to:

- describe the pathophysiology of Parkinson's disease
- understand the mechanism of action and major adverse effects of:
  - levodopa and dopamine receptor agonists
  - muscarinic antagonists
  - MAO-B inhibitors
- describe the pathophysiology of Alzheimer's disease
- understand the mechanism of action and major adverse effects of anticholinesterase drugs.

Parkinson's disease

Epidemiology

Parkinson's disease (PD) was first described in the modern context by James Parkinson in 1817, as 4–6 cycles of skeletal muscle flexion/extension per second but has been known for centuries, with one of the first written accounts described by Galen in the second century AD. It is a chronic, progressive and currently incurable disease with incidence rates of up to 19 per 100,000 inhabitants in Europe and the USA (Alves *et al.*, 2008). There is about a 1:500 chance of developing the disease in the over-60s and it is likely to have both genetic and environmental predeterminants. The cardinal symptoms of PD include resting tremor, cogwheel rigidity, bradykinesia and postural instability. Treatment of PD is for these symptoms and not the disease.

The New Prescriber. Edited by J Lymn, D Bowskill, F Bath-Hextall, R Knaggs, © 2010 John Wiley & Sons.

Table 30.1 Dopamine agonists.

Generic name	Primary receptor targets	Secondary receptor target
Pergolide	D_2	D_1, D_3, D_4, D_6
Bromocriptine	D_2, α_{1A}-antagonist	D_3, $5HT_{1A}$, α_{2A}-antagonist (D_1, D_4, D_6)
Cabergoline	D_2	
Apomorphine	D_4	D_2, D_3, D_6 (D_1, $5HT_{1A}$, α_{2A}-antagonist)
Ropinirole	D_3	D_2, D_4, $5HT_{1A}$
Rotigotine	D_3, D_4, D_6	D_1, D_2, $5HT_{1A}$ (α_{1A}, α_{2A})
Pramipexole	D_3	D_2, D_4, $5HT_{1A}$

D_1, D_2, D_3, D_4, D_6 are dopamine receptors; $5HT_{1A}$ is a serotonin receptor; alpha-1A and alpha-2A are adrenergic receptors.

Pathogenesis

Parkinson's disease is strongly associated with the degeneration of the neurons containing dopamine (DA) of the substantia nigra (SN) pathway in the midbrain (Chapter 29). Patients can lose 70–80% of these neurons before any obvious symptoms are detected. Dopamine would normally inhibit acetylcholine release from the corpus striatum but in PD, the loss of dopamine means less inhibition of acetylcholine release and hence greater activity of these cholinergic neurons. Hence PD is associated with an imbalance in the levels of dopamine and acetylcholine.

In PD there is normal synthesis of dopamine but the number of neurons available is continually decreasing. The principal targets for clinical intervention in PD are therefore associated with trying to increase the levels of dopamine in the CNS (dopamine agonists, levodopa, catechol-O-methyl transferase (COMT)) and MAO-B inhibitors) and/or reduce the effect of the increase in ACh activity (muscarinic antagonists).

Anti-parkinsonian therapy

Levodopa is the gold standard of anti-parkinsonian therapy and nearly every patient with PD will eventually receive this drug treatment (LeWitt, 2009). While initial treatment options following diagnosis also include dopamine agonists and MAO-B inhibitors, as the disease progresses the drugs used are those that increase the effectiveness of levodopa.

Dopamine agonists

Dopamine agonists (Table 30.1) are drugs that are structurally very similar to dopamine and as such they are able to mimic the action of dopamine in the body. They do not replenish the inadequate supply of dopamine in the way levodopa does but rather stimulate dopamine receptors. While some dopamine agonists are non-selective and stimulate all dopamine receptors (pergolide), others (e.g. ropinirole and pramipexole) selectively stimulate only a subset of dopamine receptors. This difference in receptor stimulation not only affects how well they work in controlling the symptoms of PD, but also accounts for the difference in side effects that a patient may experience on one particular drug compared to another.

The main side effects of all dopamine agonists include nausea and vomiting, through stimulation of dopamine receptors in the chemoreceptor trigger zone (Chapter 26), and a lowering of blood pressure caused by changes in posture (orthostatic hypotension). All dopamine agonists have the potential to induce pathological gambling, increased libido and hypersexuality. This class of drugs is used in monotherapy in early PD or added to levodopa later.

Stop and think

Both typical and atypical antipsychotic medications inhibit dopamine D_2 receptors. How would adding an antipsychotic to the drug list of someone with PD affect their treatment?

Muscarinic antagonists

Muscarinic antagonists are used to reduce the effects of overproduction of acetylcholine (in the pathways mediated by the output from the SN) by attempting to correct the balance between dopaminergic and cholinergic influences in the striatum. Specific anticholinergic agents used in PD include benzatropine, orphenadrine, procyclidine and trihexyphenidyl (benzhexol).

The usefulness of these drugs can be limited by side effects. The distribution of cholinergic receptors throughout the body means that the effects of non-selectively modifying acetylcholine action by drugs can be widespread and complex. The most common are dry mouth, mydriasis, cycloplegia, tachycardia, constipation, urinary retention; the more concerning are those associated with disruption of memory, insomnia, restlessness, delirium, paranoid reaction and hallucinations

The anticholinergic agents can be used as sole therapy or in combination with levodopa or amantadine although they may become less effective with prolonged use. They are often effective, however, for control of extrapyramidal symptoms produced by antipsychotic drugs.

Stop and think

Why are dry mouth, mydriasis, tachycardia, constipation and urinary retention side effects of muscarinic antagonists in the treatment of PD?

Monoamine oxidase-B inhibitors

Monoamine oxidase B (MAO-B) inhibitors inhibit dopamine metabolism (predominantly in the presynaptic neuron) and can be used to prolong the effect of naturally released dopamine. Dopamine is metabolised in the neuron by the enzyme MAO-B. This enzyme is distinct from the similarly named enzyme monoamine oxidase-A which is responsible for the neuronal metabolism of noradrenaline and serotonin (Chapter 29). Monoamine oxidase inhibition is therefore a strategy for the treatment of depression (Chapter 31) and the concomitant use of these inhibitors for depression in Parkinson's disease should be monitored.

Selegiline

Selegiline is a MAO-B inhibitor indicated as an adjunct in the management of patients with PD being treated with levodopa/carbidopa who exhibit deterioration in the quality of their response to this therapy. By-products of selegiline metabolism include amphetamine and

Section 3

methamphetamine which have effects of their own (CNS stimulant). Due to the relatively selective nature of selegiline as an MAO-B inhibitor, it has limited activity against MAO-A and hence causes fewer side effects than non-selective MAO inhibitors.

Practice application

Drugs which increase the effect of neurotransmitters, such as tricyclic antidepressants or serotonin reuptake inhibitors (SSRIs), may interact with selegiline, resulting in an increased risk of hypertension and serotonin syndrome (Chapter 31).

Drugs targeting dopamine synthesis and metabolism

Exogenous dopamine cannot be given to augment dopamine levels in the body as it is metabolised before it has the chance to reach the CNS. Consequently, the related drug levodopa is used.

Levodopa is the precursor for dopamine and is rapidly converted into dopamine in the body by the enzyme DOPA decarboxylase (Figure 30.1). However, levodopa is 99% metabolised outside the CNS (digestive tract (90%) and plasma (9%)), leaving only 1% of the administered dose to enter the CNS. Hence when levodopa is given for PD, it is usually given combined with a DOPA decarboxylase inhibitor such as benzerazide hydrochloride or carbidopa (Figure 30.2).

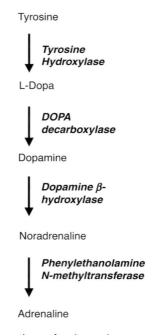

Figure 30.1 Synthesis pathway for dopamine, noradrenaline and adrenaline.

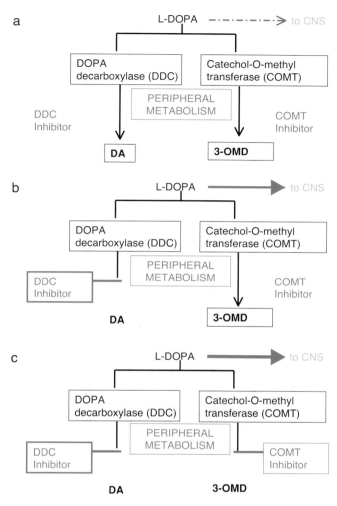

Figure 30.2 The role of peripheral DA metabolism inhibitors in raising dopamine levels in the CNS. Without enzyme inhibitors, very little levodopa reaches the CNS (a). The use of DDC inhibitors (b) and then COMT inhibitors (c) increases the available levodopa from any given oral dose.

The DOPA decarboxylase inhibitor cannot cross the blood–brain barrier and so remains in the peripheral circulation, preventing the peripheral conversion of levodopa to dopamine. The levodopa itself, however, can cross into the brain, where it is converted to dopamine by dopamine decarboxylase. This allows greater brain concentrations of dopamine to be reached with lower doses of levodopa and minimises the levodopa-related side effects. In addition to using levodopa in combination with a DOPA decarboxylase inhibitor, it is also used in combination with a decarboxylase inhibitor of another enzyme system (COMT) inhibitor such as entacapone (Figure 30.2).

Levodopa has many side effects due to its synthesis path being common with noradrenaline and adrenaline. This goes some way to explain why drugs used to treat PD symptoms can have

Table 30.2   Genetic predisposition (familial risk) and gene linkage in relation to Alzheimer's disease.

Gene name	Chromosome	Other information
Amyloid precursor protein (APP)	Ch 21	Link to Down's syndrome
Presenilin 1 (PS-1)	Ch 14	Autosomal dominant
Presenilin 2 (PS-2)	Ch 1	
Apolipoprotein E4 (ApoE4)	Ch 19	Expression suggests an increased risk
Apolipoprotein E2 (ApoE2)	Ch 19	Expression suggests a decreased risk

cardiovascular side effects. Other common side effects include nausea, depression, confusion, psychoses and dyskinesia. Over time tolerance develops, thus requiring higher doses of drug to maintain 'normality' and increasing the risk of adverse effects.

Alzheimer's disease

Epidemiology

Alzheimer's disease (AD) is defined as a progressive, irreversible, degenerative neurological disease that begins insidiously and is characterised by gradual losses of cognitive function and disturbances in behaviour and affect. AD affects about 6% of the population over 65 (Burns and Iliffe, 2009). Prevalence doubles every 5 years after 65 so that by 85+ one in three people is likely to have AD. Population statistics indicate that people aged 65 and over now represent 13% of the population but this value will be more like 18% by 2025 with 14 million cases projected by 2050 (Cowan and Kendal, 2001). Life expectancy for AD from diagnosis is generally between 8 and 12 years. It is a complex disease in terms of its diagnosis, with more women being diagnosed with AD and more men diagnosed with vascular dementia.

There is a genetic predisposition to AD (Table 30.2) as well as potential environmental triggers. Environmental factors known to increase the likelihood of AD include smoking and lifestyles that indicate an increase likelihood of developing atherosclerosis, hypertension, atrial fibrillation, hyperlipidaemia and diabetes.

Diagnosis

Alzheimer's disease has memory loss as a key feature of its diagnosis, with CNS damage occurring primarily in the cerebral cortex. This results in decreased brain size as seen in MRI scans and postmortem examination. There are other dementias that also have features of AD that can lead to misdiagnosis, such as vascular dementia, dementia with Lewy body and frontotemporal dementia.

Diagnosis for dementia involves the use of either the Bayer Activities of Daily Living Scale (Bayer-ADL) or the Neuropsychiatric Inventory with caregiver distress scale (NPI-D). Amongst the diagnostic criteria needed are an indication of multiple cognitive deficits with both memory impairment (plus one or more of aphasia, apraxia, agnosia and executive function) and impaired abstraction and/or judgement. This usually coincides with impaired social or occupational function. With these criteria, care must be taken to check that the cognitive deficits are not due to other processes (e.g. substances, systemic processes, delirium and other acute conditions). Patients will be classified as having one of three stages of dementia (Table 30.3).

Section 3

Table 30.3   Stages of dementia.

Stage 1: Mild (early)	Stage 2: Moderate	Stage 3: Late (terminal)
Routine loss of recent memory Mild aphasia or word-finding difficulty	Chronic loss of recent memory Moderate aphasia	Mixes up past and present Expressive and receptive aphasia
Seeks familiar and avoids unfamiliar places	Gets lost at times even inside home	Misidentifies familiar persons and places
Some difficulty writing and using objects	Repetitive actions, apraxia	Parkinsonism and falls risk
Apathy and depression	Possible mood and behavioural disturbances	More mood and behavioural disturbances
Needs reminders for some ADL	Needs reminders and help with most ADL	Needs help with all ADL, incontinent

Biochemical and pathological changes

Alzheimer's disease is characterised by a decrease in the number of neurons in the cerebral cortex and subcortical regions. This decrease in neurons appears to be relatively selective for cholinergic neurons, at least from measurements made postmortem on patients who suffered from AD. Alongside these losses are the appearance of histological changes described as amyloid plaques and neurofibrillary tangles at much higher levels than in non-AD patients. The most noticeable pathological lesion specific for AD is senile plaque in the cerebral cortex. AD can be described as a proteopathy or a protein misfolding disease. Plaques are composed of a protein – amyloid-beta (A-beta). Initially, A-beta aggregates into diffuse plaques that lack definite borders but later on it matures into compact plaques formed of A-beta fibrils that may be toxic to surrounding neurons. The excess production of A-beta means that it can be found in soluble form in the body fluids of patients with AD.

Also linked with AD are intracellular neurofibrillary protein tangles in the cerebral cortex. These are caused by abnormal intracellular structures caused by phosphorylation of the tau protein in the cytoskeleton of the neuron (a tauopathy). Microglial cell proliferation, especially in association with senile plaques, suggests that inflammatory processes and free radicals also play a role in the disease process.

Therapeutic interventions in Alzheimer's disease

Acetycholinesterase inhibitors

Acetycholinesterase inhibitors (Table 30.4) are approved for use with people who have been assessed as having mild to moderate AD. These drugs have a wide range of side effects due to their effect on the autonomic nervous system, increasing the available acetylcholine. Once a person starts on a drug regimen, the following cycles of treatment are often based on the monitoring of acetylcholinesterase inhibitor efficacy by caregiver report, quantified mental status examination, effects on activities related to daily living (ADL) and effects on behaviour.

There is another metabolic pathway for ACh in the periphery (butyl cholinesterase), but its role is minor in normal brain. Interestingly enough, its activity increases in AD brains.

Section 3

Table 30.4 Details of available acetylcholinesterase inhibitors.

Year available	1996	2000	2001
Drug generic	Donepezil	Rivastigmine	Galantamine
Reversible	Yes	Pseudo-irreversible	Yes
AChE	Yes	Yes	Yes
BuChE	Minimal	Yes	Minimal

Donepezil

Donepezil is indicated for mild to moderate Alzheimer's dementia. It preferentially inhibits acetylcholinesterase, which may be why it has a lower incidence of GI side effects. It also does not have hepatoxicity.

Rivastigmine

Rivastigmine is used in the treatment of mild to moderately severe AD to support cognitive and global function. It has been shown to improve ADL including eating, dressing and household chores. It also reduces behavioural symptoms, such as delusions and agitation, improves cognitive function and reduces the use of other psychotropic medications. Rivastigmine has fewer interactions with other drugs compared to other acetylcholinesterase inhibitors and has no hepatoxicity. However, it has been shown that discontinuation can lead to a more rapid decline in cognitive function within 3 weeks.

Galantamine

Galantamine is derived from the snowdrop *(Galanthus nivalis)* and is known to potentiate the effect of acetylcholine at nicotinic receptors. Galantamine may be beneficial in maintaining cognition in people with mild to moderate AD.

 Stop and think

Why might the use of acetylcholinesterase inhibitors result in diarrhoea?

Other pharmacological interventions for the treatment of AD

Glutamate receptor antagonists

Memantine is a glutamate (NMDA) receptor antagonist which reduces the effect of glutamate excitotoxicity and reduces neuronal cell death. This mechanism permits the amplification of the transmission of neuronal impulses that improve learning. Memantine is used in moderate to severe AD and may be used with donepezil as it targets a different receptor system. Side effects include hallucinations, confusion and dizziness and it should be used with caution in patients with renal impairment.

Practice application

Patients with moderate AD should be assessed every 6 months and drug treatment should normally continue only if the mini mental state examination score remains at or above 10 points and if treatment is considered to have a worthwhile effect on global, functional and behavioural condition (NICE, 2006).

Polypharmacy considerations

With AD there is a decline in the number of neurons in the CNS which affects the linking together of CNS pathways leading to neuropsychiatric features of AD which sometimes require other drugs to suppress them. These include (in order of prevalence):

● agitation
● apathy
● depression
● anxiety
● irritability
● delusional disorders and psychosis
● disinhibition
● hallucinations.

Summary

● Parkinson's disease is strongly associated with the degeneration of the dopamine-containing neurons of the substantia nigra.
● The principal targets for clinical intervention in PD are associated with trying to increase the levels of dopamine in the CNS and/or reduce the effect of the increase in ACh activity.
● Antidepressants may interact with selegiline resulting in an increased risk of hypertension and serotonin syndrome.
● Levodopa is the gold standard of therapy for PD.
● Levodopa is usually given combined with a DOPA decarboxylase inhibitor such as benzerazide hydrochloride or carbidopa.
● Drugs used to treat PD symptoms commonly have cardiovascular side effects.
● Alzheimer's disease is a progressive, irreversible, degenerative disease characterised by gradual losses of cognitive function and disturbances in behaviour.
● AD is characterised by a decrease in the number of cholinergic neurons.
● The mainstay of treatment for AD is the use of acetylcholinesterase inhibitors.
● The neuropsychiatric features of AD sometimes require other drugs to suppress them, leading to complex polypharmacy.

Section 3

Activity

1. Parkinson's disease is associated with a loss of dopaminergic neurons in the substantia nigra. True / False
2. Parkinson's disease is associated with decreased acetylcholine activity. True / False
3. Monoamine oxidase-B inhibitors inhibit the metabolism of all monoamines. True / False
4. Dopamine agonists act to replenish the body's supply of dopamine. True / False
5. Levodopa has fewer side effects if administered with a decarboxylase inhibitor. True / False
6. Levodopa can exhibit cardiovascular side effects due to the nature of its synthesis path. True / False
7. Age does not play a contributory role in the development of Alzheimer's disease. True / False
8. Acetylcholinesterase inhibitors have only limited side effects as their effects are restricted to the CNS True / False
9. Memantine is a NMDA receptor antagonist. True / False
10. All drugs used to treat Alzheimer's disease increase acetylcholine levels. True / False

Useful websites

Scottish Intercollegiate Guidelines Network (SIGN) Guide 86. Management of patients with dementia (Feb 06). www.sign.ac.uk/pdf/sign86.pdf

Health Institute of Australia. www.healthinsite.gov.au/topics/Systematic_Reviews_of_Treatments_for_Alzheimer's_Disease

NICE guidance on Alzheimer's disease – donepezil, galantamine, rivastigmine (review) and memantine. www.nice.org.uk/Guidance/TA111/Guidance/pdf/English

References

Alves, G., Forsaa, E.B., Pederson, K.F., *et al.* (2008) Epidemiology of Parkinson's disease. *J Neurol*, **255**(Suppl 5), 18-32.

Burne, A. and Iliffe, S. (2009) Alzheimer's disease. *BMJ*, **338**, 467-471.

Cowan, W.M. and Kandel, E.R. (2001) Prospects for neurology and psychiatry. *JAMA*, **285**, 594-600.

LeWitt, P.A. (2009) Levodopa therapeutics for Parkinson's disease: new developments. *Parkinsonism Relat Disord*, **15**(Suppl 1), S31-S34.

National Institute for Health and Clinical Excellence (2006) CG42 Dementia. www.nice.org.uk/nicemedia/pdf/CG042quickrefguide.pdf.

Section 3

Further reading

Bertram, L. and Tanzi, R.E. (2008) Thirty years of Alzheimer's disease genetics: the implications of systematic meta-analysis. *Nat Rev Neurosci*, **9**, 768–778.

British Geriatrics Society (2006) *Delirious About Dementia*, British Geriatric Society, London.

British Medical Association and Royal Pharmaceutical Society of Great Britain (2010) *British National Formulary*, 59th edn, BMJ Publishing, London.

Miller, D.B. and O'Callaghan, J.P. (2008) Do early-life insults contribute to the late-life development of Parkinson and Alzheimer diseases? *Metabolism*, **57**(Suppl 2), S44–S49.

Nomoto, M., Nishikawa, N., Nagai, M., *et al.* (2009) Inter- and intra-individual variation in L-dopa pharmacokinetics in the treatment of Parkinson's disease. *Parkinsonism Relat Disord*, **15**(Suppl 1), S21–S24.

Rang, H.P., Dale, M.M., Ritter, J.M. and Flower, R. (2007) *Rang and Dale's Pharmacology*, 6th edn, Churchill Livingstone, Edinburgh.

Section 3

31 Depression and anxiety

Learning outcomes

By the end of this chapter the reader should be able to:

- demonstrate an understanding of the nature of depressive illness and the monoamine theory
- demonstrate an understanding of the mechanisms of action of the major groups of antidepressants
- describe the common adverse reactions associated with antidepressant use
- identify the main groups of anxiolytic drugs
- demonstrate an understand of the mechanisms of action of anxiolytic drugs
- describe the adverse effects associated with anxiolytic use.

Both depression and anxiety are mental health states that are associated with imbalances of excitatory and inhibitory neural pathways within the CNS (Chapter 29). Depression is due to underactivity of monoamine neurotransmitter pathways, principally noradrenaline and serotonin (5HT). Anxiety-related disorders are generally the reverse of this, due primarily to the overactivity of monoamine pathways (dopamine and noradrenaline).

This chapter will initially consider depression and its treatment and then move on to anxiety disorders. It is worth remembering that overmedication for depression can produce anxiety-related side effects and overmedication for anxiety can produce depression as a side effect, and sometimes both depression and anxiety may be present in the same patient.

Depression

Depression is the most common mental illness with around one in five people experiencing an episode of depression in their lifetime. Most people have experienced the short-term effects of a 'bad day' with 'feeling down' but for our needs we must consider the differentiation of

---

Box 31.1 Symptoms of Depression (NICE Clinical Guideline 23 (Amended) 2007)

Persistent sadness or low mood
Loss of interest/pleasure in normal activities
Fatigue/low energy
Difficulty sleeping/waking early
Poor/increased appetite
Poor concentration/indecisiveness
Loss of self-confidence
Guilt/self-blame
Agitation or slowing of movements
Thinking about suicide

---

this from depression. For major depression to be diagnosed, the patient must exhibit either depressed mood and/or anhedonia (an inability to experience pleasure) for more than 2 weeks combined with several other physical and psychological symptoms (Box 31.1).

Women are twice as likely to suffer from depression than men and most people suffering with major depression have multiple episodes (Aan het Rot, Matthew and Charney, 2009; Beard, Galea and Vlahov, 2008). Depression may be triggered by stress but it is unlikely that stress alone causes depression. Data from the USA suggest that severe depression is not associated with stressful life events while moderate and mild depression are associated with a combination of stressful life events and a family history of depression (Chen *et al.*, 2000). There is evidence that some people are more vulnerable to depression and this provides a clue that there are developmental, genetic and biological components of depression.

Developmental influences linked to socio-economic disadvantage during childhood and adolescence have been linked to poor mental health in adulthood. However, the neural pathways through which socio-economic factors may exert a developmental influence on mental health remain the subject of debate and investigation.

The genetic influence on disorders is assessed by concordance rates (probability that if one twin has the disorder, the other one does too). When the concordance rate for identical twins is high and when it is significantly higher than that for fraternal twins, a disorder has a large genetic component. The concordance rates for major depression are 20% for identical twins and 14% for fraternal twins, highlighting a genetic component.

Monoamine theory of depression

This theory of depression suggests that disruptions in the serotonergic and noradrenergic systems result in depressive illness (White, Walline and Barker, 2005). These disruptions are associated with insufficient or poorly utilised noradrenaline and/or serotonin in brain synapses, which may in turn be due to insufficient production, overly rapid reabsorption and/or insensitive receptors. Areas of the brain that use noradrenaline and serotonin have links to endocrine glands that regulate metabolism, wake/sleep cycles, alertness, sex drive and appetite, all of which are disturbed in depressive illness. Current antidepressant therapies are all based around the monoamine theory of depression and all function to restore monamines to normal levels.

Section 3

Antidepressant drugs

There are a number of drug groups which can be used to treat depression.

- Selective serotonin reuptake inhibitors (SSRIs)
- Tricyclic antidepressants (TCAs)
- Serotonin and noradrenaline reuptake inhibitors (SNRIs)
- Monoamine oxidase inhibitors (MAOIs)
- Reversible inhibitors of monoamine oxidase A (RIMAs)
- Herbal products

While choice should be based on individual patient requirements, SSRIs are better tolerated and safer in overdose than other drug groups and should be considered first line for the treatment of depression (BNF, 2010; NICE, 2007).

In order to show an improvement in mood, there needs to be a prolonged enhancement of noradrenaline and serotonin levels within the synapse and hence it takes several weeks for antidepressant drugs to exert a meaningful clinical effect.

Selective serotonin reuptake inhibitors

The SSRIs inhibit the reuptake of serotonin (5HT) into the presynaptic neuron, thus increasing the amount of serotonin in the synapse and prolonging serotonin signalling. SSRIs do what their name suggests and have a much greater affinity for the serotonin transporter than the noradrenaline or dopamine transporters. SSRIs were developed with the aim of reducing the number of side effects caused by other antidepressant groups, particularly the tricyclic antidepressants and monoamine oxidase inhibitors.

Selective serotonin reuptake inhibitors can, however, interact with other receptors, such as the muscarinic acetylcholine receptor, to a limited degree and affect liver enzyme systems (Figure 31.1). The degree of interaction depends on the specific SSRI and as such, you cannot assume that they all have the same level of effect. All drugs of this class are considered to have an increased suicide risk in adolescents.

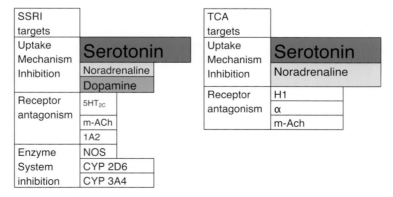

Figure 31.1   Target sites for SSRIs and TCAs. $5HT_{2C}$, serotonin type 2C receptor; H_1, histamine type 1 receptor; α, alpha-adrenoceptor; mACh, muscarininc acetylcholine receptors; 1A2, adenosine A2 receptor; NOS, nitric oxide synthetase. The size of the bar is an indication of the level of interaction.

Fluoxetine is the prototypical SSRI. It is used predominantly as an antidepressant but it is also used in the treatment of obsessive-compulsive disorder and bulimia nervosa. It is the drug of first choice in children and young people if depression is unresponsive to psychological therapy (NICE, 2007).

Side effects related to the increase in serotonin in the brain include agitation, amnesia, confusion, emotional lability and sleep disorder. Fluoxetine has a neurostimulant action and hence is taken in the morning rather than in the evening. There is an emerging view that there is increased risk of upper gastrointestinal bleeding with SSRI antidepressants, probably via an effect on systemic serotonin levels (de Abajo and Garcia-Rodriguez, 2008).

Selective serotonin reuptake inhibitors may also cause hyponatremia (low plasma sodium concentration), which is a particular problem in the elderly.

Tricyclic antidepressants

Tricyclic antidepressants are used primarily to produce non-selective inhibition of noradrenaline and serotonin reuptake systems in the CNS. These drugs have the effect of raising noradrenaline and serotonin levels throughout the body, including the CNS.

Tricyclic antidepressants exhibit substantially more side effects than SSRIs and this is related to their antagonist action at other receptors in the body, including the muscarinic acetylcholine and histamine H_1 receptors (Figure 31.1). In clinical practice, one of the major problems associated with the use of TCAs is that patients may notice side effects of these drugs within a very short space of time, long before the therapeutic effects are apparent.

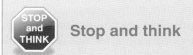

Stop and think

What side effects can you predict given that TCAs act as antagonists at muscarinic acetylcholine, histamine H_1 and alpha-adrenergic receptors?

Many tricyclic antidepressants have pharmacologically active metabolites. For example, nortriptyline, which is a drug in its own right, is actually a metabolite of amitriptyline. The presence of active metabolites may increase the severity of side effects. TCAs have a higher rate of Q-T interval prolongation than SSRIs, especially at higher doses and in overdose. They also have a narrow therapeutic index which means that when used together with drugs which inhibit cytochrome P450 activity (e.g. cimetidine), the severity of side effects may be increased, possibly leading to increased toxicity. On the other hand, when used with drugs which induce cytochrome P450 activity (e.g. rifampicin), therapeutic effect may be diminished.

Serotonin and noradrenaline reuptake inhibitors (SNRIs)

There are currently two SNRIs in clinical use: venlafaxine and duloxetine. These drugs work by selectively inhibiting the reuptake of serotonin and noradrenaline in much the same way that TCAs do. However, they do not show antagonist activity at other receptors so their side effect profile is reduced.

Section 3

Serotonin and noradrenaline reuptake inhibitors are sympathomimetic and in high dose venlafaxine has been associated with hypertensive crisis. While duloxetine has not been associated with hypertensive crisis, it should be borne in mind that this is a relatively new drug.

Monoamine oxidase inhibitors

Some MAOIs such as phenelzine, isocarboxazid and tranylcypromine produce a non-selective irreversible inhibition of the mitochondrial enzyme monoamine oxidase. By inhibiting the enzyme responsible for monoamine metabolism, they inhibit the breakdown of monoamines (e.g. serotonin and noradrenaline), resulting in enhanced levels of available monoamines in the presynaptic neuron.

 Practice application

Foods rich in the essential amino acid tyramine, such as mature cheese, pickled herring, broad bean pods, meat or yeast extract products (Bovril®, Marmite® and Oxo®), may cause a potentially fatal rise in blood pressure if taken together with an MAOI.

Reversible inhibitors of monoamine oxidase type-A

The only RIMA in clinical practice is moclobemide which produces reversible inhibition of MAO-A (Figure 31.2). As a result of this reversible effect, moclobemide does not require the dietary restrictions of the irreversible MAOIs and also has reduced incidence of hypertensive crisis. Use of moclobemide should be followed by a wash-out period before starting other antidepressant therapy.

 Stop and think

When switching from sertraline, why must you wait a period of 2 weeks before starting moclobemide therapy?

Herbal preparations

Preparations of St John's wort (*Hypericum perforatum*) are available from supermarkets, pharmacies and herbal stores and are used to treat mild depression (Linde, Berner and Kriston, 2008). The active constituents of St John's wort can both increase and decrease the activity of specific cytochrome P450 enzymes. Potentially, this may lead to a reduction in the therapeutic effect or an increase in the side effects of other prescribed drugs (Chapter 16).

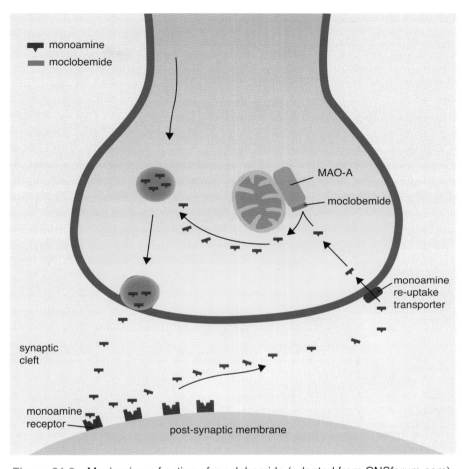

Figure 31.2 Mechanism of action of moclobemide (adapted from CNSforum.com).

Anxiety disorders

Some anxiety is an expected, normal, transient response to day-to-day stress and indeed, it is likely to be a necessary cue for adaptation and coping. Our interest in this chapter is pathological anxiety which can be manifested by the continued presence of:

- **Affective symptoms** – feelings of edginess, 'losing control', 'going to die'
- **Physiological symptoms** – tachycardia, tachypnoea, diarrhoea, diaphoresis (excessive sweating), dizziness, lightheadedness
- **Behavioural alterations** – avoidance, compulsions
- **Cognitive symptoms** – apprehension, worry, obsessions.

Pathological anxieties can be classified based on the signs and symptoms exhibited by a patient. Diagnosing pathological anxiety is a specialised area as the diagnosing clinician has

Table 31.1   Some pathological anxiety disorders.

Pathological anxiety disorder	Portrait of disorder
Panic disorder (with or without agoraphobia)	Recurrent, unexpected panic attacks, sudden onset, limited duration.
Generalised anxiety disorder (GAD)	Excessive anxiety and worry that is considered out of proportion occurring for more days than not for at least 6 months
Obsessive-compulsive disorder (OCD)	Intrusive, recurrent, unwanted thoughts, impulses, images or compulsive behaviours or rituals, that cause marked anxiety or distress.
Post-traumatic stress disorder (PSD)	Triggered by exposure of the sufferer to a traumatic event that involved the threat of death, injury, or severe harm to themselves or others.
Social phobia	A marked and persistent fear of social, or performance, situations in which the person is exposed to unfamiliar people or to possible scrutiny by others.
Simple phobia	This is a marked, persistent fear of circumscribed situations or objects.

to be able to effectively differentiate the patient's condition from a number of pathological anxiety disorders (Table 31.1).

Anxiolytic therapy

The medications used in controlling some of the symptoms of pathological anxiety fall principally into the following four categories:

1. benzodiazepines
2. azapirones
3. antidepressants
4. beta-adrenoceptor antagonists.

For current UK guidance on drug use in anxiety, please go to the NICE website (http://www.nice.org.uk/).

Benzodiazepines

Benzodiazepines are widely prescribed for all anxiety disorders (except obsessive-compulsive disorder) as they are effective and generally more rapid acting than other anxiolytic treatments.

All benzodiazepines act via the $GABA_A$ receptor (Figure 31.3) by producing changes that increase the effectiveness of the naturally produced (endogenous) GABA. Increased GABA interaction leads to an increase in chloride influx and thus prolonged hyperpolarisation (brain suppression). Benzodiazepines only work in the presence of endogenous GABA.

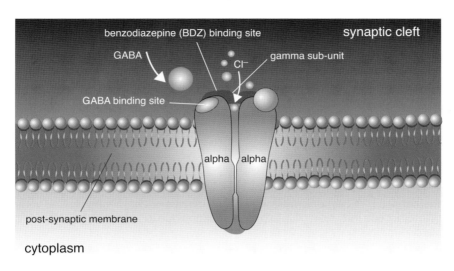

Figure 31.3 The GABA$_A$ receptor with representations of the exogenous drugs targeting the receptor (copyright CNSforum.com).

The speed of action and elimination of individual benzodiazepines varies. These differences are primarily due to variations in pharmacokinetic properties such as absorption, lipid solubility (if high then rapid onset of action), presence or absence of active metabolites, hepatic metabolism and elimination half-life. Some benzodiazepines have many active metabolites which complicates an understanding of their pharmacokinetic profile. Fast-acting benzodiazepines have higher lipid solubility and as a consequence cross cell membranes, including the blood–brain barrier, more easily than more water-soluble (hydrophilic) drugs. They are also much more addictive.

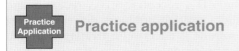 **Practice application**

In generalised anxiety disorder (GAD), benzodiazepines are generally used only in the first 2–4 weeks of treatment, switching to an SSRI antidepressant for long-term management. This combination of drugs suppresses overactive CNS pathways using the benzodiazepines and then supports recovery of monoamine levels.

Benzodiazepines have side effects that can potentially be difficult for patients to deal with. Amongst these are disinhibition (especially in children and the elderly), CNS depression, rebound insomnia, anxiety (especially for short-acting benzodiazepines such as midazolam) and respiratory depression. As well as onset adverse reactions, benzodiazepines have a complex series of withdrawal signs and symptoms that can mimic the conditions for which the drug was initially prescribed, such as 'rebound anxiety' or panic attacks. Discontinuation of benzodiazepines therefore requires tapering of the dose which allows the body to adjust to a

Section 3

reduction in GABAergic output in a way that does not precipitate rebound sympathomimetic effects, such as anxiety.

Some benzodiazepines alter the activity of cytochrome P450 enzymes in the liver and this may alter the pharmacokinetics and effects of the benzodiazepine or other drugs prescribed concomitantly. If given with other drugs that are CNS depressants, such as tricyclic antidepressants, anticonvulsants or antipsychotic drugs, there will be enhanced sedation.

 Practice application

Caution is advised when midazolam is administered concomitantly with drugs that are known to inhibit the hepatic CYP3A4 enzyme system (e.g. cimetidine, erythromycin and verapamil) as these drug interactions may result in prolonged sedation due to a decrease in plasma clearance of midazolam.

Apart from their anxiolytic properties benzodiazepines are also used in other clinical areas including:

- sedation/insomnia
- agitation
- anaesthesia induction
- akathisia (motor restlessness due to antipsychotics)
- seizures including status epilepticus.

You need to be aware of these other uses as you may have patients who receive benzodiazepines as part of other treatments.

Azapirones

Azapirones are a group of drugs that are agonists on the $5HT_{1A}$ receptor and are considered to be effective in treating GAD. The only example of this type of drug used clinically is buspirone.

Buspirone is thought to act as a partial agonist at the $5HT_{1A}$ receptor. $5HT_{1A}$ receptors are predominantly autoinhibitory presynaptic receptors and activation produces decreased firing of the serotonergic neurons on which they occur. Buspirone is effective in treating GAD and the relief of symptoms of anxiety with or without accompanying depression. It is used most commonly to augment the effect of antidepressants.

Side effects of buspirone are less problematic than those of benzodiazepines and include nausea, nervousness, restlessness and lightheadedness. Buspirone has less abuse potential than benzodiazepines and as such has been considered for substance abusers as the risk of lethality in overdose is low.

 Stop and think

What is meant by the term partial agonist? How does the efficacy of a partial agonist compare to that of a full agonist?

Antidepressants

Antidepressants are a key component in first-line treatment for anxiety disorders (especially SSRIs). Treatments for anxiety using antidepressants usually start at low dose which can cause initial 'edginess' and it can take several weeks before benefit is appreciated. In more severe cases of anxiety, the antidepressant may be combined with a benzodiazepine. Over a period of time, the dose of the antidepressant will be increased and the dose of the benzodiazepine tapered.

Selective serotonin reuptake inhibitors are commonly prescribed in anxiety (see earlier in this chapter). Trazadone may be useful in elderly patients with dementia to reduce anxiety, agitation and aggression. TCAs may also be used in anxiety management but there is a higher risk of lethality in overdose as they are cardiotoxic.

Beta-adrenoceptor antagonists

The normal function of the adrenergic beta-receptors, when stimulated by noradrenaline (and/or adrenaline), is to produce an increase in heart rate, blood pressure and respiratory rate. Blocking these receptors with a beta-adrenoceptor antagonist reduces the severity of these symptoms which may occur in anxiety, although the effect on lung smooth muscle can be a problem for asthmatics (Chapter 22). A classic example of a beta-adrenoceptor antagonist used in the treatment of anxiety is propranolol, which is primarily indicated for use in performance anxiety (e.g. for musicians and those involved in public speaking) as it acts to dull sympathetic symptoms such as palpitations and tremor.

Summary

- Depression is primarily due to underactivity of monoamine neurotransmitter pathways, principally noradrenaline and serotonin.
- Women are more likely to suffer from depression than men.
- Mild depression may be triggered by stressful life events.
- Current drug therapy for depression aims to increase levels of serotonin and noradrenaline.
- Selective serotonin reuptake inhibitors interact with other receptors and liver enzyme systems.
- Many TCAs are more active as a metabolite of the parent drug and this can lead to problems with the cardiovascular system.
- Monoamine oxidase inhibitors produce a non-selective irreversible inhibition of the mitochondrial enzyme monoamine oxidase.
- The active constituents of St John's wort can induce and inhibit drug metabolising enzymes.
- Pathological anxiety can be manifested by the continued presence of affective symptoms, physiological symptoms, behavioural alterations and cognitive symptoms.
- All benzodiazepines act via the $GABA_A$ receptor by producing changes that increase the effectiveness of the endogenous GABA.
- Some benzodiazepines alter the activity of cytochrome P450 enzymes in the liver and this may alter the pharmacokinetics of other drugs prescribed concomitantly.

Section 3

- Antidepressants are a key component in first-line treatment for anxiety disorders and are often augmented by buspirone.
- Beta-adrenoceptor antagonists reduce the severity of the symptoms which may occur in anxiety, but their effect on lung smooth muscle can be a problem for asthmatics.

✎ Activity

1. Major depression is more likely to occur in women than in men.	True / False
2. Stressful life events are a trigger for major depression.	True / False
3. The monoamine theory suggests that depression is associated with an increase in serotonin levels.	True / False
4. SSRIs preferentially inhibit the reuptake of serotonin into the presynaptic neuron.	True / False
5. Tricyclic antidepressants exhibit antimuscarinic side effects.	True / False
6. Tricyclic antidepressants have a wide therapeutic index and are safe to use across a wide range of doses.	True / False
7. Venlafaxine is a widely used SSRI.	True / False
8. SNRIs and TCAs both inhibit noradrenaline and serotonin reuptake.	True / False
9. SNRIs are sympathomimetic.	True / False
10. Moclobemide exhibits the same dietary restrictions as phenelzine.	True / False
11. St John's wort affects cytochrome P450 enzymes.	True / False
12. Anxiety is associated with increased glutamate.	True / False
13. Fast-acting benzodiazepines have high lipid solubility.	True / False
14. Buspirone is a full agonist.	True / False
15. Beta-blockers are useful in treating the underlying cause of anxiety.	True / False

---

Usefule websites

NICE CG23 Depression: quick reference guide (amended). www.nice.org.uk/Guidance/CG23/QuickRefGuide/pdf/English

NICE CG28 Depression in children and young people: quick reference guide. www.nice.org.uk/Guidance/CG28/QuickRefGuide/pdf/English

NICE CG22 Anxiety: quick reference guide (amended). www.nice.org.uk/Guidance/CG22/QuickRefGuide/pdf/English

---

References

Aan het Rot, M., Matthew, S.J. and Charney, D.S. (2009) Neurobiological mechanisms in major depressive disorder. *CMAJ*, **180**, 305–313.

Beard, J.R., Galea, S. and Vlahov, D. (2008) Longitudinal population-based studies of affective disorders: where to from here? *BMC Psychiatry*, **8**, 83.

British Medical Association and Royal Pharmaceutical Society of Great Britain (2010) *British National Formulary*, 59th edn, BMJ Publishing, London.

Chen, L.-S., Eaton, W.W., Gallo, J.J. and Nestadt, G. (2000) Understanding the heterogeneity of depression through the triad of symptoms, course and risk factors: a longitudinal, population-based study. *J Affect Disord*, **59**, 1–11

de Abajo, F.J. and Garcia-Rodriguez, L.A. (2008) Risk of upper gastrointestinal tract bleeding associated with selective serotonin reuptake inhibitors and venlafaxine therapy. *Arch Gen Psychiatry*, **65**, 795–803.

Linde, K., Berner, M.M. and Kriston, L. (2008) St John's wort for major depression. *Cochrane Database Syst Rev*, **4**, CD000448).

National Institute for Health and Clinical Excellence (2007) *Depression: Management of Depression in Primary and Secondary Care*, National Institute for Health and Clinical Excellence, London.

White, K.J., Walline, C.C. and Barker, E.L. (2005) Serotonin transporters: implications for antidepressant drug development. *AAPS J*, **7**, E421–E433.

Further reading

Bazire, S. (2007) *Psychotropic Drug Directory 2007*, Fivepin Publishing, Salisbury.

CNS Forum. http://www.cnsforum.com/educationalresources/imagebank/.

Gianaros, P.J., Horenstein, J.A., Hariri, A.R., et al. (2008) Potential neural embedding of parental social standing. *Soc Cogn Affect Neurosci*, **3**, 91–96.

Rang, H.P., Dale, M.M., Ritter, J.M. and Flower, R. (2007) *Rang and Dale's Pharmacology*, 6th edn, Churchill Livingstone, Edinburgh.

Stahl, S.M. (2000) *Stahl's Essential Psychopharmacology*, 2nd edn, Cambridge University Press, Cambridge.

Zemrak, W.R. and Kenna, G.A. (2008) Association of antipsychotic and antidepressant drugs with Q-T interval prolongation. *Am J Health Syst Pharm*, **65**, 1029–1038.

Section 3

32 Schizophrenia

Learning outcomes

By the end of this chapter the reader should be able to:

* understand the nature of schizophrenia
* identify factors which influence the development of schizophrenia
* understand the neurochemical basis of schizophrenia
* understand the mechanisms of action of neuroleptics
* describe the adverse effects associated with neuroleptic use.

Description and epidemiology

The concept of schizophrenia can be hard to understand for people who do not suffer from the disease as it may be difficult to imagine what it is like to experience a delusion or hallucination. Schizophrenia (derived from the Greek for 'split mind') is a psychotic disorder in which thinking and emotion are so impaired that the individual is seriously out of contact with reality and has trouble with social and occupational function. The life-long course of the disease coupled with the huge impact of the symptoms puts schizophrenia amongst the top ten leading causes of disease-related disability in the world (WHO, 2001).

In order to make a diagnosis of a psychotic disorder, the patient needs to have been exhibiting positive (Table 32.1) and negative (Table 32.2) psychotic symptoms for at least 1 month. The annual incidence of schizophrenia averages 15 per 100,000 (Tandon, Keshavan and Nasrallah, 2008a) and for many people the age of their first psychotic episode is between 21 and 27, being slightly later in women. Risk factors for developing schizophrenia include both genetic and environmental factors, neither of which appears to operate in isolation. Schizophrenia is heritable with genetic factors accounting for around 80% of disease liability; there is also a higher incidence of schizophrenia with male gender. Other associations include a higher incidence with urbanicity, migration and cannabis use although these remain contentious and could occur as a consequence of the mental disorder rather than being a *prima facie* cause (Tandon, Keshavan and Nasrallah, 2008b).

The New Prescriber. Edited by J Lymn, D Bowskill, F Bath-Hextall, R Knaggs, © 2010 John Wiley & Sons.

Table 32.1   Positive symptoms of schizophrenia.

Symptoms/signs	Description
Delusional thinking	Firmly held beliefs are untrue and contrary to a person's educational and cultural background. This may include elements of persecution, jealousy, sin/guilt, grandiosity, religious, somatic, reference, control, mind reading, broadcasting, thought insertion and withdrawal.
Hallucinations	Perceptions experienced without external stimuli and can be auditory (including commands and commentary), visual, tactile, olfactory and gustatory.
Disorganised speech/thought disturbances	Associative loosening, illogical thinking, over-inclusive thinking, poverty of speech, poverty of content of speech, tangential replies, perseveration, distractibility, clanging, neologisms, echolalia and blocking. This lead to problems in organising ideas and speaking so that a listener can understand. Key amongst this are loose associations (cognitive slippage) with continual shifting from topic to topic without any apparent or logical connection between thoughts.
Disorganised or bizarre behaviour	Catatonic stupor, catatonic excitement, stereotypy, echopraxia, inappropriate mannerisms, automatic obedience, negativism. Deterioration of grooming, dress, abode, social behaviour (public masturbation, shouting obscenities, etc.). Incongruity of affect (e.g. inappropriate smiling). Motor disturbances. Extreme activity levels (unusually high or low), peculiar body movements or postures (e.g. catatonic schizophrenia), strange gestures and grimaces.

Table 32.2   Negative symptoms of schizophrenia.

Symptoms/signs	Description
Anhedonia	An inability to feel pleasure along with a lack of interest or enjoyment in activities or relationships.
Avolition	An inability or lack of energy to engage in routine (e.g. personal hygiene) and/or goal-directed activities (e.g. work, school).
Alogia	A lack of meaningful speech. May take several forms, including poverty of speech (reduced amount of speech) and/or poverty of content of speech (little information is conveyed; vague, repetitive).
Asociality	Impairments in social relationships; few friends, poor social skills, little interest in being with other people.
Flat affect	No stimulus can elicit an emotional response. Patient may stare vacantly, with lifeless eyes and expressionless face. Voice may be toneless. Flat affect refers only to outward expression, not necessarily internal experience.

Section 3

Aetiology of schizophrenia

Genetic factors

While around two-thirds of cases occur sporadically, there is undoubtedly a genetic component to schizophrenia. There is a higher incidence in close relatives of schizophrenics but even in monozygotic twins there are many cases where only one sibling develops schizophrenia. There does not, however, seem to be any single major gene locus linked to the development of schizophrenia. Instead there seem to be multiple genetic polymorphisms each of which contributes a small effect (Tandon, Keshavan and Nasrallah, 2008b).

Developmental factors

There is a suggestion that there are critical periods in the development of the brain which, if adversely affected, may lead to schizophrenia. Structural magnetic resonance imaging in schizophrenia show that both whole-brain volume and grey matter volume are reduced. White matter abnormalities have also been reported and may be one of the key findings consistent with the dissociative thinking and cognitive defects observed in this illness (Keshavan *et al.*, 2008).

Biological factors

There are a variety of overlapping theories about the biological nature of schizophrenia. All of them relate to an alteration in CNS function that has a focus on the communication between the midbrain regions and the frontal cortex.

Pathogenesis of schizophrenia

The dopamine hypothesis

Dopamine excess is perhaps the most well-established theory with regard to the pathophysiology of schizophrenia, although most of the evidence for this theory is indirect. Key factors in the supporting evidence include:

- the hyperactivity found in the mesolimbic dopaminergic system, particularly the dopamine D_2 receptor linked paths
- the use of antipsychotics can produce tardive dyskinesia due to dopamine
- hypersensitivity (D_2 receptor population is upregulated by approximately 20–40%)
- antipsychotic drug efficacy is correlated to D_2 receptor blocking activity
- D_2 receptor agonists, such as amphetamine, worsen symptoms.

However, dopamine cannot be the only explanation of schizophrenia. For example, the newer 'atypical' antipsychotics have a broader range of activity including interaction with D_1, D_4 and $5HT_2$ receptors in frontal cortex and striatum. Atypical antipsychotic drugs have fewer extrapyramidal effects (similar to the effects of Parkinson's disease), because of less D_2 receptor activity. Additionally, the complete blockade of D_2 receptors does not completely alleviate all schizophrenic symptoms.

The glutamate hypothesis

In the search for other explanations for neurochemical imbalance leading to schizophrenia, researchers found decreased activity and concentration of glutamate in schizophrenic brains. This was particularly notable in drug addicts taking phenylcyclohexylpiperidine (PCP) and ketamine; these are NMDA receptor antagonists and their use causes negative schizophrenic-like symptoms and can exacerbate chronic schizophrenia. Postmortem studies have reported reduced expression of NMDA glutamate receptors in a variety of brain regions (Keshavan *et al.*, 2008). Subsequent investigations revealed that atypical antipsychotics increase NMDA receptor activity, by acting through the D_2 receptors.

 Practice application

Many schizophrenics are avid smokers, but what you may not have thought about is that nicotine increases NMDA receptor activity, and they may in fact be self-medicating.

The serotonin hypothesis

The serotonin hypothesis is closely linked with the glutamate hypothesis. This hypothesis arose from studies on interactions between the hallucinogenic drug LSD and 5HT. Both the major classes of psychedelic hallucinogens, the indoleamines (e.g. LSD) and phenethylamines (e.g. mescaline), produce their central effects through an action on $5HT_{2A}$ receptors in the locus coeruleus and the cerebral cortex which enhances glutamatergic transmission. Many atypical antipsychotic drugs show a greater affinity for $5HT_{2A}$ than D_2 receptors and the role of serotonergic antagonism in mitigating the extrapyramidal effects of antipsychotics is well established (Keshavan *et al.*, 2008).

What is clear is that the neurochemistry involved with schizophrenia is complex and multi-factorial.

Treatment of schizophrenia

The aims of treatments for schizophrenia are to minimise the impairment and achieve the best level of mental functioning. Although a range of social and psychological therapies is used in the management of schizophrenia, appropriate and timely drug treatment is essential too. There are two main types of antipsychotic drugs: the so-called 'typical' older antipsychotic drugs (such as chlorpromazine and haloperidol) and the newer 'atypical' antipsychotic drugs (like olanzapine and respiridone). The 'typical' antipsychotic drugs are predominately D_2 receptor antagonists and are most effective in the management of the positive symptoms (Table 32.1) of schizophrenia. The 'atypical' antipsychotic drugs interact with other dopamine receptor subtypes and also alter the function of other neurotransmitters (e.g. 5HT) as well as the D_2 receptors. Atypical antipsychotic drugs are more effective in treating the negative symptoms (Table 32.2) of schizophrenia than typical antipsychotic drugs.

Table 32.3   Receptor targets of typical antipsychotic drugs.

Antipsychotic	Confirmed receptor targets
Haloperidol	D_2, D_3 and D_4 receptor antagonist (primarily D_2 receptor block)
Loxapine	D_2/D_4 antagonist, $5HT_{2A/2B}$ and $5HT_7$ antagonist
Chlorpromazine	D_2 antagonist, H_1 antagonist
Fluphenazine	D_1/D_2 antagonist, H_1 antagonist
Thioridazine	D_2 receptor antagonist, with reduced extrapyramidal side effects, calcium channel blocker

Typical antipsychotics

Typical antipsychotic drugs all act as dopamine receptor antagonists and so block the action of dopamine in the brain. The therapeutic effect of antipsychotic drugs is thought to be the result primarily of D_2 receptor blockade. This does not mean, however, that antipsychotics act only to block D_2 receptors. Indeed, these drugs act as antagonists at other dopamine receptors as well as muscarinic, adrenergic, histamine H_1 and serotonergic receptors (Table 32.3), which may account for the side-effect profiles seen with these drugs.

Side effects

Interaction with D_2 receptors in other neuronal pathways in the brain results in the so-called 'extrapyramidal' side effects of antipsychotic drugs. These effects include dystonias (spasm of face and neck muscles), rigidity (slowness of movement and initiation of movement), tardive dyskinesia (repetitive 'tic'-like movements) and akathisia (motor restlessness). As dopamine usually increases the secretion of prolactin from the pituitary gland, blockade with a typical antipsychotic can lead to gynaecomastia in men and galactorrhoea.

 Stop and think

What side effects of typical antipsychotic drugs does antagonism at the alpha-1-adrenoceptor, muscarinic acetylcholine receptor and histamine H_1 receptor produce?

Neuroleptic malignant syndrome is a rare but potentially fatal side effect of antipsychotic drugs. It is characterised by hyperthermia, muscle rigidity and autonomic instability. Discontinuation of the antipsychotic drug is essential as there is no known wholly successful treatment.

Typical antipsychotics may potentiate the effects of CNS depressants such as anaesthetics, opioids and alcohol. All typical antipsychotic drugs should be administered with caution to patients with cardiovascular disorders, because of the possibility of transient hypotension and/or precipitation of angina pain.

Interactions

While there are many drug interactions listed in the British National Formulary for antipsychotic drugs, relatively few are of clinical significance. Propranolol increases the plasma concentrations of chlorpromazine and carbamazepine increases the metabolism of haloperidol. Drugs that inhibit the CYP2D6 isozyme (e.g. fluoxetine and paroxetine) and certain other drugs (e.g. fluvoxamine, propranolol and pindolol) appear to appreciably inhibit the metabolism of thioridazine. The resulting elevated levels of thioridazine would be expected to augment the prolongation of the QTc interval, leading to arrhythmia.

 Stop and think

Can you describe the mechanism by which carbamazepine increases the metabolism of haloperidol?

 Practice application

Many schizophrenic patients struggle to remember to take medication on a regular basis. Some antipsychotic medicines have been formulated as long-acting depot injections that need only be given every 2–4 weeks by deep intramuscular injection. Following injection of the drug, it is slowly released from the vehicle over a period of 2–4 weeks.

Atypical antipsychotics

Atypical antipsychotic drugs, like the typical antipsychotics, block the dopaminergic pathways but also block the serotonergic pathways from the raphe nucleus to the basal ganglia, limbic structures and the entire cortex (Table 32.4). This results in fewer extrapyramidal side effects and more effective treatment of the negative symptoms of schizophrenia. Aripiprazole differs from all other typical and 'atypical' antipsychotic drugs by acting as a partial agonist at D_2 receptors, distinguishing its action from the full antagonist profile of other antipsychotics (Mamo *et al.*, 2007).

Side effects

Atypical antipsychotics are not, however, without side effects. There are important differences between the 'atypical' antipsychotics in terms of the side effects they produce and these side effects are often dose related and can be affected by patient age and gender (Haddad and Sharma, 2007). It is important therefore to have a clear idea of the potential adverse reactions before starting treatment.

- The risk of developing acute extrapyramidal symptoms is particularly high for risperidone, with the highest risk being with high doses.

Section 3

Table 32.4 Receptor targets of atypical antipsychotic drugs.

Antipsychotic	Confirmed receptor targets
Risperidone	Antagonist with high affinity for D_2, weak affinity for D_1. Antagonist with high affinity for $5HT_2$, alpha-1 and alpha-2, and H_1. Lower affinity for $5HT_{1C}$, $5HT_{1D}$ and $5HT_{1A}$; weak affinity for haloperidol-sensitive sigma site.
Quetiapine	Antagonist at D_1 and D_2. Antagonist at $5HT_{1A}$ and $5HT_2$, H_1, plus alpha-1 and alpha-2.
Olanzapine	Antagonist with high affinity binding to D_{1-4}. Antagonist with high affinity binding to $5HT_{2A/2C}$, M_{1-5}, H_1 and alpha-1-receptors. Binds weakly to $GABA_A$, BZD and beta-adrenergic receptors.
Aripiprazole	Agonist/antagonist with high affinity for $5HT_{1A}$ and $5HT_{2A}$ receptors; moderate affinity for $5HT_{2C}$, $5HT_7$, alpha-1 and H_1 receptors, and moderate affinity for the serotonin reuptake site. Partial agonist at the $5HT_{1A}$ receptor, antagonist at $5HT_{2A}$ receptor.
Clozapine	Selective antagonist for D_4 receptor. Antagonist at $5\text{-}HT_{2A}$, $5\text{-}HT_{2C}$, $5\text{-}HT_3$, $5\text{-}HT_6$ and $5\text{-}HT_7$ receptors.

- Risk of agranulocytosis, particularly with clozapine. Patients being treated must have a baseline white blood cell and differential count before initiation of treatment as well as regular white blood cell counts during treatment and for 4 weeks after discontinuation.
- Seizures have been associated with the use of atypical antipsychotics, with a greater likelihood at higher doses; this is particularly true for clozapine.
- Prolongation of the ECG QTc interval; highest risk with ziprasidone and sertindole.
- Significant weight gain; highest risk with olanzapine and clozapine.
- Hyperprolactinaemia; highest risk with risperidone.

Interactions

There are a large number of potential drug interactions with atypical antipsychotic drugs listed in the BNF, many of which are associated with modulation of cytochrome P450 activity, including:

- fluoxetine and paroxetine increase the plasma concentration of risperidone
- plasma concentration of aripiprazole is decreased by St John's wort
- metabolism of olanzapine, quetiapine, risperidone and sertindole is accelerated by carbamazepine and phenytoin
- metabolism of aripiprazole is inhibited by ketoconazole.

Atypical antipsychotics are currently more expensive than the older typical antipsychotics and are not necessarily associated with higher quality-adjusted life-years (Davies et al., 2007). The variability in terms of pharmacodynamics and tolerability of 'atypical' antipsychotics also suggests that it may be a mistake to regard them as being a uniform drug class. Instead, selection of an antipsychotic should be on an individual patient basis.

Table 32.5   Other uses of antipsychotic drugs.

Drug	Other prescribed uses
Haloperidol	Control of motor tics including verbal tics linked with Tourette's disorder. Nausea and vomiting. Control of violent behaviour in children failing to respond to psychotherapy or other drugs.
Chlorpromazine	Treatment of mania in bipolar disorder. Control of violent behaviour in children. Control of nausea and vomiting, to relieve hiccups lasting 1 month or longer, and to relieve restlessness and nervousness that may occur just before surgery. Treatment of acute intermittent porphyria. Used along with other medications to treat tetanus.
Risperidone	Used to treat episodes of mania or mixed episodes in adults and teenagers, and children 10 years of age and older with bipolar disorder. Used to treat behaviour problems such as aggression, self-injury and sudden mood changes in teenagers and children 5–16 years of age who have autism.
Aripiprazole	Used with an antidepressant to treat depression when symptoms cannot be controlled by the antidepressant alone.

 Practice application

Atypical antipsychotics should be considered when choosing first-line treatment of newly diagnosed schizophrenia (NICE, 2009).

Other uses of antipsychotics

Many antipsychotic drugs have clinical uses other than controlling aspects of psychotic disorders (Table 32.5).

Summary

- Schizophrenia is a psychotic disorder in which thinking and emotion are impaired and the individual has trouble with social and occupational function.
- Schizophrenia is heritable, with a greater incidence in the male gender.
- Environmental risk factors for developing schizophrenia include urbanicity and migration.
- Genetic, developmental and biological factors all contribute to the development of schizophrenia.
- The three main biological hypotheses underlying schizophrenia involve alteration in dopamine, glutamate and serotonin function in the midbrain and frontal cortex.
- Antipsychotic drugs are currently classified as 'typical' (chlorpromazine, haloperidol) or 'atypical' (olanzapine, rispiridone).

Section 3

- Typical antipsychotic drugs all act as dopamine receptor antagonists.
- Typical antipsychotic drugs have more significant antagonist effects on muscarinic, histamine H_1 and alpha-1-adrenergic receptors.
- Atypical antipsychotics block the typical antipsychotic pathways plus the serotonergic pathways from the raphe nucleus to the basal ganglia, limbic structures and the entire cortex.
- Atypical antipsychotics have fewer extrapyramidal side effects.
- Atypical antipsychotics exhibit variations in tolerability and side effects and should be considered individually.

Activity

1. The more closely related a person is to someone with schizophrenia, the more likely they are to show psychoses associated with schizophrenia. True / False
2. Risk factors for schizophrenia include environmental factors such as urbanicity. True / False
3. Antipsychotic drug efficacy is correlated to D_2 blocking activity. True / False
4. The complete blockade of D_2 receptors completely alleviates all schizophrenic symptoms. True / False
5. Typical antipsychotic drugs are most effective in managing positive symptoms of schizophrenia. True / False
6. Typical antipsychotics do not antagonise muscarinic, histaminergic or adrenergic receptors. True / False
7. Typical antipsychotics do not potentiate the action of opioids. True / False
8. Atypical antipsychotics have fewer extrapyramidal side effects. True / False
9. Weight gain can be a major side effect of atypical antipsychotics. True / False
10. All atypical antipsychotics act as full antagonists at D_2 receptors. True / False

Useful websites

NICE guidance on schizophrenia – quick reference guide. http://www.nice.org.uk/Guidance/CG82/QuickRefGuide/pdf/English

Mental Health and Psychology Directory. http://www.psychnet-uk.com

References

Davies, L.M., Lewis, S., Jones, P.B., *et al.*, on behalf of the CUtLASS Team (2007) Cost-effectiveness of first- v. second-generation antipsychotic drugs: results from a randomised controlled trial in schizophrenia responding poorly to previous therapy. *Br J Psychiatry*, **191**, 14–22.

Haddad, P.M. and Sharma, S.G. (2007) Adverse effects of atypical antipsychotics: differential risk and clinical implications. *CNS Drugs*, **21**, 911–936.

Section 3

Keshavan, M.S., Tandon, R., Boutros, N.N. and Nasrallah, H.A. (2008) Schizophrenia, 'just the facts'. What we know in 2008. Part 3: Neurobiology. *Schizophr Res*, **106**, 89–107.

Mamo, D., Graff, A., Shammi, C.M., *et al.* (2007) Differential effects of aripiprazole on D2, 5-HT2 and 5-HT1A receptor occupancy in patients with schizophrenia: a triple tracer PET study. *Am J Psychiatry*, **164**, 1411–1417.

National Institute for Health and Clinical Excellence (2009) *Clinical Guideline 82: Schizophrenia. Core Interventions in the Treatment and Management of Schizophrenia in Adults in Primary and Secondary Care*, National Institute for Health and Clinical Excellence, London.

Tandon, R., Keshavan, M.S. and Nasrallah, H.A. (2008a) Schizophrenia, 'Just the Facts'. What we know in 2008. Part 2: Epidemiology and etiology. *Schizophr Res*, **102**, 1–18.

Tandon, R., Keshavan, M.S. and Nasrallah, H.A. (2008b) Schizophrenia, 'Just the Facts'. What we know in 2008. Part 1: Overview. *Schizophr Res*, **100**, 4–19.

World Health Organization (2001) *Mental Health Report 2001. Mental Health: New Understanding, New Hope*, World Health Organization, Geneva.

Further reading

Bennett, P.N. and Brown, M.J. (2003) *Clinical Pharmacology*, 9th edn, Churchill Livingstone, Edinburgh.

British Medical Association and Royal Pharmaceutical Society of Great Britain (2010) *British National Formulary*, 59th edn, BMJ Publishing, London.

Kruk, Z.L. and Pycock, C.J. (1991) *Neurotransmitters and Drugs*, 3rd edn, Chapman and Hall, London.

Rang, H.P., Dale, M.M., Ritter, J.M. and Flower, R. (2007) *Rang and Dale's Pharmacology*, 6th edn, Churchill Livingstone, Edinburgh.

Wagner, H. and Silber, K. (2004) *Instant Notes: Physiological Psychology*, BIOS Scientific Publishers, Oxford.

Webster, R.A. and Jordan, C.C. (1989) *Neurotransmitters, Drugs and Disease*, Blackwell Scientific, Oxford.

Section 3

33 Epilepsy and anticonvulsant drugs

Learning outcomes

By the end of this chapter the reader should be able to:

- understand the mechanisms of epileptic seizures
- understand the mechanisms of action, clinical uses and adverse effects of key anticonvulsant drugs including carbamazepine, sodium valproate, phenytoin, clobazam, gabapentin and pregabalin, lamotrigine, levetiracetam, topiramate and zonisamide
- describe the use and potential problems of anticonvulsant use in pregnancy
- identify other uses of anticonvulsant drugs.

The epilepsies

The plural in this heading is deliberate because epilepsy is certainly not a single disease or even group of diseases. Adding together all the many dozens of types recognised by neurologists, it has been estimated that in most countries 0.5–1% of the population is affected (Aylward, 2008). In the UK, this means 300,000 people, if not more, making it the most common serious chronic neurological disease, more frequent than Parkinson's disease and much more common than multiple sclerosis. It is very likely that anyone in whatever clinical specialty, dealing with ages from infancy to old age, will encounter patients with epilepsy. It should be appreciated that anyone can have an epileptic seizure given the right stimulus, and it can occur in previously unaffected individuals after head injury or stroke, or in the presence of a primary or secondary brain tumour (Duncan *et al.*, 2006).

In all cases the abnormality is related to unregulated electrical discharges occurring in one part of the brain, which may remain localised or become widespread. Recent research indicates that there may be abnormal electrical activity well before a seizure occurs and that some patterns are highly predictive, though the methods for recording these are not routinely available to clinicians (Dichter, 2009). In fact, it is notable that diagnosis of epilepsy is not necessarily clear-cut or straightforward, but this difficult area is (fortunately) outside the remit of this chapter. It is clear, however, that most epilepsies are idiopathic, a rather elaborate term to describe the fact that we do not know their origin.

Classification of epilepsies

Classification of the epilepsies is not straightforward in detail but can be simplified. A practical scheme is as follows.

Focal seizures

These start from one part of the brain and may be confined to that part or may become generalised. A particularly important type of complex seizure, known as temporal lobe epilepsy, can have a wide range of sensory and behavioural effects, as well as motor ones.

Generalised seizures

These are generalised from the outset. This includes the most widely known types of seizures including tonic-clonic (formerly known as grand mal) and absence seizures (petit mal). Also included are the myoclonic epilepsies, characterised by muscle jerking without necessarily impaired consciousness, many of which occur as part of complex genetic syndromes in children.

Treatment choices

There is certainly no absolute agreement on which antiepileptic (anticonvulsant) drugs are preferred in particular syndromes, though ideas are converging more than they used to and there is general consensus on some fundamental principles of treatment (Box 33.1). Unfortunately, unlike the situation in many other branches of therapeutics, it is very difficult to group anticonvulsants in classes which are of any practical use. The following is a reasonable example of current UK practice (Table 33.1) and is compatible with the relevant NICE guidelines,

---

Box 33.1 Fundamental principles of epilepsy treatment.

Discuss a management plan in detail with the patient and, if appropriate, parents, partners and carers.

Try to use a single anticonvulsant drug (monotherapy).

Start this at a low dose and increase gradually until seizures are controlled or serious side effects occur.

If the drug needs to be changed, usually establish new drug before withdrawing the previous one.

Be aware of drug interactions, even with monotherapy if the patients is on other types of medication, but especially if it is necessary to use two or very rarely more anticonvulsants.

Drug withdrawal, in seizure-free patients, must be gradual; if the patient is taking two or more drugs, only one should be withdrawn at a time.

Section 3

Table 33.1 Current UK practice for the treatment of epilepsy.

	First-line drugs	Second-line drugs	Third-line drugs
Focal (localised)	Carbamazepine Lamotrigine	Levetiracetam Topiramate Zonisamide	Gabapentin Phenytoin (+ many others)
Generalised (tonic-clonic)	Sodium valproate Lamotrigine	Levetiracetam Zonisomide	
Generalised (absence)	Ethosuximide Sodium valproate	Clobazam Topiramate	
Generalised (myoclonic)	Sodium valproate	Clobazam Lamotrigine Zonisamide	

and is certainly not an exhaustive list. Note that this chapter will not discuss the emergency management of epilepsy. There is more detailed discussion in the review of guidelines – of course, these vary from place to place and change constantly (Aylward, 2008).

Phenytoin and phenobarbital, once very widely used for many seizure types, have now been very largely relegated to third-line roles because of the introduction of newer, more effective drugs and, especially with regard to phenytoin, many serious adverse effects. Phenytoin is, however, still used for acute situations such as status epilepticus and this is unlikely to change in the near future.

The following section will consider individual drugs and their properties. The basic molecular mechanisms will be mentioned only briefly, as they rarely help in predicting the activity of the drug and in any case are often incompletely understood. There has been a very welcome increase in new drug therapies in the last decade but unlike, say, for asthma or hypertension, it is difficult if not impossible to create a coherent system for classifying both old and new drugs. This will not change, in the near future at least. There is a strong emphasis on adverse effects and interactions, as these are extremely important considerations in anticonvulsant therapy.

Summary of drug properties

The exact mechanism of action of many of the anticonvulsant drugs is not well understood but they all act to reduce abnormal neuronal excitability (Chapter 29). In the main, this is as a result of modulating voltage-gated ion channels, increasing GABA transmission and inhibiting glutamate transmission (Figure 33.1).

Carbamazepine

One of the most widely used of all anticonvulsants, for the indications already noted. The main mechanism is inhibition of sodium channels in brain nerve cells, causing them to be less active electrically. It is now commonly used in a modified-release formulation. The common adverse effects involve the brain, with drowsiness, dizziness, poor concentration and impaired co-ordination, all of which are dose dependent. The most serious, though rare, adverse effect is bone marrow suppression particularly affecting neutrophils, which can be severe and even fatal. Another uncommon but serious problem is the syndrome of inappropriate antidiuretic hormone (SIADH) secretion, when the drug stimulates the pituitary to secrete antidiuretic

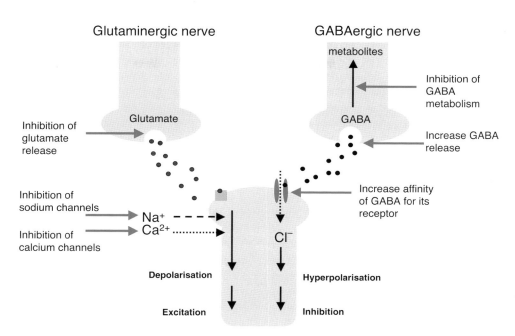

Glutaminergic nerve   GABAergic nerve

Figure 33.1   Potential targets for anticonvulsant drugs (adapted from Dawson, Taylor and Reide, 2002).

hormone, retaining water and effectively diluting the blood. The very low plasma sodium levels are potentially dangerous.

As regards interactions, this drug presents major problems. It is a very potent inducer of a number of cytochrome P450 (CYP450) enzymes in the liver, including CYP2C19 and CYP3A4. It increases the rate of its own metabolism as well as that of other drugs like the oral contraceptive pill and warfarin, making all these less effective. Co-prescribing with other drugs can therefore cause major problems. Therapeutic drug monitoring (TDM), that is, the measurement of plasma drug levels to guide treatment, may be useful.

Oxcarbazepine is a structural derivative of carbamazepine which is a less potent inducer of CYP450 enzymes and is associated with fewer side effects, making it a safer alternative to carbamazepine in some patients.

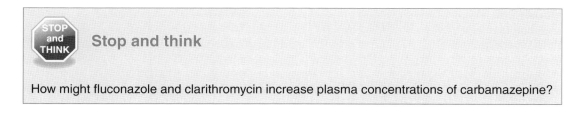

Stop and think

How might fluconazole and clarithromycin increase plasma concentrations of carbamazepine?

Sodium valproate

This chemically very simple drug is probably the nearest there is at present to a truly broad-spectrum anticonvulsant, being effective in most situations. Despite its simplicity, or more likely

Section 3

because of it, it has multiple mechanisms of action, including both sodium and calcium channel blockade and effects on the GABA system. Adverse effects are common and varied. Nausea and even vomiting usually occur early and then diminish, and the expected sedating effects are frequent. Much more serious is the very rare occurrence of liver toxicity (probably well under 1 in 10,000 patients) but this can be fatal. Other problems include thrombocytopenia, acute pancreatitis and (usually) temporary hair loss.

Interactions are less common than with, say, carbamazepine, but they are unpredictable and any combination with phenytoin should be avoided. Some increase in valproate metabolism can occur with carbamazepine.

Phenytoin

For much of the second half of the last century, phenytoin was the most widely used anticonvulsant. As other drugs have been introduced, its use has declined quite rapidly, though in its intravenous form it is still important in status epilepticus. It blocks both sodium and calcium channels, though the relevance of the latter is uncertain. One of the problems associated with phenytoin is that its rate of metabolism changes depending on the dose given and hence its half-life varies markedly. It has a quite extraordinary range of adverse effects, rivalled in their variety only by the corticosteroids. They include, apart from the expected sedation, long-term effects on learning and memory; rarely damage to the cerebellum in the brain, leading to long-term loss of co-ordination; gum hypertrophy, sometimes leading to loss of teeth; SIADH, as with carbamazepine; enlarged lymph nodes and very rarely lymphoma; megaloblastic anaemia, due to increased metabolism of folic acid; osteomalacia, due to increased metabolism of vitamin D; liver toxicity; peripheral neuropathy; skin rashes; and many more.

Interactions are also a major problem. Again like carbamazepine, it is a very potent CYP450 inducer, with effects on other drugs and itself alongside being a target for other drugs which alter the CYP450 system. Phenytoin is also highly plasma protein bound and drugs such as aspirin and sodium valproate compete for the plasma albumin binding sites and displace phenytoin. Altogether, a drug more suitable for exam questions than clinical use, if alternatives exist! However, if it is used, TDM can be useful in guiding treatment.

Practice application

If using therapeutic drug monitoring of plasma phenytoin levels, it is important to know both plasma albumin and free phenytoin levels.

Clobazam and other benzodiazepines

Clobazam and clonazepam have limited uses in oral maintenance therapy, while diazepam and lorazepam are given intravenously for severe persistent seizures (status epilepticus, usually a term for fits lasting 30 minutes or more, a medical emergency). They indirectly increase the activity of the inhibitory neurotransmitter gamma-aminobutyric acid (GABA) in the brain (Chapter 29). Adverse effects are, not surprisingly, sedation and dizziness. It is very important to remember that stopping this type of drug suddenly may trigger seizures, even in those who have never had them before, for instance in those taking benzodiazepines as sedatives rather than anticonvulsants. There are no significant interactions, except that other CNS depressants, such as alcohol, will increase the sedative effect.

Stop and think

Why might inhibition of glutamate transmission or increased GABA transmission be useful in the treatment of epilepsy?

Gabapentin and pregabalin

These are two closely related compounds, though pregabalin may have slightly better absorption properties. Although they were originally thought to mimic GABA, their mechanism is rather more complex, but involves reduction in the amount of excitatory transmitters in the brain; that is, those that may activate seizures. In general, they have not proved quite as effective as had been hoped and are now probably more often used for non-anticonvulsant indications (see below). Adverse effects are again related to sedation and dizziness and interactions are not relevant except with other CNS depressants.

Lamotrigine

Although it is a relatively new drug, lamotrigine is very widely prescribed in several types of epilepsy. It also affects sodium channels in the brain. It is exceptionally well absorbed and generally well tolerated, apart from the usual dose-related sedation, but with one important adverse reaction: up to 30% of patients, regardless of dose, are affected by a generalised rash. The drug must be stopped if this happens, as in a minority of cases the rash can develop into a very serious and potentially lethal condition called the Stevens-Johnson syndrome which can cause multiorgan failure. Lamotrigine is metabolised by the CYP450 system, though it neither inhibits nor induces it. However, interactions can occur as it is affected by drugs which do alter the system, such as carbamazepine or inhibitors like the macrolide antibiotics.

Practice application

Dosing of lamotrigine varies according to the other drugs a patient is currently taking.

Levetiracetam

This is an even more recent anticonvulsant, but it is increasingly regarded as very promising in a range of epilepsies. At the moment, this is mostly as add-on therapy but it is likely to become more prominent as monotherapy. It appears to have a unique mechanism of action,

Section 3

modulating neurotransmitter release. As usual, adverse effects include sedation and dizziness but there appear to be no unusual ones. Interactions are also lacking.

Topiramate

This relatively new drug has attracted interest for both its efficacy and its unusual spectrum of side effects. It interacts with sodium channels, potentiates the effects of GABA and blocks the glutamate receptors, an excitatory neurotransmitter that can destabilise neurons. Adverse effects include sedation, as might be expected, but also more serious impairment of memory and concentration, acute glaucoma, renal stones, reduced sweating and anorexia with weight loss. Although some patients might welcome this, in fact it can be very severe and potentially dangerous. With respect to interactions, it is a weak CYP450 inducer but paradoxically increases plasma concentrations of phenytoin.

Zonisamide

This again is a chemically unusual anticonvulsant, related to the sulphonamides which were once used as antibiotics and more distantly to diuretics like the thiazides. Again, its action involves blockade of sodium channels, reduction of voltage-dependent calcium channels and reduction of glutamate-induced transmission (Macleod and Appleton, 2007) and its use is increasing in several types of epilepsy. Although it is structurally quite different, several of the adverse effects resemble those of topiramate, though it does not cause acute glaucoma. It is also subject to numerous interactions, particularly with enzyme inducers such as carbamazepine which will reduce its concentration: interaction with enzyme inhibitors is less well documented.

Anticonvulsants and pregnancy

This is a very difficult and sensitive topic, and is of obvious relevance as many patients with epilepsies are women of child-bearing age. A recent systematic review summarises current views (Meador *et al.*, 2008). The use of anticonvulsant drugs increases the risk of congenital malformations 2–3-fold; those associated with neural tube defects such as spina bifida were most prominent compared to mothers not on anticonvulsants. The incidence of facial malformations, such as cleft palate, was also increased. The figures show an increase in incidence of birth defects from 2–3% to about 7% overall. In terms of monotherapy, sodium valproate and carbamazepine are associated with the highest risks, while low-dose lamotrigine appears to be safest. Combination drug therapies also considerably increase risk. These risks may be reduced by high-dose folic acid supplements before and during pregnancy.

 Practice application

The increased risk of teratogenicity associated with antiepileptic drugs requires detailed and careful discussion with women who are pregnant or may conceive, bearing in mind that the great majority of babies are entirely normal and that failure to control seizures is a very serious risk to mother and especially the baby.

Uses of anticonvulsant drugs in non-epileptic conditions

There is increasing use of the drugs described above for conditions totally unrelated to epilepsy. These currently include the following main categories, with the main drugs listed for each.

● Neuropathic pain syndromes, such as trigeminal neuralgia, postherpetic neuralgia and diabetic neuropathy (gabapentin, pregabalin, carbamazepine). These are conditions where conventional analgesics, including non-steroidal anti-inflammatory drugs and even opioids, are of limited efficacy.
● Mood stabilisation in bipolar affective disorders, often as a substitute for lithium, particularly for preventing the manic phase of this condition (carbamazepine, lamotrigine and sodium valproate).
● Migraine prophylaxis in patients with frequent attacks not prevented by beta-blockers or tricyclic drugs, or patients who cannot tolerate these (topiramate, sodium valproate).

Other possible indications include anxiety, depression and addictive states (Chapter 31). In most of these situations, even with quite well-established indications, the clinical trial evidence does need to be expanded if possible. A summary of drug action, interactions and other uses is shown in Table 33.2.

Future prospects

Anyone reading this chapter up to this point will appreciate that developing new antiepileptic drugs is of very real current interest. Even when existing drugs are effective, they often have severe and even dangerous adverse effects and may be prone to interactions with other anticonvulsants or many other drugs. There is also a minority of patients, possibly as many as 30% of the total, in whom none of the current drugs effectively suppress seizures even when used in combination. Some of these need radical and potentially damaging brain surgery. At any one time 15–20 new drugs may therefore be in development.

One area of research which should help in the better use of existing drugs is pharmacogenetics. Probably the simplest application of this concerns metabolism of drugs, particularly by the CYP450 system, where this information can help to individually adjust dosage to for maximum efficacy and minimal side effects. There are now increasing data on the genetics of one particular type of sodium channel which is involved in the mechanism of action of many anticonvulsants and may predict response to these. More surprisingly, patients with one tissue (HLA) type common in the Far East seem much more susceptible to a rare hypersensitivity reaction to carbamazepine (Löscher et al., 2009).

Summary

● Epilepsy is a serious, chronic neurological disease affecting around 1% of the population.
● Most epilepsies are idiopathic but they may also be the result of head injury, stroke and brain tumours.
● Epilepsies can be classified as either focal or generalised.

Section 3

Table 33.2 Summary of mechanism of action, drug interactions and other uses of antiepileptic drugs.

Drug	Proposed mechanism of action	Drug interactions	Other uses
Carbamazepine	Inhibition of voltage-activated sodium channels	Induces CYP2C19 and CYP3A4 Affected by drugs which induce and inhibit CYP3A4 activity	Bipolar disorder Neuropathic pain
Clonazepam	Increases GABA activity	Affected by drugs which induce and inhibit CYP450 activity	Anxiety
Gabapentin	Inhibits glutamate release Inhibition of calcium channels		Neuropathic pain Migraine
Lamotrigine	Inhibition of voltage-activated sodium channels. Inhibition of calcium channels and thus exocytosis	Affected by drugs which induce and inhibit CYP450 activity	Bipolar disorder Neuropathic pain
Levetiracetam	Inhibits the exocytosis of glutamate		Neuropathic pain
Phenytoin	Inhibition of voltage-activated sodium channels Inhibition of calcium channels	Induces CYP3A4 Affected by drugs which induce and inhibit CYP2C9 and CYP2C19 activity	
Sodium valproate	Increases GABA synthesis Inhibits GABA metabolism	Affected by drugs which induce and inhibit CYP2C9 activity	Bipolar disorder Neuropathic pain Migraine
Topiramate	Inhibition of voltage-activated sodium channels Potentiates effects of GABA Glutamate receptor antagonist	Weak inducer of CYP3A4	Migraine
Zonisamide	Inhibition of voltage-activated sodium channels Inhibition of calcium channels Enhances GABA release	Affected by drugs which induce and inhibit CYP3A4 activity	

- Treatment of epilepsy may require the use of more than one anticonvulsant drug, thereby increasing the likelihood of drug interactions and side effects.
- Anticonvulsant drugs reduce abnormal neuronal excitability.
- The main mechanism of action of anticonvulsant drugs is via an inhibition of sodium and/or calcium channels, inhibition of glutamate transmission and/or increasing GABA transmission.
- Some anticonvulsant drugs, including carbamazepine and phenytoin, are potent inducers of the cytochrome P450 system of enzymes.
- Plasma concentrations of many anticonvulsant drugs, including carbamazepine, phenytoin, lamotrigine, sodium valproate and zonisamide, are affected by CYP450 enzyme inducers and inhibitors.
- The use of anticonvulsant drugs in pregnancy has been linked to an increased risk of congenital malformations.
- Anticonvulsant drugs are also used for the treatment of neuropathic pain, bipolar disorder and migraine prophylaxis.

Activity

1. The most important neurotransmitters in epilepsy are GABA and glutamate.   True / False
2. Carbamazepine is recommended for use in absence seizures.   True / False
3. Phenytoin is a potent inducer of cytochrome P450.   True / False
4. The benzodiazepines such as clobazam act through the GABA system.   True / False
5. Anticonvulsant drugs rarely cause sedation.   True / False
6. Carbamazepine can increase the metabolism of sodium valproate.   True / False
7. The most common adverse reaction associated with lamotrigine is a generalised rash.   True / False
8. Sodium valproate and phenytoin are frequently used in combination.   True / False
9. Which of the following statements is most accurate with regard to anticonvulsant drugs in pregnancy?
   A. The use of anticonvulsants increases the rate of birth defects tenfold.
   B. Vitamin C may reduce the risk of foetal malformations.
   C. Sodium valproate is most likely to cause urinary tract abnormalities.
   D. Lamotrigine is relative safe in pregnancy at low doses.
   E. The withdrawal of anticonvulsants is generally recommended in the first trimester of pregnancy.
10. Anticonvulsant drugs can be used to treat trigeminal neuralgia.   True / False

Useful websites

NICE guidance: epilepsy in adults and children. www.guidance.nice.org.uk/index.jsp?action=download&o=29531

Epilepsy Action. www.epilepsy.org.uk/

Section 3

References

Aylward, R.L.M. (2008) Epilepsy: a review of reports, guidelines, recommendations and models for the provision of care for patients with epilepsy. *Clin Med*, **8**, 433-438.

Dichter, M.A. (2009) Emerging concepts in the pathogenesis of epilepsy and epileptgenesis. *Arch Neurol*, **66**, 443-447.

Duncan, J.S., Sander, J.W., Sisodiya, S.M. and Walker, M.C. (2006) Adult epilepsy. *Lancet*, **367**, 1087-1100.

Löscher, W., Klotz, U., Zimprich, F. and Schmidt, D. (2009) The clinical impact of pharmaco-genetics on the treatment of epilepsy. *Epilepsia*, **50**, 1-23.

Macleod, S. and Appleton, R.E. (2007) The new antiepileptic drugs. *Arch Dis Child Ed Pract*, **92**, 182-188.

Meador, K., Reynolds, M.W., Crean, S., *et al.* (2008) Pregnancy outcomes in women with epilepsy: a systematic review and meta-analysis of published pregnancy registries and cohorts. *Epilepsy Res*, **81**, 1-13.

Further reading

British Medical Association and Royal Pharmaceutical Society of Great Britain (2010) *British National Formulary*, 59th edn, BMJ Publishing, London.

Cader, S. and Cockerell, C. (2008) Epilepsy: current drug options and their recommended use. *Prescriber*, **5**, 31-47.

Dawson, J.S., Taylor, M.N.F. and Reide, P.J.W. (2002) *Pharmacology*, 2nd edn, Mosby, London.

Ettinger, A.B. and Argoff, C.E. (2007) Use of antiepileptic drugs for nonepileptic conditions: psychiatric disorders and chronic pain. *Neurotherapeutics*, **4**, 75-83.

Landmark, C.J. (2007) Targets for antiepileptic drugs in the synapse. *Med Sci Monit*, **13**, RA1-RA7.

Landmark, C.J. and Johanessen, S.I. (2008) Pharmacological management of epilepsy: recent advances and future prospects. *Drugs*, **68**, 1925-1939.

Perucca, E. (2005) Clinically relevant drug interactions with antiepileptic drugs. *Br J Clin Pharmacol*, **61**, 246-255.

Perucca, E., French, J. and Bialer, M. (2007) Development of new antiepileptic drugs: chal-lenges, incentives, and recent advances. *Lancet Neurol*, **6**, 793-804.

Pollard, J.R. and French, J. (2006) Antiepileptic drugs in development. *Lancet Neurol*, **5**, 2064-2067.

Rang, H.P., Dale, M.M., Ritter, J.M. and Flower, R. (2007) *Rang and Dale's Pharmacology*, 6th edn, Churchill Livingstone, Edinburgh.

34 Pain and analgesia

Learning outcomes

By the end of this chapter the reader should be able to:

- define pain and distinguish between the different types of pain
- briefly describe the processes involved in pain transmission
- outline the major steps in prostaglandin biosynthesis
- describe the gate control theory of pain and discuss its significance
- understand the basic and clinical pharmacology of simple analgesics, non-steroidal anti-inflammatory drugs and opioids
- understand the principles of the World Health Organization ladder for pain.

Pain, more than any other topic in this book, is something that we have all experienced. Persistent pain is a massive problem; in 2003 a Europe-wide telephone survey suggested that between 12% and 30% of people had persistent pain, defined as pain lasting for longer than 6 months (Breivik *et al.*, 2006), and this causes a great deal of suffering, which in turn affects quality of life. Before thinking about the drugs used to control pain in more detail, it is important to think about what pain actually is and how pain signals are transmitted in the body.

What is pain?

Put most simply, pain is what the patient says it is. Unlike many illnesses, there is no biochemical or physiological test that tells us how much pain someone is experiencing.

The International Association for the Study of Pain defines pain as 'An unpleasant sensory and emotional experience associated with actual or potential tissue damage or described in terms of such damage'. This helpful definition reminds us that pain is usually associated with some form of tissue damage and that although pain is predominantly a sensory phenomenon, emotion contributes to the degree of pain that someone is experiencing. In a report on the provision of acute pain services, the Royal College of Surgeons goes further, stating 'Pain does not occur in isolation but in a specific human being in psychosocial, economic and cultural contexts that influence the meaning, experience and verbal and non-verbal expression of pain'.

The New Prescriber. Edited by J Lymn, D Bowskill, F Bath-Hextall, R Knaggs, © 2010 John Wiley & Sons.

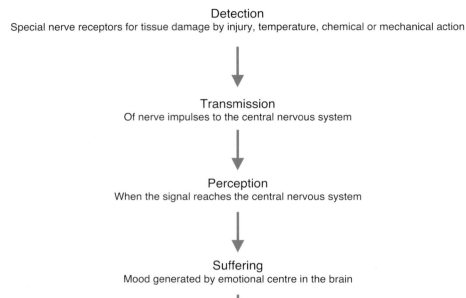

Detection
Special nerve receptors for tissue damage by injury, temperature, chemical or mechanical action

↓

Transmission
Of nerve impulses to the central nervous system

↓

Perception
When the signal reaches the central nervous system

↓

Suffering
Mood generated by emotional centre in the brain

↓

Outward behaviour

Figure 34.1   Physiology of pain.

Acute pain is something that we have all experienced and usually signals impending or actual tissue damage, allowing the individual to avoid further injury. Persistent pain is much harder to define. Previously it was defined as pain that lasts for longer than 6 months. More recently, it is thought of as pain that persists longer than normal healing; usually this is considered to be 3 months.

Pain physiology

The processes by which the body understands that someone is in pain can be thought of in a series of steps (Figure 34.1).

Pain detection

Initially, tissue damage is detected by special nerve receptors (nociceptors). There are different receptor types according to what has caused the injury. This may be because of temperature changes (too hot or cold), mechanical damage (pressure) and chemical changes (as occur in inflammation). The severity of the pain is influenced by the relative number of nociceptors (some areas of the body, such as the head and neck, have many more than others, the limbs for example) and by the frequency with which nerve impulses are generated by them. Damaged

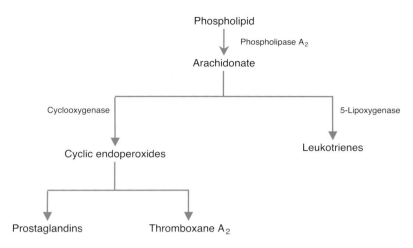

Figure 34.2   Synthesis of prostaglandins.

tissue releases many chemicals, including prostaglandins, histamine, bradykinin and serotonin, that increase the sensitivity of the nociceptors and act as mediators of inflammation.

Inflammatory mediators

Prostaglandins are a family of chemicals that are produced by phospholipids, found in the cell membrane of all human cells (Figure 34.2). Initially, arachidonic acid is formed from phospholipids found in cell membranes using the enzyme phospholipase A_2. Arachidonate is metabolised by two enzymes, lipoxygenase and cyclooxygenase (COX), to produce leukotrienes and endoperoxides respectively. Leukotrienes are inflammatory chemicals causing narrowing of the airways and blood vessels and increased capillary permeability but have little effect on pain. Prostaglandins and thromboxane A_2 are produced from the very unstable endoperoxides.

Prostaglandins, along with other hormones and chemicals, control a large number of normal physiological functions, including secretion of gastric acid, renal blood flow, salt and water excretion by the kidney, temperature regulation (Table 34.1). In addition, prostaglandins have been found to play an important role in local sensitisation of tissues to inflammatory mediators and pain perception.

In 1991, scientists discovered that two different genes code for cyclooxygenase enzymes and the enzymes were named COX-1 and COX-2. COX-1 is present in most tissues and is responsible for maintaining normal homeostasis and tissue function in many organs, such as the GI tract, kidney, lung and platelet. On the other hand, COX-2 is only produced in inflammatory states (Box 34.1). More recently, another form of the COX enzyme (COX-3) has been found in some animal models. The relevance of COX-3 to humans is still unclear.

Pain transmission

Once a painful stimulus has been generated, the signals are passed from the area of tissue damage to the spinal cord and ultimately to the brain. Individual nerve fibres covering the

Table 34.1 Physiological functions of prostaglandins.

Prostaglandin	Physiological function
PGD_2	Inhibits platelet aggregation
	Vasodilator
	Relaxation of GI and uterine smooth muscle
PGE_2	Vasodilator
	Increases gastric acid secretion
	Decreases mucus production in stomach
	Controls renal blood blow
	Alters Na^+ and water excretion from kidney
	Bronchoconstrictor
$PGF_{2\alpha}$	Bronchoconstrictor
	Myometrial contractions
PGI_2	Vasodilator
	Inhibition of gastric acid secretion
	Decreases mucus production in stomach
	Inhibits platelet aggregation
	Controls renal blood blow
	Alters Na^+ and water excretion from kidney

same area of skin join to make a single spinal nerve that enters the spinal cord. In the spinal cord these signals are processed before being sent to the brainstem. There is another synapse in the brainstem and a third neuron sends the signal to the cortex where the brain is able to determine where the pain is coming from (Figure 34.3).

There are relatively few places where drugs may modify transmission of pain signals:

● site of tissue damage or inflammation
● peripheral nerves carrying pain signals
● spinal cord
● brain.

Box 34.1 **Functions of different forms of COX enzyme.**

COX-1	COX-2	COX-3
Always present in most cells (constitutive)	Only induced in inflammatory cells	Normally present in the brain of some animals
Required for normal homeostasis:	Important in pain and inflammatory states	Involved in sensing pain
GI tract		
		Little involvement in inflammation
Kidney		
Platelet		

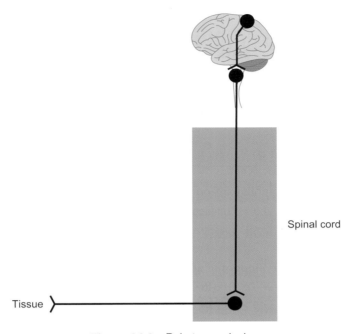

Figure 34.3   Pain transmission.

Gate control theory

The 'gate control' theory of pain suggests that the spinal cord has a key role in determining why some people develop persistent pain and takes into account both the physiological and psychological components of pain. The key principle of gate control theory is that impulses flow from the periphery to the brain through a 'gate' in the spinal cord, which may be opened or closed by other nerve circuits (Figure 34.4).

Put simply, the amount of stimulation passing through the gate is dependent upon the relative activities in large-diameter myelinated A-beta nerve fibres, smaller diameter A-delta nerve fibres and unmyelinated C nerve fibres. When the amount of information passing through the gate (i.e. C fibre activity is greater than A-beta fibre and A-delta fibre) reaches a critical level, there is increased activity in areas of the brain associated with pain experience and increases in the level of pain that a patient is experiencing. The gate is closed by increased stimulation of ascending A-beta nerves and descending signals from several brainstem areas.

Pain perception

In the brain there are many different nerve pathways that are activated when a painful stimulus is detected. These activate memories of previous painful experiences, interact with the emotional centres in the brain and are modified by cultural influences. The brainstem also probably helps initiate the response of the autonomic nervous system to pain, including the initiation of nervous impulses resulting in muscular contraction so that you move away from the source of the pain.

Section 3

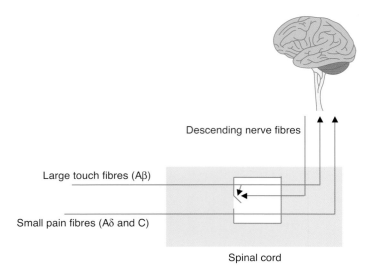

Descending nerve fibres

Large touch fibres (Aβ)

Small pain fibres (Aδ and C)

Spinal cord

Figure 34.4   Gate control theory (adapted from Stannard and Booth, 2005).

Analgesic pharmacology

Paracetamol

Paracetamol is regarded as the mainstay analgesic for almost all types of acute and persistent pain.

Mechanism of action

Despite being used in clinical practice for over 50 years, it is still unclear how paracetamol exerts its pharmacological effect, although it is thought that its mechanism of action is within the central nervous system as it has antipyretic effects (fever reducing) as well as being a painkiller. It has been suggested that possibly paracetamol interacts with the COX-3 enzyme (Chandrasekharan *et al.*, 2002), although other evidence suggests the neurotransmitter serotonin (5HT) may also be involved (Pelissier *et al.*, 1996).

Pharmacokinetics

Following oral administration, the bioavailability of paracetamol is around 60%. If given by the rectal route, bioavailability is much lower and much more variable. Therapeutic plasma levels are reached within 30 minutes of oral administration. The elimination half-life of paracetamol is relatively short ($t_{1/2} = 2$–4 hours), so frequent dosing is required to maintain its analgesic effect.

Paracetamol metabolism and toxicity

With normal doses the majority of paracetamol is metabolised and inactivated in the liver, undergoing a phase II conjugation reaction with glucuronic acid (Figure 34.5). A small proportion of a dose is metabolised using a CYP450-mediated reaction that forms a reactive intermediate, *N*-acteyl-*p*-benzoquinimine (NAPQI). Usually NAPQI can be deactivated by conjugation with

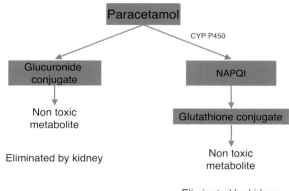

Figure 34.5 Paracetamol metabolism in liver. CYP450, cytochrome P450; NAPQI, *N*-acteyl-*p*-benzoquinimine.

glutathione in the liver. However, following ingestion of a large amount of paracetamol, the hepatic stores of both glucuronic acid and glutathione become depleted, leaving free NAPQI to cause liver damage. Toxicity may occur following ingestion of approximately twice the normal daily dose (14–16 paracetamol 500 mg tablets).

 Stop and think

Liver damage following paracetamol overdose occurs because the liver's supplies of glutathione are depleted. How is the paracetamol overdose treated?

Side effects

Thankfully, given the availability of paracetamol, side effects are uncommon. Occasionally rash, jaundice or an anaphylactic type reaction may occur.

Combination products

There are many over-the-counter preparations and several prescription products that contain paracetamol in addition to other products. These must always be considered prior to recommending and/or prescribing a paracetamol product.

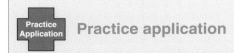 **Practice application**

Combination analgesic preparations (e.g. co-codamol and co-dydramol) containing varying amounts of paracetamol and a weak opioid are not recommended for routine prescribing as

Section 3

the opioid content is generally too low to be effective as an analgesic but is sufficient to cause opioid side effects. Co-proxamol was withdrawn from the UK market in 2007 because it was implicated in a significant number of suicides.

Non-steroidal anti-inflammatory drugs (NSAIDs)

Non-steroidal anti-inflammatory drugs are particularly effective in acute pain, such as tension headache and postoperative pain, and where the disease process produces significant inflammation (e.g. rheumatoid arthritis). Commonly prescribed NSAIDs include aspirin, ibuprofen, diclofenac, naproxen and indometacin.

Mechanism of action

Non-steroidal anti-inflammatory drugs are effective painkillers as they inhibit the enzyme cyclooxygenase, responsible for arachidonate metabolism to cyclic endoperoxides (Figure 34.2). By doing this, the production of prostaglandins and thromboxane A_2 is reduced.

 Stop and think

Given the normal physiological roles of prostaglandins, what potential side effects of NSAIDs can you predict?

Pharmacokinetics

All NSAIDs are almost completely absorbed after oral absorption, but the rate of absorption may be altered by changes in gastrointestinal (GI) blood flow or motility or if taken with food. Some NSAIDs have been formulated with an enteric coat that is only broken down in the small intestine to reduce the direct irritant effect on the GI mucosa. Most NSAIDs are weak organic acid compounds, so absorption does begin in the stomach but due to a much increased surface area, the majority occurs in the small intestine.

Following absorption, there is significant binding of NSAIDs to plasma proteins, including albumin (>95% in most cases). Reduction in the amount of serum albumin will result in more unbound drug in the systemic circulation, with potential additional harm. Because there is only a limited amount of plasma proteins, other drugs (e.g. oral anticoagulants such as warfarin) that are also highly bound to plasma proteins may compete for the albumin-binding sites and hence cause drug interactions.

Side effects

The side effects of NSAIDs are produced as a result of decreasing prostaglandin production required for normal body function, particularly in the GI and respiratory tracts, kidneys and platelets.

Although effective in conditions in which there is an inflammatory contribution to pain, NSAIDs have serious, potentially fatal side effects that may be remembered by the acronym 'GRAB'.

G – gastrointestinal

Gastrointestinal side effects are the most common unwanted effects of NSAIDs. These may be non-specific and less serious (e.g. dyspepsia, diarrhoea, nausea and vomiting) or more serious (e.g. ulceration, bleeding, intestinal obstruction). Each year there are around 2500 deaths in the UK directly related to NSAID use (Blower et al., 1997).

R – renal

In susceptible individuals, especially the elderly, NSAIDs may cause acute renal failure. Also, NSAIDs alter salt and water homeostasis which may worsen heart failure and produce a small increase in blood pressure.

A – asthma

Non-steroidal anti-inflammatory drugs, particularly aspirin, may worsen asthma in some patients.

B – blood disorders

All NSAIDs reduce platelet aggregation and increase the risk of bleeding, not just from the gastrointestinal tract.

Probably the safest NSAID as an analgesic is ibuprofen (200–400 mg three times daily). At higher doses (up to 800 mg three times daily) the incidence of side effects increases to levels similar to other NSAIDs.

 Stop and think

What is the underlying mechanism for NSAIDs to worsen control of asthma symptoms?

Cautions and contraindications

Non-steroidal anti-inflammatory drugs should be used with caution in patients with many other conditions.

Cardiac disease

Patients with hypertension, congestive heart failure, ischaemic heart disease, peripheral arterial disease or cerebrovascular disease need careful assessment before considering NSAID therapy due to an increased risk of thromboembolic events with some NSAIDs. Similar consideration should be made before initiating longer term treatment of patients with risk factors for cardiovascular events.

Section 3

Impaired cardiac or renal function, including patients being treated with diuretics
Non-steroidal anti-inflammatory drugs have the opposite effect to diuretics on salt and water elimination in the kidney, hence acting as physiological antagonists.

Haematological disorders
Due to an increased risk of bleeding.

Elderly
Increased incidence of gastrointestinal, renal and cardiac side effects.

Children under the age of 16 years
There is an increased chance of developing Reye's syndrome if aspirin is given to children.

Other contraindications
Due to the potential for side effects, NSAIDs are contraindicated in:

- active, or history of, gastrointestinal ulcers, bleeding or perforation
- previous hypersensitivity reactions (e.g. asthma, angio-oedema, urticaria or acute rhinitis) to ibuprofen, aspirin or other NSAIDs
- severe hepatic, renal or heart failure
- pregnancy (especially third trimester).

Routes of administration

Non-steroidal anti-inflammatory drugs have been formulated for administration by a variety of routes. The oral route is the most common and is the preferred route for both acute and chronic administration. If the area of inflammation is relatively localised, a topical NSAID may be considered (see The care and management of osteoarthritis in adults: NICE clinical guideline 59). A smaller number of NSAIDs (e.g. diclofenac, ketorolac, parecoxib) have been marketed as injections for parenteral administration, but serious side effects (e.g. abscess formation) have limited their routine use.

COX-2 selective drugs

Cyclooxygenase-2 selective inhibitors, or coxibs, were developed in an attempt to reduce the gastrointestinal side effects of NSAIDs. Clinical experience has demonstrated that coxibs are as effective as full NSAID comparators, but are no better. Gastrointestinal side effects are reduced but not eliminated and hence these drugs are best reserved for patients who have more significant risk factors for a GI bleed.

It now appears that COX-2 is important in normal physiology as well as pain and that a balance between COX-1 and COX-2 is necessary for optimum NSAID activity. Concern has been expressed about the cardiovascular safety of coxibs, and an increased incidence of myocardial infarction and stroke led to the withdrawal of rofecoxib in September 2004.

Those coxibs still available (celecoxib, etoricoxib) should not be given to patients with established ischaemic heart disease, cerebrovascular disease or symptomatic heart failure. Caution should be exercised if patients have risk factors for developing ischaemic heart disease (hypertension, hyperlipidaemia, diabetes mellitus and smoking).

Section 3

Practice application

The MHRA guidance on NSAID use suggests that the lowest effective dose of NSAID or COX-2 selective inhibitor should be prescribed for the shortest time necessary. The need for long-term treatment should be reviewed periodically.

- Prescribing should be based on the safety profiles of individual NSAIDs or COX-2 selective inhibitors, on individual patient risk profiles (e.g. gastrointestinal and cardiovascular).
- Prescribers should not switch between NSAIDs without careful consideration of the overall safety profile of the products and the patient's individual risk factors, as well as the patient's preferences.
- Concomitant aspirin (and possibly other antiplatelet drugs) greatly increases the gastrointestinal risks of NSAIDs and severely reduces any gastrointestinal safety advantages of COX-2 selective inhibitors. Aspirin should only be co-prescribed if absolutely necessary.

Opioids

Opioids have been used for thousands of years although morphine and other active constituents of the opium poppy were only extracted in the early 19th century. An opioid is any substance that produces morphine-like effects.

Opioids traditionally have been classified as either weak or strong (Box 34.2). Weak opioids have a lower analgesic potency, but are capable of producing profound side effects, including constipation and respiratory depression.

Mechanism of action

The human body has specific protein receptors for naturally occurring opioid compounds (the enkephalins and endorphins). Opioid drugs act by augmenting, or increasing, the effects of the enkephalins and endorphins in the spinal cord and brain. In the spinal cord, opioids prevent the transmission of pain signals through the 'gate' mechanism in the dorsal horn

Box 34.2   Opioid classification.

Weak opioids	Strong opioids
Codeine	Morphine
Dihydrocodeine	Oxycodone
Dextropropoxyphene	Fentanyl
Tramadol	Buprenorphine
	Methadone

Section 3

Table 34.2 Opioid receptor subtypes.

Receptor	Site of action	Physiological effects
MOP (OP$_3$) (μ)	Brainstem Spinal cord	Analgesia at spinal level Analgesia at supraspinal level Respiratory depression Sedation Euphoria Constipation
KOP (OP$_2$) (κ)	Cortex Brainstem Spinal cord	Analgesia at spinal level Sedation
DOR (OP$_1$)(δ)	Spinal cord	Analgesia Alteration of mood

and spinal reflexes. Descending signals from the brainstem back to the spinal cord are also modified.

Three types of opioid receptor have been identified, each contributing to the overall pharmacological effects observed (Table 34.2). Although predominantly found within areas of the CNS associated with processing of pain signals, opioid receptors are found in other CNS areas (e.g. those associated with control of breathing and the cough and vomiting reflexes) and other tissues, such as gastrointestinal tract.

Pharmacokinetics

The physical and chemical properties, and hence pharmacokinetics of opioids, vary considerably. A comprehensive description of the pharmacokinetics of individual opioids is beyond the scope of this book. If information is required, specialist data should be consulted.

Side effects

Side effects with opioids are numerous and include the following.

Nausea and vomiting
Brain areas associated with the regulation of vomiting (chemoreceptor trigger zone) can be stimulated when an opioid is given.

Constipation
Opioids increase smooth muscle tone and reduce motility in the GI tract, leading to constipation. Unlike other side effects, constipation tends to persist with prolonged opioid therapy. Prophylactic treatment with a stimulant laxative (e.g. senna) and faecal softener (e.g. docusate sodium) should be considered.

Sedation
Sedation and drowsiness are common on initiation of opioid therapy and on dose escalation. Most patients develop tolerance to these effects within days to weeks.

Respiratory depression

Breathing is controlled by several areas in the brainstem. These areas contain opioid receptors and are stimulated when a patient is given an opioid, leading to decreased frequency (i.e. respiratory rate) and depth (i.e. tidal volume) of breathing.

Hypotension

Opioids cause vasodilation by reducing tone of vascular smooth muscle and through local histamine release at the site of administration.

Urinary retention

Opioids cause urinary retention because of loss of the natural voiding reflex.

Other problems

Concerns regarding tolerance, dependence and addiction with long-term opioid use continue to trouble public and healthcare professionals alike and sometimes are barriers to effective pain relief.

Cautions and contraindications

Thankfully, there are relatively few cautions and contraindications when using opioids. In the treatment of pain, morphine should be used with caution in the following situations.

Hypotension

As opioids produce vasodilation, blood pressure may be lowered further.

Asthma/COPD, although not an absolute contraindication

Opioids cause central respiratory depression and may compromise breathing. For patients with existing respiratory disease, this may be problematic.

Ileus

If large quantities of oral opioid are given in the early postoperative period, significant amounts of morphine may be absorbed from the small intestine when gastrointestinal transit returns to normal. This has been implicated in deaths in the United Kingdom and other countries.

Hepatic and/or renal impairment

Empirical dose reduction or conversion to an alternative opioid may be necessary.

Pregnancy/breastfeeding

Lipophilic opioids may be transferred to the foetus and neonate in substantial quantities.

Routes of administration

Almost all routes of drug delivery have been used at some point with opioids. Patients who experience inadequate pain relief or intolerable side effects with one opioid often may be successfully treated with another opioid or with the same opioid delivered by a different route.

Practice application

Common routes of opioid administration include:

- oral (liquid, tablet, capsule)
- rectal
- parenteral (intramuscular, subcutaneous, intravenous)
- transdermal
- buccal
- spinal (epidural, intrathecal).

Other analgesics

A wide variety of other drugs (e.g. antidepressants, antiepileptics and muscle relaxants) may have a role in the management of specific types of persistent pain, but this is beyond the scope of this discussion. If further information is required, it is recommended to consult a specialist information source (Dickman and Simpson, 2008).

Practice application

Other drugs used for pain:

- antidepressants (e.g. amitriptyline, nortriptyline)
- antiepileptics (e.g. carbamazepine, gabapentin, pregabalin)
- corticosteroids
- nefopam
- local anaesthetics
- $5HT_1$ agonists (e.g. sumatriptan).

World Health Organization pain ladder

In 1986 the World Health Organization (WHO) proposed an analgesic ladder for use in cancer pain (Figure 34.6). One of the intentions of developing this ladder was to increase the availability and appropriate use of opioid analgesics in developing countries. Although not intended for use in other pain conditions, it provides a good basis for safe prescribing in other types of pain. In acute, severe pain (e.g. postoperative pain) it may be more appropriate to consider the ladder in reverse.

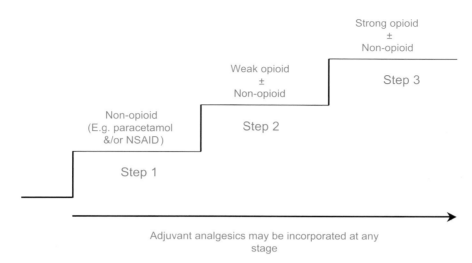

Figure 34.6   World Health Organization analgesic ladder.

Summary

- To feel a painful stimulus requires:
  - detection using specific receptors
  - transmission of the signals to the spinal cord and brain, and
  - interpretation and perception of those signals once they have reached the brain.
- The gate control theory recognises the importance of the spinal cord in interpreting painful stimuli and how physiological and psychological factors contribute to pain.
- Paracetamol is the mainstay of analgesia although its mechanism of action is not fully understood. To prevent liver and kidney damage, it is important that the maximum recommended dose is followed.
- Non-steroidal anti-inflammatory drugs are effective analgesics, inhibiting the production of the inflammatory prostaglandins. Despite their efficacy, side effects are relatively common and must be monitored.
- Opioids interact with specific opioid receptors.
- The WHO pain ladder provides a step-wise approach to analgesic use.

 Activity

For each of the statements in 1–10 choose the most appropriate option from A to L. Each option may be used once, more than once or not at all.

Section 3

Options

A.	Morphine	B.	Dihydrocodeine
C.	Ibuprofen	D.	Amitriptyline
E.	Gabapentin	F.	Paracetamol
G.	Glyceryl trinitrate	H.	Aspirin
I.	Buprenorphine	J.	Tramadol
K.	Diamorphine	L.	Oxycodone

1. A drug which should not be given to children under the age of 16 due to the risk of Reye's syndrome.
2. A drug that treats the pain associated with angina pectoris by producing vasodilation of coronary arteries.
3. A drug which would be appropriate to reduce fever in a 10-year-old boy.
4. A drug which would be appropriate to prevent further ischaemic events in a 65-year-old woman who has recently suffered a myocardial infarction.
5. An opioid drug used in the immediate treatment of a myocardial infarction.
6. A drug which would be appropriate to treat a 36-year-old man suffering from tennis elbow.
7. An opioid that is formulated for transdermal administration.
8. An opioid drug that is contraindicated in epilepsy.
9. An antiepileptic drug used in the management of neuropathic pain.
10. An opioid used almost exclusively in palliative care because of high water solubility that allows smaller volumes to be infused by the subcutaneous route.

Useful websites

MHRA guidance on use of coxibs and NSAIDs www.mhra.gov.uk/Safetyinformation/Generalsafetyinformationandadvice/Product-specificinformationandadvice/CardiovascularsafetyofCOX-2inhibitorsandnon-selectiveNSAIDs/CON019582

NICE. Osteo-arthritis and rheumatoid arthritis. COX-II inhibitors (review). www.nice.org.uk/guidance/index.jsp?action=byID&o=11687

Oxford pain website. www.medicine.ox.ac.uk/bandolier/booth/painpag/

References

Blower, A.L., Brooks, A., Fenn, G.C., *et al.* (1997) Emergency admissions for upper gastrointestinal disease and their relation to NSAID use. *Aliment Pharmacol Ther*, **11**, 283–291.

Breivik, H., Collett, B., Ventafridda, V., *et al.* (2006) Survey of chronic pain in Europe: prevalence, impact on daily life, and treatment. *Eur J Pain*, **10**, 287–333.

Chandrasekharan, N.V., Dai, H., Roos, K.L., *et al.* (2002) COX-3, a cyclooxygenase-1 variant inhibited by acetaminophen and other analgesic/anti-pyretic drugs: cloning, structure and expression. *Proc Natl Acad Sci*, **99**, 12926–12931.

Dickman, A. and Simpson, K. (2008) *Oxford Pain Library Series: Chronic Pain*, Oxford University Press, Oxford.

NICE (2004) The care and management of osteoarthritis in adults. www.nice.org.uk/Guidance/CG59

Pelissier, T., Alloui, A., Caussade, F., *et al.* (1996) Paracetamol exerts a spinal antinociceptive effect involving an indirect interaction with 5-hydroxytryptamine: in vivo and in vitro evidence. *J Pharmacol Exp Ther*, **278**, 8–14.

Stannard, C. and Booth, S. (2005) *Churchill's Pocketbook of Pain*, 2nd edn, Churchill Livingstone, Edinburgh.

Further reading

Dickenson, A.H. (2002) Gate control theory stands the test of time. *Br J Anaesth*, **88**, 755–777.

Melzack, R. and Wall, P.D. (1965) Pain mechanisms: a new theory. *Science*, **150**, 971–979.

Melzack, R. and Wall, P.D. (1988) *The Challenge of Pain*, 2nd edn, Penguin, Harmondsworth.

Royal College of Surgeons of England and the College of Anaesthetists (1990) *The Commission on the Provision of Surgical Services*. Report of the Working Party. Royal College of Surgeons, London.

Twycross, R. and Wilcock, A. (2009) *Symptom Management in Advanced Cancer*, 4th edn, Palliativedrugs.com, Oxford.

Twycross, R. and Wilcock, A. (2007) *Palliative Care Formulary*, 3rd edn, Palliativedrugs.com, Nottingham.

Section 3

35 Antibacterial chemotherapy

Learning outcomes

By the end of this chapter the reader should be able to:

- understand the differences between gram-positive and gram-negative and anaerobic and aerobic bacteria
- understand the difference between bactericidal and bacteristatic action
- understand what is meant by broad- and narrow-spectrum antimicrobials
- describe the four principal mechanisms of action of antibacterial agents and suggest examples of classes of drugs that utilise these mechanisms
- describe the principal clinical uses of major classes of antibiotics.

General principles of antimicrobial chemotherapy

Antimicrobials act by exploiting the differences between how micro-organisms and mammalian cells function, to either kill or inactivate the micro-organism without harming us. This is called selective toxicity.

Bacterial classification

Bacteria are prokaryotes or single-celled organisms which contain proteins and genetic information (in the form of RNA and DNA). The DNA is generally confined to a central region, known as the nucleoid, but is not contained within a membrane. Bacteria are surrounded by a cell wall and sometimes a capsule. Bacteria can be described in terms of their cell wall structure, shape and oxygen requirements. Classification is important as some antibiotics affect only certain types of bacteria.

The New Prescriber. Edited by J Lymn, D Bowskill, F Bath-Hextall, R Knaggs, © 2010 John Wiley & Sons.

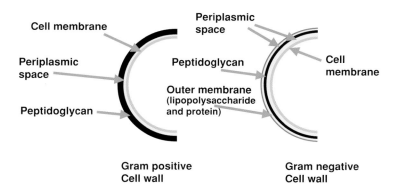

Figure 35.1 The differences in cell wall structure between a gram-positive and gram-negative bacterium. Note the thicker peptidoglycan layer in the gram-positive cell and the additional outer membrane in gram-negative cells.

Gram stain

Gram staining is a basic laboratory staining process performed on most grown cultures. It separates bacteria into two groups (gram positive and gram negative) depending on their cell wall structure (Figure 35.1). Gram-positive bacteria have cell walls which contain more peptidoglycan than gram-negative bacteria and it is this additional peptidoglycan which allows these bacteria to take up the crystal violet stain so the cells appear deep purple. Gram-negative cell walls have less peptidoglycan so stain poorly; they are viewed by the addition of a counterstain to give a red colour.

Cell shape and arrangement

The shape of a bacterium can give you a hint of what it might be. The majority of bacterial cells are shaped like a grape (cocci) or are more cylindrical (rods or bacilli). Cocci can be arranged in pairs (e.g. *Neisseria* species), chains (e.g. *Streptococcus* species) or clusters, like a bunch of grapes (e.g. *Stapylococcus* species).

Aerobic/anaerobic

Cultures are grown in the presence and absence of oxygen. Some bacteria prefer, or only grow in, conditions either containing oxygen (aerobic) or that are oxygen free (anaerobic).

These initial tests give the microbiologist an idea of what the bacteria involved might be (Table 35.1). They allow an informed decision about the appropriateness of empirical therapy before a definitive identification is made.

Further tests

The bacterium is grown on various selective media and/or is subjected to various tests that can further differentiate it into species (e.g. *Streptococcus*) and make a formal identification (e.g. *Streptococcus pyogenes*). It is also cultured with antibiotic discs to see if they inhibit bacterial growth and identify which antibiotics can be used to treat the infection (sensitivities) and

Section 3

Table 35.1 Bacterial classification by gram stain, shape and aerobic/anaerobic nature.

| Gram +ve | | | | Gram −ve | | | |
| Cocci | | Bacilli | | Cocci | | Bacilli | |
Aerobic	Anaerobic	Aerobic	Anaerobic	Aerobic	Anaerobic	Aerobic	Anaerobic
Staphylococcus spp *Streptococcus pneumoniae*	*Peptostreptococcus*	*Listeria*	*Clostridium* spp	*Neisseria*	Rare	*Pseudomonas* spp *Escherichia coli* 'Coliforms' Legionella	Bacteroides

to determine the lowest concentration of an antibiotic that will inhibit the bacteria's growth (minimum inhibitory concentration or MIC).

Choosing empirical antibiotic therapy

There are a number of factors which should be considered when deciding which antibiotics to use and these can be remembered using the acronym CLEFS.

- **Cost** – whilst it may be less important, if the differences between antibiotics are small, cost should be considered.
- **Local** resistance patterns – Different hospitals will have different problems, for example *C. difficile*, MRSA infections, and hospital policies will vary.
- **Environment** – what are the likely bugs in this environment? Is this a hospital- or community-acquired infection? What is the risk of MRSA? How severe is the disease?
- **Patient factors** – co-morbidity (e.g. myasthenia gravis, epilepsy), other medication/interactions (erythromycin/rifampicin). What routes of administration are available? Are there any physiological changes such as pregnancy?
- **Site** – the antibiotics chosen must be able to penetrate into the area where the infection occurs.

Practice application

Most of the hard work will be done for you. Microbiologists and local experts will take most of these factors into account when producing your local acute/primary care trust guidelines. If you plan to prescribe antibiotics, it is essential that you obtain your trust's antibiotic guideline.

Stop and think

What route of administration would be most appropriate for a deep-seated infection (e.g. bone and joint infection, endocarditis) which requires high blood levels for effective antibiotic penetration and treatment?

Antibiotics – key descriptions

Before moving on to the mechanism of action of antibiotics, it is necessary to describe a few key terms which are important in antimicrobial chemotherapy.

Does the antibiotic kill bacteria or stop their growth?

Bactericidal antibiotics kill the bacteria while *bacteriostatic* antibiotics stop bacterial growth, thus allowing host defences to kill them. Generally, these differences do not matter. There are situations where bactericidal antibiotics are considered superior, however, and these include

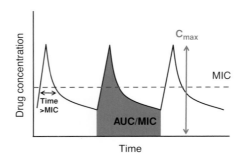

Figure 35.2   An example drug concentration against time graph for three drug doses.

where the host defences are compromised (e.g. neutropenia) and when the host defences struggle to get to the site of the infection (e.g. central nervous system, endocarditis).

What is most important for efficacy? (Figure 35.2)

- **Time-dependent killing (time > MIC)** – the time for which the antibiotic concentration is above the MIC is the most important; how high above the MIC does not make a lot of difference (e.g. penicillins).
- **Concentration-dependent killing (C_{max})** – the greater the concentration above the MIC, the more effective the bactericidal effect but the duration for which the concentration remains high is less important (e.g. aminoglycosides).
- **Area under the curve divided by the MIC (AUC/MIC)** – most antibiotic classes fit into this group the best. Here a mixture of concentration- and time-dependent aspects is important for efficacy.

Spectrum of activity

You may have heard of 'broad-spectrum' and 'narrow-spectrum' antibiotics. What this means exactly is not strictly defined but the broader the spectrum, the more species of bacteria the antibiotic can treat. Usually a broad-spectrum antibiotic would be able to treat a range of gram-positive and gram-negative organisms.

 Practice application

The use of empirical broad-spectrum antibiotics is essential when the patient is septic and the range of possible pathogens is wide (e.g. ventilator-associated pneumonia). It is usually possible to change to more targeted narrow-spectrum therapy once the results are available.

Mechanism of action of antibacterial drugs

There are four key mechanisms of action employed by antibacterial drugs, all of which are based around the concept of selective toxicity. The main pharmacodynamic properties of the major classes of antibiotics are summarised in Table 35.2.

Section 3

Table 35.2 A summary of the major antibiotic classes with example drugs and main pharmacodynamic features.

Class	Examples	Action	Effect	Notes
Aminoglycosides	Gentamicin Tobramycin	Inhibit ribosomal protein synthesis	-cidal	Synergy with antibiotics that act on cell walls, antagonised by bacteriostatic agents (e.g. tetracycline, chloramphenicol)
Carbapenems	Imipenem Meropenem	Inhibit peptidoglycan formation in cell wall	-cidal	8% cross-over allergy risk with penicillin-allergic patient
Cephalosporins	Cefuroxime Ceftriaxone	Inhibit peptidoglycan formation in cell wall	-cidal	2–16% cross-over allergy risk (often quoted as 10%) with penicillin-allergic patient
Glycopeptides	Vancomycin Teicoplanin	Inhibit peptidoglycan formation in cell wall	-cidal (-static at low concentration)	
Macrolides	Clarithromycin Erythromycin	Inhibit ribosomal protein synthesis	-static except at high concentration	Competes in binding on the ribosome with chloramphenicol, streptogamins and lincosamides – antagonistic and cross-resistance
Nitrofurantoin + nitroimidazoles	Nitrofurantoin Metronidazole	Free radical damage to DNA, RNA and proteins.	Probably -cidal	Only useful for UTIs (excluding pyelonephritis)
Quinolones	Fluroquinolones Nalidixic acid	Inhibit topoisomerases and DNA replication	-cidal	
Penicillins	Benzylpenicillin	Inhibit Peptidoglycan formation in cell wall	-cidal	
Rifamycins	Rifampicin	Interfere with DNA transcription to mRNA and thus protein synthesis.	-cidal	Resistance occurs quickly: NOT to be used as monotherapy
Sulphonamides + diaminopyrimidines	Sulphadimidine Sulphathiazole Trimethoprim	Interfere with folate synthesis	-static; combination treatment can be -cidal	There is synergy between trimethoprim and sulphonamides → bactericidal
Tetracyclines	Doxycycline Oxytetracycline	Inhibit ribosomal protein synthesis.	-static	Stop the iron tablets with most!

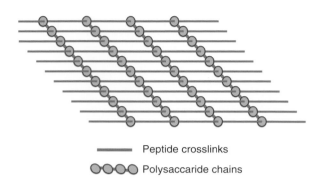

Peptide crosslinks

Polysaccharide chains

Figure 35.3   Structure of peptidoglycan.

Inhibition of cell wall synthesis

Bacterial cells all have a cell wall while mammalian cells do not, making this is an ideal target for antibacterial therapy. Peptidoglycan is a major constituent of many bacterial cell walls. It is made up of polysaccharide chains with peptide cross-links and provides structure and strength to the cell (Figure 35.3). As mammalian cells do not contain peptidoglycan, antibiotics that target its formation will have selective toxicity.

Peptidoglycan synthesis is inhibited by beta-lactam antibiotics (penicillins and cephalosporins) and glycopeptides (vancomycin).

Beta-lactam antibiotics

The beta-lactam ring is the core active component for a number of antibiotics with various properties and spectra, including penicillins, cephalosporins, monobactams and carbapenems.

The mechanism of action of these antibiotics is related to the beta-lactam ring itself. This acts as a false substrate for a bacterial transpeptidase enzyme (penicillin binding protein (PBP)), which is involved in the final peptide cross-links of the peptidoglycan in the bacterial cell wall. The beta-lactam ring mimics the structure of the natural substrate of PBP. While the bond between PBP and its natural substrate is temporary, beta-lactam antibiotics form an irreversible bond, neutralising the transpeptidase enzyme and interrupting peptidoglycan synthesis and thus causing cell lysis.

Penicillins

No other antibiotic has been more important than penicillin, which was discovered by Alexander Fleming in 1928. Benzylpenicillin (penicillin G) and the orally active phenoxymethylpenicillin (penicillin V) are the original penicillins. Both are rapidly cleared by the kidneys, resulting in a short half-life and frequent dosing regimens (every 6 hours). They were originally active primarily against gram-positive organisms including staphylococci and streptococci and are therefore useful in treating skin and soft tissue infection. However, resistance in staphylococci has emerged so these drugs can only be relied on now to cover streptococci. Over time, the structure of penicillin has been changed to develop semi-synthetic penicillins such as amoxicillin and flucloxacillin with a broader spectrum of activity but with a similar short half-life (Table 35.3).

Table 35.3   Clinical uses of semi-synthetic penicillins.

Drug	Amoxicillin	Flucloxacillin
	An aminopenicillin that is better absorbed than phenoxymethylpenicillin but still broken down by all beta-lactamases	A beta-lactamase resistant penicillin
Oral dose	500 mg tds (sometimes increases to 1 g tds)	500 mg qds (sometimes increases to 1 g qds)
PO bioavailability	75–89% and unaffected by concurrent food	50–70% and reduced by concurrent food (advise taking on an empty stomach)
Main uses	Otitis media Bacterial sinusitis Infective exacerbations of chronic bronchitis (although see above re *H. influenzae* resistance) Non-severe community-acquired pneumonia Sensitive urinary and biliary infections (not blind therapy)	Skin and soft tissue infections (e.g. impetigo, cellulitis) Bone and joint infections (under a specialist) Most sensitive *Staphylococcus aureus* infections
Other notes	Clavulanic acid- A beta-lactamase inhibitor Irreversibly inactivates beta-lactamase 'protecting' the penicillin Extends spectrum of activity of amoxicillin. =>increased activity vs beta-lactamase producing *Staphylococcus aureus*/gram-negative enteric organisms (e.g. *E.coli*/anaerobes) to give a 'similar' spectrum to using cefuroxime (see cephalosporins below) and metronidazole Risk of cholestatic jaundice if use exceeds 14 days and in elderly patients	Risk of cholestatic jaundice especially with use >14 days or in elderly patients

Penicillins are well known for causing 'allergy'. What this means varies greatly, ranging from diarrhoea to anaphylaxis. Nausea, vomiting and diarrhoea are adverse drug reactions that can occur with any antibiotic and would not contraindicate its use. Patients describing minor non-confluent, non-pruritic rash of delayed onset, emerging over 72 hours after starting the drug, are probably not allergic. Penicillins can be used with caution in serious infections where alternatives are inferior or have other disadvantages. Patients describing severe reactions such as anaphylaxis, angio-oedema and systemic rashes including urticaria should not receive a penicillin again as these reactions are life-threatening.

Cephalosporins

Another group of beta-lactam antibiotics, cephalosporins are subdivided into first, second and third generation. Drugs within the same generation tend to have similar spectra of activity (Table 35.4).

Table 35.4 Cephalosporins in current UK practice.

Generation	First	Second	Third
Oral	Cefalexin Cefradine Cefadroxil	Cefaclor Cefuroxime	Cefixime Cefpodoxime
Parenteral	Cefradine	Cefuroxime	Cefotaxime Ceftriaxone Ceftazidime
Spectrum of activity	Good gram-positive activity Unreliable gram-negative activity	Good gram-positive activity Improved gram-negative activity (more resistant to beta-lactamase)	Reduced gram-positive activity Broad-spectrum gram-negative activity

Most cephalosporins, with the notable exception of ceftriaxone, have short half-lives and thus require frequent dosing regimens.

Upto 6.5% of patients allergic to a penicillin will also have a reaction with a cephalosporin. Cross-reactivity is thought to be due to the side-chains rather than the beta-lactam ring and is much more likely with first-generation cephalosporins. Patients who are severely allergic to penicillins (immediate-onset rash, urticaria, angio-oedema, anaphylaxis, etc.) should not generally receive a cephalosporin. However, in the case of life-threatening infections, where alternatives are inferior and where resuscitation/anaphylaxis management facilities are available (e.g. inpatient treatment of meningitis), third- (and more rarely second-) generation cephalosporins are sometimes used.

Cephalosporins have fallen out of favour in recent years due to their capacity for inducing *Clostridium difficile* diarrhoea (DH, 2007).

The clinical use of selected cephalosporins is shown in Table 35.5.

Glycopeptides

Glycopeptides also inhibit peptidoglycan synthesis. They bind to the growing peptide chain and prevent cross-link formation. The key glycopeptides in clinical use are vancomycin and teicoplanin. Both have very good gram-positive cover (including MRSA) but are inactive against gram-negative bacteria. Resistance to these antibiotics in *Staphylococcus aureus* is still quite rare, especially considering that vancomycin has been in use since the 1950s (Hiramatsu *et al.*, 1997).

Vancomycin has a narrow therapeutic window so, when given intravenously, requires close monitoring in order to ensure efficacy and prevent toxicity.

Glycopeptides are not significantly absorbed orally. Systemic infections require parenteral treatment. Oral therapy is used for treating *C. difficile* (Chapter 36) as the infection is within the GI tract.

Table 35.5 Clinical uses of common cephalosporins.

	Cefradine (first generation)	Cefaclor (second generation)
Oral dose	500 mg qds	500 mg tds
PO bioavailability	90% and unaffected by concurrent food	93% and unaffected by concurrent food
Main uses	Generally not used first line Alternative for UTI Soft tissue infections Sometimes used in surgical prophylaxis *Not* suitable for respiratory infections (doesn't cover *H. influenzae*)	Alternative for UTI Alternative for respiratory infection (e.g. allergy)
Other notes	Higher risk of *C. difficile* diarrhoea than penicilllins	Higher risk of *C. difficile* diarrhoea than penicilllins Limited clinical advantages over first-generation cephalosporins within the context of UTI

Inhibition of bacterial protein synthesis

Bacterial cells, like mammalian cells, synthesise proteins by transcribing genes into messenger RNA that is translated by ribosomes into an amino acid chain and then folded into a protein.

There are many antibiotic classes that act by inhibiting protein synthesis, so why do they not harm us? Fortunately, the structure and size of the bacterial ribosomes are sufficiently different from those of mammalian ribosomes. Antibiotics preferentially bind to the bacterial version whilst not affecting ours, thus allowing selective toxicity. Many antibiotics interfere with protein synthesis, including aminoglycosides, macrolides, tetracyclines and chloramphenicol (Figure 35.4).

Macrolides

The key macrolides in clinical use are erythromycin, clarithromycin and azithromycin. All can be given orally whilst erythromycin and clarithromycin are also available in intravenous form.

Macrolides are especially useful for their activity against atypical pathogens such as *Chlamydia, Mycoplasma* and *Legionella*. They are also active against most streptococci and *Staphylococcus aureus* and are often used either as an alternative to penicillin, in allergic patients, for mild respiratory tract infection or skin/soft tissue infection or when atypical cover is required, for example in combination with a penicillin/cephalosporin in community-acquired pneumonia. Resistance does occur, so it is important that culture results are reviewed and patients are followed up.

All the macrolides inhibit enzymes in the cytochrome P450 system. Erythromycin and clarithromycin are potent inhibitors and have more clinically significant drug interactions than azithromycin. Clinical uses of erythromycin are shown in Table 35.6.

Section 3

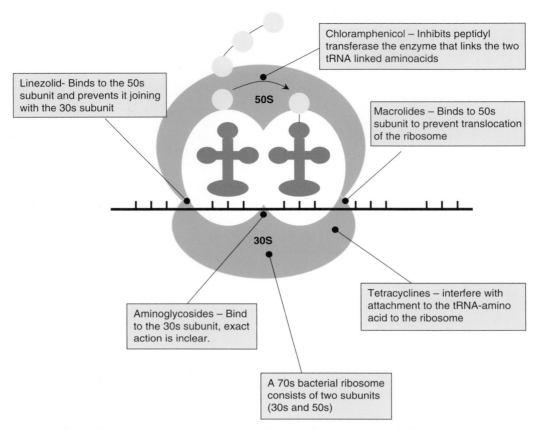

Figure 35.4 Antibiotic classes that inhibit protein synthesis and where they act.

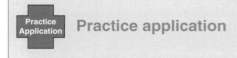 **Practice application**

It is always important to check the BNF for interactions when prescribing erythromycin and clarithromycin as many are clinically significant and contraindicate concurrent use.

Tetracyclines

The key tetracyclines in clinical use are tetracycline, oxytetracycline, doxycycline and minocycline. All are only available orally in the UK and have quite a broad spectrum of activity.

Most tetracyclines bind with divalent ions in the gut. These complexes cannot be absorbed by the body and so the antibiotic is rendered ineffective. For this reason, tetracyclines should not be taken at the same time as indigestion remedies or taken at all in patients taking iron supplements; some tetracyclines should not be taken at the same time as dairy products because of the calcium ions they contain. The affinity of tetracyclines for calcium is the reason

Table 35.6   Clinical uses of erythromycin and doxycycline, both of which act by inihibiting bacterial protein synthesis.

Drug	Erythromycin	Doxycycline
Oral dose	500 mg qds	200 mg loading dose then 100 mg od. 100 mg bd for STDs and more serious infections
PO bioavailability	18–45%; varies on the salt form	93%
Main uses	First choice for some STDs, for example *Chlamydia* First choice for legionnaire's disease, usually in combination Used in combination with aminopenicillins for respiratory infection As an alternative in skin/soft tissue infections	Used to treat some STDs, for example *Chlamydia* Respiratory infections As an oral alternative in sensitive MRSA infections
Other notes	Nausea and vomiting are sometimes troublesome; in these patients clarithromycin may be used	Stop iron tablets whilst treating with doxycycline! Restart after course Sensitises the skin to sunlight

why these drugs should not be used at all in children under 12 as they can lead to discoloured teeth. Apart from minocycline and doxycycline. tetracyclines should not be used in patients with kidney disease as they can cause renal impairment. The clinical uses of doxycycline are shown in Table 35.6.

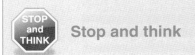

Stop and think

The interaction between tetracyclines and indigestion remedies is an example of which type of drug antagonism?

Aminoglycosides

The key aminoglycosides in clinical use are gentamicin, amikacin and tobramycin. None are absorbed orally so must be given intravenously for treating systemic infection. All aminoglycosides require close monitoring to ensure efficacy (from high enough peak levels) and avoid nephrotoxicity and ototoxicity (by ensuring low enough trough levels).

Aminoglycosides can exhibit synergy when used with beta-lactams (lower doses/peak levels required for efficacy).

Over the last decade there has been a move towards giving the total dose of aminoglycoside as a single daily infusion in an attempt to maximise efficacy and minimise toxicity. A number of meta-analyses have shown reduced nephrotoxicity with trends towards improved efficacy and similar ototoxicity (Barza *et al.*, 1996).

Section 3

Table 35.7 Clinical uses of ciprofloxacin and metronidazole, both of which act by inihibiting bacterial DNA synthesis.

Drug	Ciprofloxacin	Metronidazole
Oral dose	250–750 mg bd	400 mg tds
PO bioavailability		100%
Main uses	Alternative for UTI Sometimes used for pseudomonal infection	Anaerobes (including *Clostridium difficile*) Some protozoa Often used as part of a combination to cover anaerobes (GI, gynae, etc.)
Other notes	Oral gives as good a level as IV 400 mg IV = 500 mg PO => 80% bioavailability (IV gives high levels more rapidly). Usually give 750 mg bd as equivalent to 400 mg bd IV	Avoid alcohol whilst taking and for 72 hours after

Inhibition of bacterial DNA synthesis

DNA synthesis is fundamental to growing life and hence antibiotics that interfere with DNA synthesis tend to be bactericidal. Obviously, mammalian cells also need to synthesise DNA and so these drugs have to be designed carefully to achieve selective toxicity. Key antibiotics which act by inhibiting bacterial DNA synthesis are the quinolones, metronidazole, nitrofurantoin and rifampicin.

Quinolones

The key quinolones in clinical use are ciprofloxacin (Table 35.7), levofloxacin, ofloxacin and moxifloxacin. Quinolones are very well absorbed orally and distribute extensively throughout the body so intravenous preparations are rarely necessary. Although the half-life varies, most quinolones can be given as once- or twice-daily regimens.

Resistance seems to occur rapidly and resistance to one fluoroquinolone generally means resistance to all.

Quinolone antibiotics inhibit DNA gyrase and topoisomerase IV, enzymes involved in the coiling of bacterial DNA and which are essential for DNA replication in bacteria. Mammalian cells do not contain DNA gyrase and so selective toxicity is assured.

 Practice application

Although very effective, quinolones have fallen out of favour in recent years due to being highlighted as a risk factor for MRSA colonisation, extended-spectrum beta-lactamase infections and *Clostridium difficile* infection.

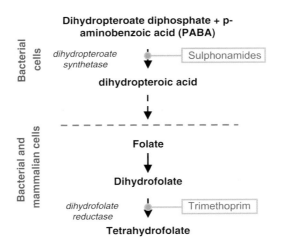

Figure 35.5 Action of antibiotics on bacterial folate synthesis.

Metronidazole and nitrofurantoin

Metronidazole (Table 35.7) and nitrofurantoin are reduced intracellularly to reactive metabolites that interact with and cause direct damage to DNA, with bactericidal effect.

Inhibition of folate synthesis

Folate is essential for DNA synthesis. Mammals obtain folate from their food while bacterial cells synthesise their own. Both mammals and bacteria have to reduce folate into its active form, tetrahydrofolate, before it can be used for DNA synthesis. Key antibiotics which act by inhibiting folate synthesis are trimethoprim and the sulphonamides.

Figure 35.5 highlights the two enzymes in folate metabolism inhibited by sulphonamides and trimethoprim.

For the sulphonamides, achieving selective toxicity is obvious as their target is not found in mammalian cells. For trimethoprim, it is more complicated. Dihydrofolate reductase (DHFR) is an enzyme common to both bacteria and mammals so why doesn't trimethoprim harm us? The reason is that whilst trimethoprim could inhibit mammalian DHFR, it is much less active against this than it is against the bacterial version (Table 35.8). The IC_{50} is the concentration necessary to inhibit 50% of the enzyme; the lower the IC_{50}, the more active the drug. Hence trimethoprim is about 50,000 times more active against bacteria than humans. Methotrexate is most active against the human DHFR and hence is a useful cytotoxic. Pyrimethamine is an antiprotozoal drug.

Sulphonamides

Sulphonamides are now rarely used as monotherapy due to growing resistance. However, they are still used in combination with DHFR inhibitors. Separately, sulphonamides and trimethoprim are bacteriostatic. Combined as co-trimoxazole, they work synergistically and are usually bactericidal with enhanced activity against rarer organisms such as *Pneumocystis jiroveci* (formerly *Pneumocystis carinii*) which is an important opportunistic pathogen in the immunosuppressed. Sulphonamides (and co-trimoxazole) have a poor side-effect profile, including serious

Section 3

Table 35.8 The relative potency of DHFR inhibitors.

	IC$_{50}$ for DHFR		
	Human	Protozoal	Bacterial
Trimethoprim	260	0.07	0.005
Pyrimethamine	0.7	0.0005	2.5
Methotrexate	0.001	Approx. 0.1	Inactive

blood dyscrasias and frequent rashes, so co-trimoxazole is usually restricted to infections where other options are not suitable.

Trimethoprim
The clinical uses of trimethoprim are shown in Box 35.1.

Summary

- Antimicrobials exploit differences between humans and micro-organisms to cause selective toxicity.
- Bacteria are divided into gram positives and gram negatives based on their cell wall structure.
- Bacteria are divided into cocci or bacilli based on their shape under a microscope and into anaerobic and aerobic, depending on whether they can grow in the presence or absence of oxygen.
- Broad-spectrum antibiotics treat lots of types of bacteria; narrow-spectrum agents are more targeted to specific species.
- Antibiotics either kill the bacteria (bactericidal) or prevent them from multiplying (bacteriostatic), allowing the host defences to kill them.
- Use your local antibiotic guidelines when deciding on empirical (blind) therapy.

Box 35.1 **Clinical uses of trimethoprim.**

Spectrum	Generally active	*E.coli*
		Most other urinary pathogens
		Some strains of *Staph. aureus* (inc. some MRSA)
	Generally inactive	Anaerobic bacteria
Oral dose	200 mg bd	
PO bioavailability	90–100%	
Main uses	First line for UTI	
Other notes	Resistance is growing	

- Review antibiotic choice with the results of microbiology cultures.
- Antibiotics within the same class have the same mechanism of action and, generally, a similar spectrum of activity.
- There are four principal mechanisms of antibacterial action: damaging the bacterial cell wall, inhibiting bacterial protein synthesis, inhibiting bacterial DNA synthesis and inhibiting bacterial metabolic pathways.
- Beta-lactam antibiotics and glycopeptides inhibit bacterial cell wall synthesis.
- Aminoglycosides, macrolides and tetracyclines all inhibit bacterial protein synthesis.
- Quinolones, metronidazole, nitrofurantoin and rifampicin all inhibit bacterial DNA synthesis.
- Trimethoprim and sulphonamides inhibit bacterial metabolic pathways.

 Activity

1. Which of the following statements regarding bacteria and antibiotics are correct?
   A. Ciprofloxacin is the first-line antibiotic to treat uncomplicated urinary tract infection.
   B. Augmentin® can be used in patients allergic to a penicillin.
   C. Trimethoprim and sulphonamides act on the same metabolic pathway and have synergy when used in combination.
   D. *Staphylococcus aureus* is a gram-positive organism.
   E. Gentamicin's efficacy is linked to the amount of time its concentration is above the bacteria's MIC.
2. Which two of the following antibiotics would be effective against respiratory atypicals?
   A. Co-amoxiclav
   B. Cefuroxime
   C. Clarithromycin
   D. Doxycycline
   E. Vancomycin
3. Which three of the following antibiotics act by inhibiting peptidoglycan synthesis?
   A. Co-amoxiclav
   B. Cefuroxime
   C. Clarithromycin
   D. Doxycycline
   E. Vancomycin
4. Which two of the following organisms commonly cause skin and soft tissue infections (e.g. cellulitis)?
   A. *Staphylococcus aureus*
   B. *Haemophilus influenzae*
   C. *Moraxella catarrhalis*
   D. *Streptococcus pyogenes* (group A beta-haemolytic Strep.)
   E. *Bacteroides* spp
5. Which of the following bacteria can be treated by metronidazole?
   A. *Staphylococcus aureus*
   B. *Haemophilus influenzae*
   C. *Moraxella catarrhalis*
   D. *Streptococcus pyogenes* (group A beta-haemolytic Strep.)
   E. *Bacteroides* spp

Section 3

Useful websites

Management of hospital infection. www.bsac.org.uk/pyxis

The Prudent Antibiotic User website. www.pause-online.org.uk/

Reusable learning objects

Pharmacokinetic and pharmacodynamic influences of aminoglycoside dosing. www.nottingham.ac.uk/nursing/sonet/rlos/bioproc/aminoglycosides/

References

Barza, M., Ioannidis, J.P., Cappelleri, J.C. and Lau, J. (1996) Single or multiple daily doses of aminoglycosides: a meta-analysis. *BMJ*, **312**, 338–345.

Department of Health (2007) *Saving Lives: Antimicrobial Prescribing, A Summary of Best Practice*, Department of Health, London.

Hiramatsu, K., Hanaki, H., Ino, T., *et al.* (1997) Methicillin-resistant Staphylococcus aureus clinical strain with reduced vancomycin susceptibility. *J Antimicrob Chemother*, **40**, 135–136.

Further reading

Abbanat, D., Morrow, B. and Bush, K. (2008) New drugs in development for the treatment of bacterial infections. *Curr Opin Pharmacol*, **8**, 582–592.

British Medical Association and Royal Pharmaceutical Society of Great Britain (2010) *British National Formulary*, 59th edn, BMJ Publishing, London.

Page, C.P., Curtis, M.J., Sutter, M.C., *et al.* (2006) *Integrated Pharmacology*, 3rd edn, Mosby, London.

Pai, M.P., Momarry, K.M. and Rodvold, K.A. (2006) Antibiotic drug interactions. *Med Clin North Am*, **90**, 1223–1255.

Rang, H.P., Dale, M.M., Ritter, J.M. and Flower, R. (2007) *Rang and Dale's Pharmacology*, 6th edn, Churchill Livingstone, Edinburgh.

Ranji, S.R., Steinman, M.A., Shojania, K.G. and Gonzales, R. (2008) Interventions to reduce unnecessary antibiotic prescribing: a systematic review and quantitative analysis. *Med Care*, **46**, 847–862.

Thethi, A.K. and van Dellen, R.G. (2004) Dilemmas and controversies in penicillin allergy. *Immunol Allergy Clin North Am*, **24**, 445–461.

36 Antibiotic resistance and *Clostridium difficile*

Learning outcomes

By the end of this chapter the reader should be able to:

- demonstrate an understanding of how antibiotic resistance emerges and spreads
- discuss the main mechanisms of antibiotic resistance that bacteria employ
- describe how *Clostridium difficile* infection occurs
- outline the main risk factors associated with contracting *Clostridium difficile* infection
- describe the treatment of *Clostridium difficile* infection and know when to refer patients for specialist care.

Bacteria and the human body

The human body is a bacterial ecosystem. There are ten times more bacterial cells on, or in, our body than human cells (most live within the bowel). Whilst some of these are pathogenic and cause infection, most do no harm and many live alongside us performing useful functions such as synthesising vitamins (such as vitamin K) or aiding digestion. Moreover, our natural flora helps prevent overgrowth of pathogenic micro-organisms by providing competitive pressure for space and nutrients. The use of antibiotics alters this natural human flora by killing off the sensitive bacteria, allowing the resistant species that are left to multiply with less competition. The broader the spectrum of antibiotic, the more species of bacteria affected and the more chance of a resistant colonisation occurring.

For example, if a patient has cellulitis in their right leg, most likely to be either haemolytic streptococci or *Staphylococcus aureus* (Figure 36.1a), one could treat with a narrow-spectrum antibiotic such as flucloxacillin. This will treat the infection; it will also kill the other haemolytic streptococci or *Staphylococcus aureus* (and other sensitive bacteria) on the body that are not

The New Prescriber. Edited by J Lymn, D Bowskill, F Bath-Hextall, R Knaggs, © 2010 John Wiley & Sons.

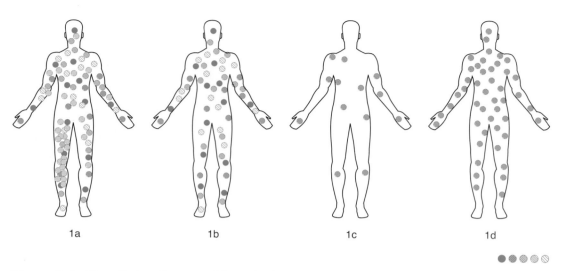

Figure 36.1   The effect on the natural flora of using narrow- and broad-spectrum antibiotics to treat a patient with cellulitis of the right leg (different shade spots represent different populations of bacteria).

causing the infection (so-called 'innocent bystanders') but this is unavoidable (Figure 36.1b). Alternatively one could choose to treat the infection with the broader spectrum antibiotic cefuroxime. It would still treat haemolytic streptococci or *Staphylococcus aureus* but also covers a range of gram-negative enteric bacteria. Hence, it would select for resistance in more species of bacteria and have a greater impact on the natural flora, leaving only the resistant micro-organisms (Figure 36.1c). With less competition for space and nutrients, these resistant micro-organisms grow, colonise the patient (Figure 36.1d) and pass to another person. For this reason, it is generally best to use the most narrow-spectrum antibiotic available that will treat the infection effectively.

It is also important to use the antibiotics for the shortest duration that will effectively treat the infection (Haider, Saeed and Bhutta, 2008; Michael *et al.*, 2002; El Moussaoui *et al.*, 2008). Longer durations of antibiotic therapy will suppress the natural flora for longer and increase the risk of acquiring a multiresistant colonisation.

 Stop and think

Can you think of examples of broad-spectrum antibiotics that have been used unnecessarily?

 Practice application

If initial broad-spectrum antibiotic therapy is necessary (e.g. for neutropenic sepsis) it is important that microbiology cultures are taken and therapy reviewed in light of the results.

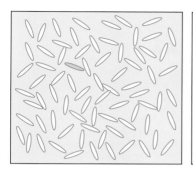 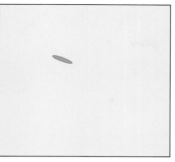 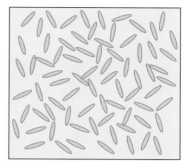

Figure 36.2 About every one in 10^7 bacteria will have a mutation (green). If this confers new resistance to an antibiotic that is used, the sensitive population is killed, leaving the resistant organism to multiply and cause a resistant colonisation which may then be passed on to another patient.

Antibiotic resistance

Antibiotic resistance is a well-documented problem both within secondary care and, increasingly, in the community. Resistance to an antibiotic varies between species and strains, being either native or following a mutation in the antibiotic's target.

Native resistance

Some bacteria or strains were always resistant to the antibiotic even before it was introduced these are called natively resistant. They either naturally contain an enzyme conferring resistance (e.g. some strains of *E. coli* and beta-lactamase) or their structure is such that the antibiotic cannot reach its target or the target does not exist (e.g. *Mycoplasma* sp. does not have peptidoglycan in its cell wall and therefore beta-lactam antibiotics would never work against it).

Resistance acquired following mutation

Point mutations tend to occur within the genome of one in about every 10^7 bacterial cells (Figure 36.2). If the mutation is part of the gene that encodes for the antibiotic's target, it may lead to resistance.

Genes that code for resistance may be positioned on a bacterial chromosome or contained on a plasmid (a separate ring of DNA that can be transferred to other bacteria). Resistance genes on a chromosome are spread clonally (Figure 36.2). Dividing bacteria colonise and may spread from patient to patient where infection control precautions are not perfect. A good example of this is meticillin-resistant *Staphylococcus aureus* (MRSA) where two very successful epidemic clones account for the vast majority of UK healthcare-associated infections (Johnson *et al.*, 2001).

Resistance genes on a plasmid spread clonally but can also be easily shared between strains and even species. For example, vancomycin resistance in enterococci (VRE) has been transferred *in vitro* to MRSA to produce a vancomycin-resistant MRSA (VRSA). The first report of a clinical infection with vancomycin-resistant MRSA was in a patient co-colonised with VRE and MRSA (Chang *et al.*, 2003).

Potentially, resistance genes can also spread following cell lysis as some bacteria can scavenge DNA lying around the environment and incorporate it into their chromosome. Bacteriophages

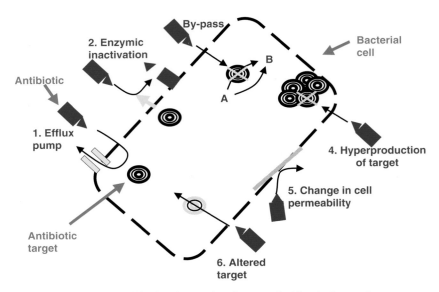

Figure 36.3   Mechanisms of resistance that bacteria employ.

(viruses that infect bacteria) may also extract DNA from one bacterium and inject it into another one.

Mechanisms of resistance

The mechanisms of resistance that bacteria employ are varied but most fit into one of six categories (Figure 36.3).

Efflux pumps

The antibiotic enters the cell but is actively pumped out by efflux pumps so that intracellular concentration does not become high enough to affect the target. Tetracycline resistance is often mediated through efflux pumping. Multidrug efflux pumps are sometimes expressed by *Pseudomonas aeruginosa* and are able to excrete a variety of antibiotics including quinolones, beta-lactams, trimethoprim, sulphonamides and aminoglycosides.

Enzymic degradation

The bacterial cell secretes an enzyme that is capable of inactivating the antibiotic before it is able to reach the target. The best-known example is beta-lactamase which can hydrolyse the beta-lactam ring of some penicillins, cephalosporins and carbapenems. Aminoglycosides can also be degraded by specific secreted enzymes.

Bypass

The antibiotic inhibits an essential enzyme in a cell metabolic pathway. The bacteria manage to bypass this to produce the required metabolite using another pathway. This type of resistance can occur against sulphonamides.

Hyperproduction of target

The bacteria produce so much of the target enzyme that the antibiotic is unable to inhibit it all. Hyperproduction of dihydrofolate reductase can confer resistance to trimethoprim in some bacteria.

Change in cell permeability

Many antibiotics enter cells through porins in the cell wall. Alterations in these porins reduce the amount of antibiotic that enters the bacteria. Consequently, a higher concentration of antibiotic is necessary to obtain sufficient concentrations within the cell and leads to an increase in the minimum inhibitory concentration (MIC) and resistance. Cephalosporins can sometimes be affected by porin alteration. Gentamicin resistance is sometimes conferred by alterations in the cell wall uptake mechanism.

Altered target

Direct mutations to the antibiotic target can led to decreased affinity and reduced antibiotic efficacy. Many antibiotics are potentially susceptible to mutation in their targets, including aminoglycosides, macrolides, clindamycin and quinolones.

Multiresistant bacteria

Meticillin-resistant Staphylococcus aureus (MRSA)

The original 'superbug', MRSA is resistant to all current beta-lactam antibiotics (penicillins, cephalosporins and carbapenems). Different strains have variable resistance to other anti-staphylococcal antibiotics. All antibiotics that can treat *Staphylococcus aureus* have the potential to select for MRSA although quinolones have been highlighted as particularly high risk for MRSA colonisation. This is probably because they are excreted in sweat (MRSA colonises the groin, axillae and nose) and can induce the expression of *Staphylococcus aureus* adhesion factors (Weber *et al.*, 2003). Several new antibiotics have recently become available that are active against MRSA (and VRSA), including linezolid, daptomycin and tigecycline, and more are in development.

Extended-spectrum beta-lactamase producers (ESBLs)

A gram-negative bacterium (e.g. *E. coli*) that produces an enzyme that inactivates a wider range of beta-lactam antibiotics, including cephalosporins. Unfortunately, as well as cephalosporin resistance, these bacteria also tend to carry resistance to quinolones, gentamicin, trimethoprim, co-amoxiclav, piperacillin/tazobactam and in some cases nitrofurantoin. This can leave the carbapenems as the only option. With few antibiotics in the development pipeline that will treat ESBL producers, and *E. coli* being such a successful pathogen, these are likely to be one of the major problem organisms in the near future.

Vancomycin-resistant enterococcus (VRE)

Although a lower-grade pathogen than *E. coli* or *Staph. aureus*, enterococci still cause infections such as endocarditis in susceptible patients. Depending on the strain, VRE may be

Section 3

sensitive to amoxicillin, although nearly all are sensitive to the new anti-MRSA drugs linezolid, tigecycline and daptomycin.

Acinetobacter baumannii

Another low-grade pathogen that tends to affect immunocompromised patients or those who have had numerous antibiotics. Hospital strains tend only to be sensitive to colistin, tigecycline and sometimes the carbapenems.

Antibiotic-associated diarrhoea and *clostridium difficile*

Diarrhoea is one of the most common adverse effects with antibiotic use. It can occur with any antibiotic and is often attributed to *Clostridium difficile*.

Clostridium difficile (*C. diff*) is a gram-positive spore-forming bacterium. Bacterial spores are like seeds – they can survive for months in the environment and are very hard to kill, even with disinfectants. If ingested, these spores move through the GI tract to the lower bowel where they germinate into vegetative bacteria. The patient's normal bowel flora is a useful defence but if it is disrupted by antibiotic, then the Clostridia are allowed to proliferate, colonise and, if the strain is able, produce toxin. Additionally, it appears that some antibiotics may actually encourage spore germination and/or toxin production and disease.

 Practice application

C. diff spores are not reliably killed by alcohol handrubs. When caring for patients with C. diff infection (CDI) or diarrhoea, it is important to use soap and water to clean hands.

Clostridium difficile can produce three types of toxin which together cause gut mucosal inflammation, epithelial cell apoptosis and fluid and electrolyte leakage into the lumen, leading to offensive diarrhoea.

 Practice application

The severity of disease that CDI causes varies from patient to patient. A few will be asymptomatic carriers but may act as a reservoir for further spread. Some will only experience mild diarrhoea, while for others profuse diarrhoea may follow infection; these will require active treatment. In its severest form, CDI may cause life-threatening pseudomembraneous colitis (PMC). What determines the severity of disease is unclear but in part it may be due to the patient's ability to mount an immune response to the toxins and certainly the elderly and the immunosuppressed are at greatest risk of severe disease.

Treatment of Clostridium difficile infection (CDI)

With confirmed or highly suspected CDI, the first job is to review and stop the causative antibiotic if at all possible. Mild CDI is often self-limiting and treatment consists of stopping the causative antibiotic and ensuring adequate hydration and nutrition. Those with moderate disease will require active treatment with metronidazole or vancomcyin.

 Stop and think

As *C. diff* causes infection within the gut lumen, which route of administration would be most appropriate for treatment of this infection?

The two therapies are similar in terms of overall symptomatic cure or bacteriological recurrence. However, vancomycin's greater cost and concerns about selecting out VRE have lead metronidazole to be used first line for moderate disease (Wilcox, 1998). More recent studies have shown that patients with severe disease had a better overall outcome with vancomycin. This has been reflected in the new national guidance that recommends using oral vancomycin first line for patients with severe or life-threatening disease (DH, 2008).

A particular problem of treating CDI is the rate of symptom recurrence. Approximately 20–30% of patients who initially respond to therapy will experience recurrence, mostly within the first month. Half of these can be attributed to a different *C. diff* strain and are therefore reinfections rather than relapses. For this reason, the first relapse is usually treated with the same regimen that the patient's diarrhoea originally responded to (unless the recurrence is severe infection in which case vancomycin should always be used). Further relapses would generally be treated with oral vancomycin under the supervision of a specialist.

Modulation of CDI risk

Antibiotics

Many factors have been identified that increase the risk of contracting CDI ,the most obvious being antibiotic usage. Antibiotics disrupt the normally protective gut bacteria flora and all are considered potential risk factors for CDI (including, paradoxically, oral vancomycin and metronidazole!). Some groups have been shown to offer increased risk over others; these are generally the broad-spectrum agents (Table 36.1).

Using more than one antibiotic at once appears to increase the CDI risk although it is difficult to say how much. What is clear is that extending the duration of the treatment course increases the risk of contracting CDI. With a more sustained disruption to bowel flora, the patient is without their natural defence for longer and there is more chance that if *C. diff* spores are ingested, they will germinate (Pépin *et al.*, 2005).

Age and immune system

With the exception of the under-2s, the patient's CDI risk increases as their age increases, with those over 65 being especially at risk. The reason for this is probably multifactorial; older people

Table 36.1 Examples of antibiotic classes and their risk of CDI.

Risk of *C. diff*	Antibiotic	Comment
High risk	Cephalosporins	Particularly third generation. Also been linked to promoting MRSA and VRE colonisation.
	Quinolones	A recent study suggested that quinolones were the highest independent risk factor of all the antibiotic classes. Also been linked to encouraging MRSA colonisation.
	Clindamycin	Implicated as the major causative antibiotic in many of the early CDI outbreaks. Anecdotally some centres report seeing less CDI associated with higher (e.g. 600 mg qds) compared with lower doses.
Moderate risk	Macrolides and aminopenicillins	Studies have linked macrolides, amoxicillin and co-amoxiclav to CDI, with co-amoxiclav expected to be higher risk due to its broader spectrum of activity and greater disruption of anaerobic bacteria.
Lower risk	Narrow-spectrum penicillins Tetracyclines Metronidazole Trimethoprim Rifampicin	Benzylpenicillin, flucloxacillin.
	Glycopeptides (intravenous)	Glycopeptides do not distribute into the gut lumen and therefore do not disrupt gut flora when given intravenously.
	Aminoglycosides (parenteral)	Aminoglycosides have broad-spectrum gram-negative activity but do not partition across the gut mucosa and cause limited disruption of bowel flora when given parenterally.
	Topical antibiotics (e.g. eye drops)	The risk of disrupting gut flora is low regardless of the class of antibiotic they contain.

often have more co-morbidities coupled with longer hospital stays, and their immune systems also tend to be poorer. Patients who are unable to mount a significant immune response to *C. diff* toxin are at much greater risk from recurrent CDI and are likely to experience more severe disease.

Characteristics of hospital stay

As a patient's stay in hospital continues, their risk from CDI increases. Some studies have also suggested that a stay on the intensive care unit increases risk. Patients who are sicker also tend to be more susceptible to CDI. Similarly, the presence of a nasogastric tube appears to increase the risk of contracting CDI, probably as this by-passes the protective stomach.

Proton pump inhibitors (PPIs)

The theory is that increasing gastric pH reduces the protection that the stomach offers, allowing more spores through into the bowel, although current clinical evidence regarding PPI use is conflicting. Until subsequent evidence clarifies the situation, the prudent approach is to ensure that PPI use is in line with NICE guidance and ensure that patients are regularly reviewed to prevent CDI, with strong consideration to stopping them in patients with recurrent disease.

Probiotics

Probiotics are living micro-organisms taken to promote a 'good' or 'friendly' gut flora. Although they have provoked much interest in the media, most preparations have not been tested in controlled trials. *Saccharomyces boulardii*, a non-pathogenic yeast, has shown promise in preventing CDI recurrence in patients who have had at least one recurrence (McFarland *et al.*, 1994). Most interest has been surrounding the use of Actimel® which in a placebo-controlled trial appeared to reduce the risk of diarrhoea and CDI. However, it has been suggested that the 'placebo' used may actually have induced diarrhoea and hence confounded the results (Hickson *et al.*, 2007). Similar studies are planned in an attempt to determine whether a real benefit exists.

Summary

- Inappropriate use of antimicrobials does not just affect the patient (through side effects), but also impacts the community by encouraging resistance.
- Always use antibiotics in line with local guidelines and for the shortest duration that will treat the infection.
- If antibiotics are indicated, narrow down the spectrum in line with microbial sensitivities to reduce the impact on natural flora.
- Bacteria may have native resistance to antibiotics or acquire resistance following mutation.
- The mechanisms of resistance employed by bacteria fall into six categories including efflux pumps, enzymic degradation, bypass, hyperproduction of target, change in cell permeability and altered target.
- Most antibiotic-resistant bacteria are spread clonally; excellent infection control reduces their spread.
- Diarrhoea is one of the most common adverse effects seen with antibiotics and is often attributed to *Clostridium difficile*.
- Risk factors for CDI include antibiotic use, particularly broad-spectrum antibiotics and use of multiple antibiotics.
- Other risk factors for CDI include age, length of hospital stay, severe co-morbidities, the presence of feeding tubes and possibly acid-suppressing agents.
- Mild CDI is generally self-limiting and may not require treatment.
- Moderate CDI is treated with oral metronidazole and severe infection with oral vancomycin.

Section 3

 Activity

1. Using a broader-spectrum antibiotic reduces the risk of resistance as it can treat more infections. True / False
2. *Clostridium difficile* infection can be induced by the use of any antibiotic. True / False
3. The risk of contracting *Clostridium difficile* infection increases with age. True / False
4. The risk of relapse following *Clostridium difficile* infection is low (<5%). True / False
5. An extended-spectrum beta-lactamase producer (ESBL) is:
   A. an antibiotic that kills most types of bacteria (e.g. meropenem)
   B. a gram-negative bacteria with resistance against all current cephalosporins and penicillins
   C. a strain of *Clostridium difficile* that produces more toxin causing more severe disease
   D. a form of MRSA that is particularly difficult to eradicate
6. Which of these antibiotics are considered higher risk for inducing *Clostridium difficile* infection?
   A. Ciprofloxacin
   B. Doxycycline
   C. Piperacillin/tazobactam
   D. Gentamicin IV
7. Which of these is NOT a resistance mechanism employed by bacteria to evade antibiotic attack?
   A. Hyperproduction of the target
   B. Efflux pumps
   C. Ribosomal inhibition
   D. Changing the cell permeability

Useful website

Department of Health and the Health Protection Agency. *Clostridium difficile* infection: how to deal with the problem. www.hpa.org.uk/web/HPAwebFile/HPAweb_C/1204186175140

References

Chang, S., Sievert, D.M., Hageman, J.C., *et al.* (2003) Vancomycin-resistant Staphylococcus aureus investigative team: infection with vancomycin-resistant Staphylococcus aureus containing the vanA resistance gene. *N Engl J Med*, **348**, 1342–1347.

Department of Health and the Health Protection Agency (2008) *Clostridium Difficile Infection: How to Deal With the Problem*, Department of Health, London.

El Moussaoui, R., Roede, B.M., Speelman, P., *et al.* (2008) Short-course antibiotic treatment in acute exacerbations of chronic bronchitis and COPD: a meta-analysis of double-blind studies. *Thorax*, **63**, 415–422.

Section 3

Haider, B.A., Saeed, M.A. and Bhutta, Z.A. (2008) Short-course versus long-course antibiotic therapy for non-severe community-acquired pneumonia in children aged 2 months to 59 months. *Cochrane Database Syst Rev*, 2, CD005976.

Hickson, M., D'Souza, A.L., Muthu, N., *et al.* (2007) Use of probiotic Lactobacillus preparation to prevent diarrhoea associated with antibiotics: randomised double blind placebo controlled trial. *BMJ*, **335**, 80–83.

Johnson, A.P., Aucken, H.M., Cavendish, S., *et al.*, UK EARSS Participants (2001) Dominance of EMRSA-15 and -16 among MRSA causing nosocomial bacteraemia in the UK: analysis of isolates from the European Antimicrobial Resistance Surveillance System (EARSS). *J Antimicrob Chemother*, **48**, 143–144.

McFarland, L.V., Surawicz, C.M., Greenberg, R.N., *et al.* (1994) A randomized placebo-controlled trial of Saccharomyces boulardii in combination with standard antibiotics for Clostridium difficile disease. *JAMA*, **271**, 1913–1918.

Michael, M., Hodson, E.M., Craig, J.C., *et al.* (2002) Short compared with standard duration of antibiotic treatment for urinary tract infection: a systematic review of randomised controlled trials. *Arch Dis Child*, **87**(2), 118–123.

Pépin, J., Saheb, N., Coulombe, M.A., *et al.* (2005) Emergence of fluoroquinolones as the predominant risk factor for Clostridium difficile-associated diarrhea: a cohort study during an epidemic in Quebec. *Clin Infect Dis*, **41**, 1254–1260.

Weber, S.G., Gold, H.S., Hooper, D.C., *et al.* (2003) Fluoroquinolones and the risk for methicillin-resistant Staphylococcus aureus in hospitalized patients. *Emerg Infect Dis*, **9**, 1415–1422.

Wilcox, M.H. (1998) Treatment of Clostridium difficile infection. *J Antimicrob Chemother*, **41** (Suppl C): 41–46

Further reading

Cunningham, R. and Dial, S. (2008) Is over-use of proton pump inhibitors fuelling the current epidemic of Clostridium difficile-associated diarrhoea? *J Hosp Infect*, **70**, 1–6.

Monaghan, T., Boswell, T. and Mahida, Y.R. (2008) Recent advances in Clostridium difficile-associated disease. *Gut*, **57**, 850–860.

Zar, F.A., Bakkanagari, S.R., Moorthi, K.M. and Davis, M.B. (2007) Comparison of vancomycin and metronidazole for the treatment of Clostridium difficile-associated diarrhea, stratified by disease severity. *Clin Infect Dis*, **45**, 302–307.

Section 3

37 Antifungal and antiviral drugs

Learning outcomes

By the end of this chapter the reader should be able to:

- understand the aetiology of fungal diseases
- discuss the use, mechanism of action and problems associated with the following antifungal drugs:
  - nystatin
  - azole antifungals
  - terbinafine
- understand the nature of viruses and viral infections
- discuss the use, mechanism of action and problems associated with the use of the following antiviral drugs:
  - aciclovir
  - zanamivir/oseltamivir.

Mycology and classification

Fungi are eukaryotes with a rigid cell wall, like plants but without the chlorophyll. Pathogenic fungi occur in two forms: unicellular yeasts (e.g. *Candida*) and filamentous moulds (e.g. *Aspergillus*). Some fungi are capable of growth in either form depending on the conditions and are called dimorphic. Fungi are able to reproduce independently of any host organism. Yeasts do so asexually through budding, whereas moulds produce airborne spores.

Fungi are generally seen as opportunistic pathogens. In normal hosts disease tends to be superficial, mostly occurring if the normal flora has been altered, for example by the use of broad-spectrum antibiotics (Chapter 35). In immunocompromised patients, however, fungi can cause difficult-to-treat deep and/or invasive infections which are often life-threatening (Lass-Flörl, 2009).

The New Prescriber. Edited by J Lymn, D Bowskill, F Bath-Hextall, R Knaggs, © 2010 John Wiley & Sons.

Pathogenic moulds

Dermatophytes

These are a group of more than 30 species of fungi that live in the dead layers of nails and skin. Most are spore-forming moulds. Dermatophytes produce keratinase, an enzyme that digests keratin, the tough protein that provides structure. Keratin is the main component of nails and the top layer of the skin (stratum corneum). Dermatophytes cause a group of diseases known as ringworm. Ringworm, despite its name, has nothing to do with worms but derives its name from a moth (*Tinea*) whose worms produce similar shaped holes when they grow in woollen blankets! Ringworm infections are also known as the 'tineas'.

Aspergillus spp

Aspergillus is a naturally occurring spore-forming fungus. These spores are very common and can be found in decaying vegetation, soil, potted plants, pepper and spices. Whilst there are many species of *Aspergillus* (>250), only a few actually cause disease.

Aspergillus-related disease occurs in three forms.

- Colonisation and allergic response, for example allergic bronchopulmonary aspergillosis.
- Colonisation of pre-existing cavities, for example an aspergilloma in the sinuses or in the lungs after tuberculosis infection.
- Invasive disease – generally only seen in the immunocompromised.

Pathogenic yeasts

Candida spp

This is the most common pathogenic yeast. It is found in small numbers in the normal skin flora and in the flora of the gastrointestinal and genitourinary tracts. Candidal overgrowth and mucocutaneous infection occur when the normal body microbial flora is altered (e.g. by broad-spectrum antibiotics). Infection develops as discrete small white patches on the mucosal surface which can join to form a pseudomembrane (e.g. oral thrush). Cutaneous infections present as spreading erythema, sometime with pustules or macerated skin. Cutaneous candidiasis only occurs in warm moist areas. In immunocompromised patients, invasive systemic infection involving any organ in the body may occur.

 Practice application

Patients may be immunocompromised for a variety of reasons.

- **Cancer patients** – cytotoxic chemotherapy leading to neutropenia.
- **Transplant patients** – immunosuppressive therapy to prevent organ rejection.
- **Intensive care unit** – many patients with multiple organ failure have a reduced immune response and have often received multiple courses of antibiotics and venous cannulae.

Section 3

Cryptococcus neoformans

Cryptococcus is a yeast-like fungus and is found naturally in bird faeces (especially pigeons!). It is the most common cause of life-threatening fungal infection in people with HIV infection, probably 6–10% in the pre-HAART (highly active antiretroviral therapy) era. Most common sites for infection are the lungs and the CNS, where *Cryptococcus* meningitis has been well studied.

Antifungal drugs

Fungi, being eukaryotes, are fundamentally more similar to mammalian cells than bacteria. However, there are still plenty of targets for selective toxicity, particularly the fungal cell wall and the fungal cell membrane. There are fewer drugs available to treat fungal infections than bacterial ones and many of these seem to have quite toxic side effects.

Cell wall active drugs

Echinocandins

Echinocandins, such as caspofungin, prevent the synthesis of 1,3 beta-glucan, an essential component of fungal cell walls. Remember, mammalian cells do not have a cell wall and hence antifungal drugs which target this structure will only act on the fungal cells and not on our cells. Prevention of the synthesis of 1,3 beta-glucan renders the fungal cell vulnerable to osmotic changes and is often fungicidal. Caspofungin is active against *Candida* spp and *Aspergillus* spp and is licensed in adult and paediatric patients for:

- treatment of invasive candidiasis
- treatment of invasive aspergillosis in patients who are refractory to or intolerant of amphotericin B, lipid formulations of amphotericin B and/or itraconazole. Refractoriness is defined as progression of infection or failure to improve after a minimum of 7 days of prior therapeutic doses of effective antifungal therapy
- empirical therapy for presumed fungal infections (such as *Candida* or *Aspergillus)* in febrile, neutropenic adult patients.

Anidulafungin and micafungin are recently licensed echinocandins although their indications are currently more limited than those of caspofungin.

Cell membrane active drugs

Ergosterol is the main sterol in the fungal cell membrane; the mammalian equivalent sterol is cholesterol. Targeting ergosterol is therefore an ideal example of selective toxicity and as such it is a target for a variety of antifungal drug classes.

Interactions with ergosterol

The polyenes are a class of fungicidal drugs which act by disrupting the fungal cell membrane, the best known of which are nystatin and amphotericin B. Eight polyene drug molecules

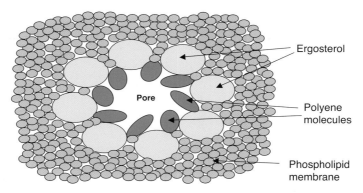

Figure 37.1 Polyene antifungal molecules combine with ergosterol to form a hydrophilic pore through the fungal cell membrane.

combine with eight molecules of ergosterol to form a hydrophilic pore lined with hydroxyl groups (Figure 37.1). This pore allows the movement of intracellular ions and water across the membrane and leads to membrane depolarisation and cell death. While mammalian cell membranes do not contain ergosterol, polyenes have been shown to form pores with cholesterol. Fortunately, this is not a significant issue because polyenes complex preferentially with ergosterol rather than cholesterol and the pores formed with cholesterol are less stable and are smaller and less effective carriers of cations (Baginski *et al.*, 2005). The clinical uses of nystatin are outlined in Box 37.1.

Amphotericin B is a broad-spectrum antifungal that is given intravenously in the treatment of life-threatening infections. Its usefulness is limited by dose-related nephrotoxicity. Toxicity is reduced by combining amphotericin B in a lipid formulation (as AmBisome®, Abelcet® or Amphocil®) although these are very expensive.

Box 37.1 Clinical uses of nystatin.

Activity spectrum	Both moulds and yeasts inc. *Candida* spp, *Aspergillus* spp and *Cryptococcus neoformans.*
Oral dose	For oral candida 100,000 units qds, usually for 7 days.
Bioavailability	Insignificant absorption currently only available in topical preparations.
Excretion	N/A
Main uses	Cutaneous and mucocutaneous candidal infections.
Other notes	An IV lipid-based preparation is likely to be available soon for systemic infection.

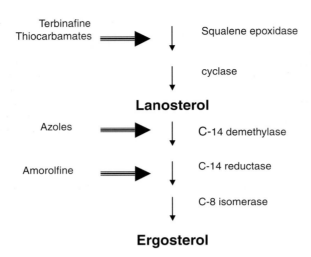

Figure 37.2 Many drugs interfere with ergosterol biosynthesis with actions at various enzymes within the biosynthetic pathway.

 Practice application

With all ampthotericin B preparations, it is important to give the patient an initial test dose and monitor them for 30 minutes for infusion-related reactions (fever, headache, chills, allergic reactions). These reactions are far less common with the lipid-associated preparations but if they do occur, symptoms can often be managed with paracetamol, antiemetics and antihistamines or by slowing the speed of the infusion. As well as renal function, patients should be closely monitored for changes in potassium, magnesium and calcium (initially daily).

Inhibitors of ergosterol biosynthesis

Several of the enzymes involved in ergosterol synthesis are major targets for antifungal drug classes (Figure 37.2), including the azoles and terbinafine. The clinical uses of fluconazole and terbinafine are outlined in Table 37.1. Ergosterol is essential for maintaining the fluidity and permeability of the cell. Inhibition of these enzymes prevents the formation of ergosterol and compromises the cell. The azoles are the most numerous group of antifungal drugs (e.g. fluconazole). Most, when used systemically, are inhibitors of the cytochrome P450 group of metabolising enzymes causing numerous drug interactions.

 Stop and think

Have you checked your patient's current medication before prescribing an azole? Is the azole likely to inhibit the metabolism of other prescribed medication?

Section 3

Table 37.1 Clinical uses of antifungal drugs which act by inhibiting ergosterol biosynthesis.

Drug	Fluconazole	Terbinafine
Activity spectrum	*Candida albicans* and *Cryptococcus neoformans*	Active against most dermatophytes. Also active against *Candida* spp and *Aspergillus* spp but not used for systemic infections.
Oral dose	Various depending on indication	Various depending on indication.
Bioavailability	90% absorbed. Little need of IV unless 'nil by mouth'	~40%
Excretion	Mostly renally excreted (60–90%)	Mixed excretion – requires dose reduction in renal impairment. Avoid in liver impairment.
Main uses	Cutaneous and mucocutaneous candidal infections that fail topical treatment. Deep infections caused by *Candida albicans* or other known sensitive *Candida* spp, especially as 'step-down' oral therapy following initial treatment with intravenous antifungals.	Drug of choice for treating fungal nail infections. Cutaneous fungal infection when oral therapy appropriate.
Other notes	Hepatotoxic – not to be used in patients with liver impairment.	Hepatotoxic – not to be used in patients with chronic or active liver impairment.

Practice application

Resistance to one azole does not necessarily imply resistance to all. Voriconazole is a broad-spectrum azole antifungal which, although expensive, can still be used to treat fluconazole-resistant *Candida* strains.

Viruses

Viruses contain at least two types of macromolecules: proteins and genetic information contained in nucleic acid (either DNA *or* RNA but not both). They differ from the other major groups of micro-organisms in that they require a living eukaryotic or prokaryotic host cell for replication, attaching and entering the cell with specific receptor-binding proteins. There are many types of virus but this section will concentrate on two of the more common pathogens: herpes and influenza virus.

Anti-herpes virus drugs

Herpesviridae is a large family of viruses many of which cause human disease. The most common are herpes simplex virus (HSV) which causes oral (HSV-1) and genital (HSV-2) herpes,

Section 3

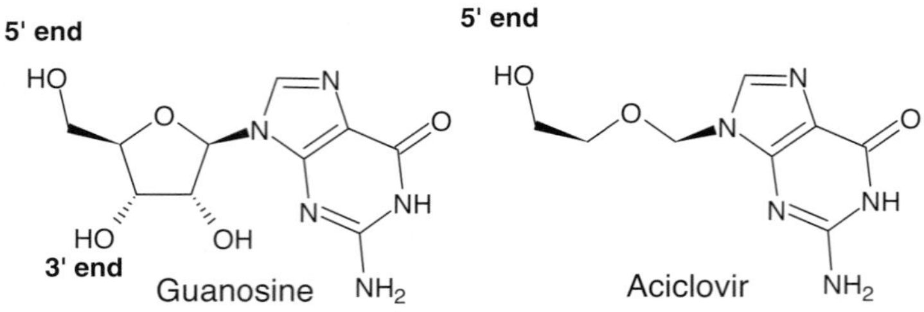

Figure 37.3   The structures of guanosine and aciclovir.

varicella zoster virus (VZV) which causes chickenpox and shingles, Epstein–Barr virus (EBV) which causes glandular fever and cytomegalovirus (CMV). These viruses contain their genetic information in the form of DNA.

DNA is made up of a series of four 'bases', one of which is guanosine. Aciclovir is very similar in structure to guanosine (Figure 37.3) and, within cells infected with the herpes family of viruses, it actually acts as a guanosine analogue. After being activated by the addition of phosphate groups, aciclovir is incorporated into the viral DNA strands by the enzyme DNA polymerase. Once incorporated, it acts as a DNA chain terminator as there is nowhere to attach the next base.

Mammalian cells also use DNA polymerase in DNA synthesis but selective toxicity is assured because aciclovir is activated by viral enzymes and is much more effective at inhibiting viral DNA polymerase compared to the cellular version DNA polymerase (Elion, 1983). The clinical uses of aciclovir are shown in Box 37.2.

Anti-influenza virus drugs

The influenza virus contains eight segments of single-stranded RNA, the genetic code for making new virus/enzymes contained in a capsid. On the virus surface are two protruding glycoproteins: haemagglutinin and neuraminidase.

Box 37.2   Clinical uses of aciclovir.

Activity spectrum	Herpesviruses family. Most active against herpes simplex, good activity against varicella zoster, slight activity against Epstein–Barr virus, very slight activity against cytomegalovirus.
Oral dose	Varies with indication.
Bioavailability	20%
Excretion	Mostly renally excreted.
Main uses	Infections caused by herpes simplex and varicella zoster viruses. Prophylaxis of infection in immunocompromised.
Other notes	Valaciclovir and famaciclovir are pro-drugs of aciclovir with better bioavailability. They are, however, more expensive.

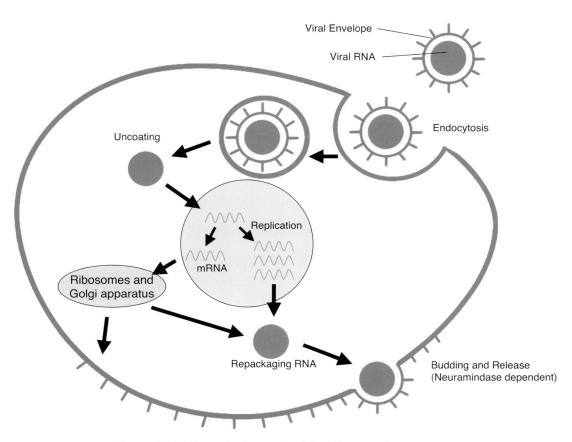

Figure 37.4 Reproduction cycle of the influenza virus.

Haemagglutinin aids the adhesion and phagocytosis of the virus into the host cell. Once inside, the viral RNA uses the host's organelles to manufacture further copies of the RNA viral code and the protein capsid, which together are packaged into new viral particles. These bud at the surface of the cell and, with the help of neuraminidase, are released to infect other host cells (Figure 37.4).

Oseltamivir and zanamivir are neuraminidase inhibitors and prevent the release of the viral particles from the infected cell and hence the spread of infection within the body. As most of the spread occurs early in the infection, the drugs are more effective the sooner they can be started after symptoms appear. Both zanamivir and oseltamivir are licensed for the treatment of patients who present with flu-like illness, when influenza A or B is circulating in the community, and can start taking the medicine within 48 hours of the onset of symptoms. Oseltamivir is additionally indicated for postexposure prevention in adults and adolescents 13 years of age or older following contact with a clinically diagnosed influenza case when influenza virus is circulating in the community.

NICE (www.nice.org.uk/or see BNF) has evaluated both neuraminidase inhibitors and suggested that their use be restricted to the treatment of at-risk patients and post-exposure prophylaxis of at-risk patients or residents of care establishments (regardless of vaccination status).

Section 3

'At-risk' individuals are those who are not effectively protected by influenza vaccination and have one of the following conditions:

- chronic respiratory disease, including asthma and COPD
- significant chronic heart disease (excluding hypertension)
- chronic renal disease
- chronic liver disease
- diabetes mellitus
- chronic neurological conditions
- immunosuppression
- patients over 65.

Summary

- Invasive fungal infections usually affect compromised patients. In normal hosts fungal infections tend to be superficial.
- The most common invasive fungal pathogens are *Candida* spp, *Aspergillius* spp and *Cryptococcus neoformans*.
- The dermatophytes cause superficial skin and nail infections.
- Polyene antifungals (amphotericin B and nystatin) punch holes through the fungal cell membrane by forming a complex with ergosterol.
- Azole antifungals (e.g. fluconazole, voriconazole) and terbinafine inhibit the biosynthesis of ergosterol.
- Azole antifungals inhibit cytochrome P450 enzymes and have numerous drug–drug interactions.
- Terbinafine is particularly useful for the treatment of fungal nail infections. It can be hepatotoxic.
- Viruses need to enter a eukaryotic or prokaryotic cell in order to replicate.
- Aciclovir prevents viral DNA synthesis in cells infected by the herpes viruses, particularly herpes simplex and varicella zoster viruses.
- Oseltamivir and zanamivir inhibit neuraminidase to prevent the spread of influenza A and B virus.

Activity

1. Invasive fungal infections only affect patients who have recently received chemotherapy.   True / False
2. The dermatophytes are a group of fungi that cause fungal lung infections.   True / False
3. Voriconazole is a broad-spectrum antifungal with good activity against *Candida* and *Aspergillus*.   True / False
4. Aciclovir has poor bioavailability, so the intravenous route should be used for treating life-threatening viral infections such as herpes simplex encephalitis.   True / False
5. Oseltamivir should be started as soon as possible after flu symptom onset but certainly within the first 48 hours.   True / False

Section 3

6. Lipid-associated formulations of amphotericin B are more effective for treating fungal infections. True / False
7. Fluconazole is the drug of choice for treating fungal nail infections. True / False

Useful website

NICE technology appraisals for the prevention and treatment of influenza infection by zanamivir, amantadine and oseltamivir (TA168). www.nice.org.uk

References

Baginski, M.J., Sternal, K., Czub, J. and Borowski, E. (2005) Molecular modelling of membrane activity of amphotericin B, a polyene macrolide antifungal antibiotic. *Acta Biochim Polon*, **52**, 655–658.

Elion, G.B. (1983) The biochemistry and mechanism of action of acyclovir. *J Antimicrob Chemother*, **12**(Suppl B), 9–17.

Lass-Flörl, C. (2009) The changing face of epidemiology of invasive fungal disease in Europe. *Mycoses*, **52**, 197–205.

Further reading

Cappelletty, D. and Eiselstein-Mckitrick, K. (2007) The echinocandins. *Pharmacotherapy*, **27**, 369–388.

Chapman, S.W., Sullivan, D.C. and Cleary, J.D. (2008) In search of the holy grail of antifungal therapy. *Trans Am Clin Climatol Assoc*, **119**, 197–215.

Pappas, P.G., Rex, J.H., Sobel, J.D., *et al.*, Infectious Diseases Society of America (2004) Guidelines for treatment of candidiasis. *Clin Infect Dis*, **38**, 161–189.

Reece, P.A. (2007) Neuraminidase inhibitor resistance in influenza virus. *J Med Virol*, **79**, 1577–1586.

Wainberg, M.A. (2009) Perspectives on antiviral drug development. *Antiviral Res*, **81**, 1–5.

Walsh, T.J., Anaissie, E.J., Denning, D.W., *et al.*, Infectious Diseases Society of America (2008) Treatment of aspergillosis: clinical practice guidelines of the Infectious Diseases Society of America. *Clin Infect Dis*, **46**, 327–360.

Section 3

Section 3: Pharmacology activity answers: Chapters 14–37

Chapter 14: General principles underlying drug action

1. C
2. B
3. D
4. C
5. A
6. D

Chapter 15: Pharmacokinetics 1 – absorption and distribution

1. True, False, True, True, True
2. False, True, False, False, True
3. False, True, True, False, True
4. False, True, True, False, True

Chapter 16: Pharmacokinetics 2 – metabolism and excretion

1. True, False, True, True, True
2. True, False, True, True, True
3. True, False, False, False, True
4. False, True, True, False, True
5. True, False, True, True, True

The New Prescriber. Edited by J Lymn, D Bowskill, F Bath-Hextall, R Knaggs, © 2010 John Wiley & Sons.

Chapter 17: Routes of drug administration

1. True, True, False, False, True

2. True, False, True, True, True

3. True, False, True, True, True

4. False, True, False, True, True

Chapter 18: Variations in drug handling

1. True, False, True, True, False

2. True, True, True, False, True

3. True, False, False, True, True

4. False, False, False, False, True

5. False, False, False, False, True

Chapter 19: Adverse drug reactions and interactions

1. True, False, True, True, False

2. True, True, True, False, True

3. False, False, False, False, True

4. False, False, True, True, True

5. True, False, True, False, False

Chapter 20: Introduction to the autonomic nervous system

1. False

2. True

3. False

4. True

5. True

6. False

7. True

8. True

9. False

10. True

11. True

12. False

13. False

14. True

15. False

Chapter 21: Clinical application of the principles of the autonomic nervous system

1. Tropicamide will bind to muscarinic receptors in the eye, preventing the binding of acetylcholine to these receptors. This will block the contraction of the ciliary muscle and resulting constriction of the pupil usually stimulated by acetylcholine binding. This will effectively result in dilation of the pupil, allowing eye examination to be performed.

2. B

3. Anticholinesterase drugs will further reduce the heart rate by stimulating the activation of muscarinic receptors in the heart by acetylcholine. May therefore result in heart block.

4. C

5. If overused, salbutamol can be absorbed into the systemic circulation and act on other beta-2-adrenoreceptors in the body, including those located on the skeletal muscle. Stimulation of these receptors on skeletal muscle results in tremor.

6. Beta-adrenoceptor antagonists will compete with salbutamol for binding to the beta-2-adrenoreceptors in the lungs, thus reducing the ability of salbutamol to promote bronchodilation.

7. Ephedrine constricts the blood vessels in the nasal mucosa and therefore results in reduced oedema (same as phenylephrine).

Chapter 22: The respiratory system

1. False

2. True

3. True

4. False

5. False, False, True, True, True

6. True

7. False

8. False

9. True

10. False

Chapter 23: The cardiovascular system

1. True, True, False, True, True

2. True, True, False, False, True

3. True, True, False, True, True

4. True, False, True, True, True

Chapter 24: Haemostasis and thrombosis

1. False

2. True

3. False

4. False

5. True

6. False

7. True

8. True

9. True

10. False

11. False

12. False

Chapter 25: The renal system

1. True

2. False

3. True

4. True

5. False

6. True

7. False

8. True

9. False

10. False

Chapter 26: The gastrointestinal system

1. C

2. A

3. B

4. C

5. A

6. B

7. D

Chapter 27: The endocrine system

1. C

2. True

3. True

4. B

5. B

6. True

7. B

Chapter 28: Contraception

1. B

2. True

3. False

4. False

5. B

Chapter 29: Introduction to the central nervous system

1. True
2. False
3. True
4. True
5. False
6. False
7. False
8. False
9. False
10. True

Chapter 30: Neurodegenerative disorders

1. True
2. False
3. False
4. False
5. True
6. True
7. False
8. False
9. True
10. False

Chapter 31: Depression and anxiety

1. True
2. False
3. False
4. True
5. True

6. False

7. False

8. True

9. True

10. False

11. True

12. True

13. True

14. False

15. False

Chapter 32: Schizophrenia

1. True

2. True

3. True

4. False

5. True

6. False

7. False

8. True

9. True

10. False

Chapter 33: Epilepsy and anticonvulsants

1. True

2. False

3. True

4. True

5. False

6. True

7. True

8. False

9. d

10. True

Chapter 34: Pain and analgesia

1. Aspirin (H)

2. Glyceryl trinitrate (G)

3. Paracetamol (F)

4. Aspirin (H)

5. Morphine (A)

6. Ibuprofen (C)

7. Buprenorphine (I)

8. Tramadol (J)

9. Gabapentin (E)

10. Diamorphine (K)

Chapter 35: Antibacterial chemotherapy

1. False, False, True, True, False

2. C and D

3. A, B and E

4. A and D

5. E

Chapter 36: Antibiotic resistance and *Clostridium difficile*

1. False

2. True

3. True

4. False

5. B

6. A

7. C

Chapter 37: Antifungal and antiviral drugs

1. False
2. False
3. True
4. True
5. True
6. False
7. False

Section 3: Pharmacology Glossary

Absorption: The passage of a drug from its site of administration to the plasma. Important for all drugs except those given IV (not strictly required for inhalation of bronchodilators.

Acetylcholine: Neurotransmitter in both the autonomic nervous system and central nervous system.

Acetylcholinesterase: Enzyme present in synaptic cleft which inactivates acetycholine by breaking it down into acetate and choline.

Acid-glycoprotein: An example of a plasma protein; binds basic drugs (particularly propranolol, tricyclics and lidocaine).

Adenosine diphosphate (ADP): Pro-aggregatory chemical released by activated platelets.

Adrenaline: Endocrine hormone produced by the adrenal medulla following stimulation by the sympathetic nervous system.

Adrenergic receptors (adrenoceptors): Receptors of the sympathetic nervous system. Stimulated by endogenous adrenaline and noradrenaline. Can be divided into alpha- and beta-receptors which have differential affinity for A and NA.

Adverse drug reaction (ADR): A noxious or unintended reaction to a drug that is administered in standard doses by the proper route for the purpose of prophylaxis, diagnosis or treatment (WHO definition).

Affinity: Likelihood of drug binding to a receptor.

Afterload: The force against which the heart has to pump (peripheral vascular resistance).

Agonist: Binds to a receptor and elicits a response (has affinity and efficacy). Full agonists induce a maximal tissue response.

Albumin: An example of a plasma protein; binds mainly acidic drugs. Most important plasma-binding protein, binds warfarin, aspirin, phenytoin, furosemide and so on.

Aldosterone: Hormone produced by the action of angiotensin II on the adrenal cortex. Promotes the retention of sodium ions in the plasma.

Angiotensin II: Potent vasoconstrictor produced by the action of angiotensin-converting enzyme on angiotensin I.

Antagonist: Binds to a receptor but does not elicit a response (has affinity but no efficacy).

The New Prescriber. Edited by J Lymn, D Bowskill, F Bath-Hextall, R Knaggs, © 2010 John Wiley & Sons.

Autocrine hormone: Hormone which is released from and acts upon the same cell.

Autonomic nervous system: The nervous system responsible for regulating involuntary body systems.

Beta-globulin: An example of a plasma protein; binds basic drugs.

Biliary excretion: Major route of excretion of large ionised molecules (often glucuronide or sulphate conjugates).

Bioavailability: Indicates the proportion of administered drug that passes into the systemic circulation and can therefore have a therapeutic effect, taking into account absorption and first-pass metabolism. Important for orally administered drugs.

Blood pressure (BP): BP = cardiac output × peripheral vascular resistance.

Bradykinin: Inflammatory mediator.

Cardiac output (CO): Cardiac output = heart rate × stroke volume.

Carrier protein: One of the four groups of protein drug targets.

Central nervous system (CNS): The brain and the spinal cord.

Chemical antagonism: Binding of 'antagonist' and drug in solution to produce an inactive complex.

Cholesterol: Lipid produced by the liver which is a key component of cell membranes and forms the basis of a number of hormones.

Clearance: Rate of drug elimination divided by plasma concentration. Concerned with the rate at which an active drug is removed from the body. Involves metabolism and excretion.

Cockcroft–Gault equation: This equation allows for rapid estimation of creatinine clearance. Incorporates patient's weight.

Competitive antagonism: Antagonist competes with agonist for receptor binding. Binding is only weak (hydrogen bonds, etc.). Agonist receptor occupancy is reduced in the presence of competitive antagonist, can be overcome by increasing agonist concentration. Inhibition is surmountable.

Creatinine clearance: $\frac{U \times V}{P} \times 100$ where U = urine concentration of creatinine, V = rate of urine flow, P = plasma concentration of creatinine. Is an estimation of GFR.

Cyclooxygenase: Enzyme which is important in the production of prostaglandins from arachidonate. Activity is inhibited by NSAIDs.

Cytochrome P450: Large family of drug-metabolising enzymes found mainly in the liver.

Distribution: Refers to the localisation of drug throughout the body. Each drug has a specific pattern of localisation/distribution.

DNA: Long threadlike molecule made up of a large number of deoxyribonucleotides (themselves made up of a base (ATCG), a sugar and a phosphate). The bases carry the genetic information, found in the cell nucleus.

Dopamine: One of the principal neurotransmitters in the CNS.

Efficacy: The likelihood of drug binding to activate the receptor resulting in an effect.

E_{max}: The maximal response to a drug.

Endocrine hormone: Hormone released into the bloodstream which acts on distant targets.

Endocrine system: Diverse range of organs, tissue and cells, which release hormones to regulate most body systems.

Endogenous: Naturally occurring (within the body) product or mediator.

Enterohepatic recycling: Recycling of metabolised drugs in the bile. Transported from the liver to the gut, drugs are then hydrolysed in the gut, releasing parent drug which is then reabsorbed into the hepatic portal system and transported back to the liver where it is metabolised again.

Enzyme: A protein which speeds up chemical reactions within the body without being chemically altered itself. Enzymes are one of the four groups of protein drug targets.

Estimated GFR (e-GFR): Prediction of patient's GFR based on formula which takes into account patient's age, gender, ethnicity and creatinine levels.

Excretion: The removal of drug from the body.

Exocrine secretions: Secretions stimulated by the parasympathetic nervous system (with the exception of sweat which is a sympathetic response).

Fibrin: An insoluble protein which cross-links platelets and stabilises the platelet plug. The end-product of the coagulation cascade.

First-pass metabolism: Metabolism that occurs in the liver and gut wall prior to drug reaching systemic circulation. Significant feature of orally administered drugs. Reduces bioavailability.

Forebrain: Largest part of the brain. Area where conscious thought and action are initiated.

Full agonist: Binds to a receptor and induces a maximal tissue response.

Gamma-amino butyric acid (GABA): The major inhibitory neurotransmitter in the CNS.

Gastrin: Endocrine hormone which stimulates gastric acid production.

Glial cells: Cell type found in the brain. Do not directly take part in electrical communication but can modulate and support neuronal function.

Glomerular filtration: Fundamental process of drug excretion. Diffusion of drug through glomerular capillaries into filtrate.

Glomerular filtration rate (GFR): A measure of the rate at which blood is filtered by the kidneys.

Glutamate: The major excitatory neurotransmitter in the CNS.

Glycogenolysis: Breakdown of glycogen to glucose for energy.

Glycolipids: Lipids contained in the plasma membrane of the cell.

Section 3

Haemostasis: Arrest of blood loss from damaged blood vessels. Normal physiological response.

Half-life ($t_{1/2}$): The half-life of a drug is the time taken for the plasma concentration to fall by 50%.

Heart rate (HR): Measure of cardiac activity. CO = HR × stroke volume.

Hindbrain: Located at the top of the spinal cord. Consists of three structures (medulla oblongata, pons, cerebellum).

Histamine: Inflammatory mediator, released from mast cells.

Hydrophilic: Water loving. Drugs that are hydrophilic do not readily cross cell membranes (polar, ionised, lipophobic).

Hydrophobic: Water hating. Hydrophobic drugs readily cross cell membranes (unionised, non-polar, lipophilic).

Inducers: Drug/chemical which speeds up the activity of specific cytochrome P450 enzymes.

Inhibitors: Drug/chemical which inhibits the activity of specific cytochrome P450 enzymes.

Inotrope: Acts directly on the heart muscle.

Ion channels: Proteins which act as gated tunnels allowing passage of ions across cell membranes. Ion channels are one of the four groups of protein drug targets.

Ionised: Drug that is charged, lipophobic, hydrophilic. Will not readily cross cell membranes.

Irreversible antagonist: A drug which binds to the receptor using strong covalent bonds. Dissociates from the receptor only slowly or not at all.

Leukotrienes: Inflammatory mediators which cause bronchoconstriction.

Lipolysis: The breakdown of fats to produce fuel molecules.

Lipophilic: Lipid loving. Lipophilic drugs can readily cross cell membranes (unionised, non-polar, hydrophobic).

Lipophobic: Lipid hating. Lipophobic drugs do not readily cross cell membranes (ionised, polar, hydrophilic).

Mediators: Chemicals/drugs which modulate biological processes, for example neurotransmitters, hormones, inflammatory mediators.

Metabolism: The enzymatic conversion of one chemical entity to another. Transformation of drugs within the body with the purpose of making them more hydrophilic.

Midbrain: Smallest processing region of the brain. Connects hindbrain to forebrain.

Monoamine oxidase: Enzyme which acts to break down monoamines once they have been taken back up into the presynaptic nerve cell.

Muscarinic receptors: Postsynaptic cholinergic receptors of the parasympathetic nervous system. Also found in the CNS.

Neonate: Newborn infant (particularly less than 1 month old).

Neuron: Nerve cell.

Neurotransmitter: Chemical which is released from nerve cells and transmits signal either to another nerve cell or to an effector organ.

Nicotinic acetylcholine receptors: Presynaptic cholinergic receptors of the autonomic nervous system. Also found in the CNS.

Non-competitive antagonist: 'Antagonist' does not act at receptor level but instead interferes with the cellular response to an agonist.

Non-polar: Substances which dissolve freely in lipids, move readily across cell membranes (unionised, lipophilic, hydrophobic).

Noradrenaline: Neurotransmitter released from postganglionic neurons in the sympathetic system and in the CNS.

Paracrine hormone: Local hormone which is released from specialised cells and acts on neighbouring cells.

Parasympathetic nervous system: Branch of the autonomic nervous system, usually active during satiation and repose (rest and digest system).

Parenteral: Describes the route of administration of drugs given by injection (subcutaneous, intramuscular, intravenous).

Partial agonist: Binds to receptor and induces a submaximal tissue response. Less efficacious than full agonists.

Passive diffusion: Fundamental process of drug excretion. Reabsorption of plasma and drug as it passes through renal tubule.

Peripheral nervous system: Connects the central nervous system and body tissues. Made up of the autonomic nervous system and the somatic nervous system.

Peripheral vascular resistance (PVR): Degree of vasoconstriction /vasodilation of the peripheral arteries. BP = CO × PVR.

pH: Measure of acidity or alkalinity of a solution.

Pharmacogenetics: Clinically important hereditary variation in response to drugs. May result, for example, in increased or decreased activity of cytochrome P450 enzyme activity.

Pharmacokinetics: How the body handles the drug (absorption, distribution, metabolism, excretion).

Pharmacokinetic antagonism: Situation where 'antagonist' acts to either reduce absorption of the drug or increase its metabolism and/or excretion.

Phase I metabolism: Consists of three types of chemical reaction (oxidation, reduction, hydrolysis). Often involves the cytochrome P450 family of enzymes. Phase I metabolites may still be active.

Phase II metabolism: Involves the process of conjugation. Phase II metabolites are generally inactive.

Phospholipids: Lipids contained in the plasma membrane of cells.

Physiological antagonism: Situation where 'antagonist' has the opposite effect to the drug such that they cancel each other out. Occurs more frequently in polypharmacy.

pKa: The pH at which a drug exists in a 50:50 equilibrium between unionised and ionised forms.

Plasma proteins: Proteins found in the plasma that bind drugs. Drug–protein binding interaction is rapid, reversible and saturable. Does not represent a drug target. Non-selective. Has no physiological effect.

Plasmin: The end-product of the fibrinolytic cascade. Acts to break down fibrin.

Polar: Drug that is ionised, lipophobic, hydrophilic. Will not readily cross cell membranes.

Postganglionic neuron: The second neuron in the autonomic nervous system.

Potency: Affinity × efficacy.

Preganglionic neuron: The first neuron in the autonomic nervous system. Has its cell body in the CNS.

Preload: Volume load of the heart.

Pro-drug: Drug that is not active until it has been metabolised.

Prostaglandins: Lipid-derived mediators which have a wide variety of roles within the body.

Proton pump: K^+/H^+ ATP-ase which actively pumps hydrogen ions into the lumen of the stomach.

Receptor: Naturally occurring body protein which acts as a recognition site for the body's normal mediators. Found either within the cell (nuclear receptors) or on the cell surface. Receptors are one of the four groups of protein drug targets.

Renin: Enzyme secreted from the juxtaglomerular cells of the kidney. Acts to convert angiotensinogen to angiotensin I.

Serotonin (5HT): One of the principal neurotransmitters of the CNS.

Smooth endoplasmic reticulum: Large membranous structure and, in hepatocytes, the location of the cytochrome P450 enzyme system.

Somatic nervous system: Relays messages from the central nervous system to the skin and skeletal muscles. Regulates voluntary responses.

Specificity: Describes the likelihood of a drug acting on a subsection of targets.

Stroke volume (SV): The volume of blood pumped from the heart. CO = HR × SV.

Sympathetic nervous system: Branch of the autonomic nervous system, activity increased during times of stress (fight/flight/fright system).

Synapse: Gap between two nerve cells or between a nerve cell and an effector organ.

Therapeutic index: The ratio between the minimum effective dose and the maximum tolerated dose of a drug.

Thrombosis: The pathological formation of a blood clot in the absence of bleeding.

Thromboxane A_2 (TXA$_2$): Pro-aggregatory chemical secreted from platelets.

Tubular secretion: Fundamental process of drug excretion. Drug molecules are carried into tubular lumen by carrier systems.

Type A ADR: Adverse drug reaction which represents an augmented, or exaggerated, response to the pharmacological action of the drug. Predictable, usually dose related and known prior to marketing.

Type B ADR: Bizzare effects which can occur at any dose, not predictable, usually immunologically mediated.

Unconjugated: Free drug which is released following hydrolysis of conjugated drug by bacteria in the small intestine.

Unionised: Substances which dissolve freely in lipids, move readily across cell membranes (non-polar, lipophilic, hydrophobic).

Volume of distribution (Vd): Volume of plasma that would be required to contain the total body content of a drug at the same concentration as that present in the plasma.

Index